Second Edition

Textbook of
Forensic
Pharmacy

for Pharmacy Students and Professionals

IM
V

Second Edition

Textbook of Forensic Pharmacy

for Pharmacy Students and Professionals

Guru Prasad Mohanta MPharm, PhD

Professor of Pharmacy
Annamalai University
Annamalai Nagar
Tamil Nadu

Former WHO Officer at Country Office for India

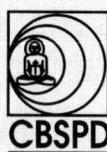

CBSPD

CBS Publishers & Distributors Pvt Ltd

New Delhi • Bengaluru • Chennai • Kochi • Kolkata • Lucknow • Mumbai
Hyderabad • Jharkhand • Nagpur • Patna • Pune • Uttarakhand

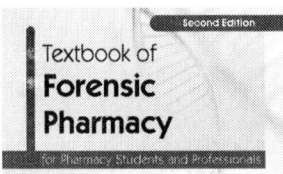

ISBN: 978-93-87085-97-8

Copyright © Author and Publisher

Second Edition: 2018

Reprint: 2019, 2023, 2025

First Edition: 2013

Published by Satish Kumar Jain and produced by Varun Jain for

CBS Publishers & Distributors Pvt Ltd

4819/XI Prahlad Street, 24 Ansari Road, Daryaganj, New Delhi 110 002, India
Ph: 011-23289259, 23266838   Website: www.cbspd.com
                                    e-mail: delhi@cbspd.com
Corporate Office: 204 FIE, Industrial Area, Patparganj, Delhi 110 092
Ph: 011-4934 4934   Fax: 011-4934 4935   e-mail: publishing@cbspd.com; publicity@cbspd.com

Branches

- **Bengaluru:** Seema House 2975, 17th Cross, K.R. Road, Banasankari 2nd Stage, Bengaluru 560 070, Karnataka, India
  Ph: +91-80-26771678/79   Fax: +91-80-26771680   e-mail: bangalore@cbspd.com
- **Chennai:** 18/8B, Subbarayan Street, Shenoy Nagar, Chennai 600 030, Tamil Nadu, India
  Ph: +91-44-42032115, 26681266   e-mail: chennai@cbspd.com
- **Kochi:** 42/1325, 1326, Power House Road, Opp KSEB, Power House, Ernakulam 682 018, Kerala, India
  Ph: +91-484-4059061-65   Fax: +91-484-4059065   e-mail: kochi@cbspd.com
- **Kolkata:** 147, Hind Ceramics Compound, 1st Floor, Nilgunj Road, Belghoria, Kolkata-700056, West Bengal, India
  Ph: 033-25633055, 033-25633056   e-mail: kolkata@cbspd.com
- **Lucknow:** Basement, Khushnuma Complex, 7-Meerabai Marg (Behind Jawahar Bhawan), Lucknow 226001, India
  Ph: 0522-4000032   e-mail: tiwari.lucknow@cbspd.com
- **Mumbai:** PWD Shed. Gala no. 25/26, Ramchandra Bhatt Marg, Next to JJ Hospital Gate no. 2 Opp. Union Bank of India Noorbaug Mumbai-400009, Maharashtra, India
  Ph: 022-66661880/89   e-mail: mumbai@cbspd.com

Representatives

- **Hyderabad** 0-9885175004 • **Jharkhand** 0-9811541605 • **Nagpur** 0-8692091830
- **Patna** 0-9334159340 • **Pune** 0-9664372571 • **Uttarakhand** 0-9716462459

Printed at Mudrak, Noida, UP, India

to

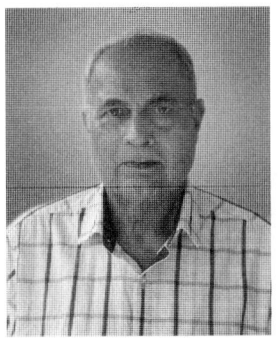

Sri Parameswar Mohanta, my childhood school teacher,
who laid the foundation of my learning process.
A personality who is ahead of his timings and
teacher par excellence has been the inspiration for me and
perhaps for many others. His blessings have made me what
I am today and I am grateful to the Almighty for
blessing me to have this wonderful teacher.

Directorate General of Health Services
Central Drugs Standard Control Organization
Ministry of Health & Family Welfare
FDA Bhawan, Kotla Road,
New Delhi – 110002
Tel: +91-11-23216367/23236975
Fax: +91-11-23236973
E-mail: vksmani@gmail.com

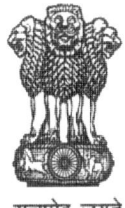

सत्यमेव जयते

Foreword

"One of the greatest delusions in the world is the hope that the evils in this world are to be cured by legislation"
— *Thomas Brackett Reed*

Drugs are special commodities and perhaps the greatest weapons of the mankind to fight against diseases. If drugs are not of standard quality, they will harm the user. The Government makes legislation to control the manufacture and distribution of medicines to ensure the availability of quality products.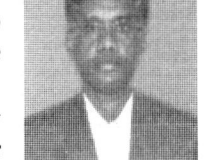

Pharmaceutical jurisprudence is an important subject as per the new syllabus of AICTE and PCI that deals with the laws related to drugs and other related products/services.

Dr Guru Prasad Mohanta of Department of Pharmacy, Annamalai University, is a well-known teacher and researcher with credible publications in peer reviewed reputed journals. I appreciate his attempt of revising the popular *Textbook of Forensic Pharmacy* making it up to date. As the regulations change with time, the revision is a necessity.

Textbook of Forensic Pharmacy covers almost all the Acts related to pharmaceutical sciences and pharmaceutical profession. There is separate chapter for each Act and each chapter is also short, to the point and crispy. Another feature is that it has a lot of case studies which the readers may find interesting. I am sure this book will be very student friendly.

Any person who is involved in manufacturing, storing, distributing, dispensing or marketing any pharmaceutical product should know about the government regulations related to that and he is also expected to fulfil the required regulatory norms. The book can be a ready reckoner to all of them.

It is good to know that even Glossary has been written chapterwise in a simple language for easy and quick understanding. His vast experience as a teacher, as a positive thinker and as a National Technical Officer—WHO Country Office for India, has helped him to bring out this book in the best possible way.

I believe this revised textbook would be a good companion for pharmacy students and pharmaceutical and other related healthcare professionals.

S Manivannan MPharm, PhD
Deputy Drugs Controller (India)
Central Drugs Standard Control Organization
Ministry of Health & Family Welfare
Government of India

Preface to the Second Edition

"At his best, man is the noblest of all animals; Separated from law and justice, he is the worst".

The subject 'Jurisprudence' is very dynamic in nature and so as 'Pharmaceutical Jurisprudence'. There are many new developments in rules and regulations related to pharmaceutical profession. Some of them are: Improved price control system for drugs and other products; easing rules for promoting pharmaceutical business; remarkable changes in clinical trial regulations: Registration of ethics committee and payment of compensation; generic promotion through making bioequivalency mandatory based on biopharmaceutical classification system; asserting the validity of 3(d) of Patent Act preventing ever greening patents, and New National Intellectual Property Rights Policy; improving the availability of opioids through concept of essential narcotic drugs; introduction of pharmacy practice regulation; and so on. These all necessitate the need of revision of the text written some five years back.

The text is revised to meet the new B Pharm. syllabus of Pharmacy Council of India and PharmD programmes. The book is also of reasonable reference for the students of Regulatory Affairs. The new text retained the original style of discussing the regulatory provisions covering the genesis and prospects of the regulations besides updated case studies.

I appreciate a student, Mr D Varun, who wrote me on the need of revision narrating how the students value it. In his language, it is "We debate in classes almost always referencing your text". I value his opinion. Similarly, I acknowledge with thanks many teachers who have liked the text and given their suggestion and appreciation. The timely reminder of Mr YN Arjuna of CBS Publishers and Distributors is thankfully acknowledged.

I am grateful to Professor Prabal Kumar Manna, Head of the Department of Pharmacy, Annamalai University, who has been my guiding force for over three decades. He always extends the helping hand whether it is personal, official or professional. I am thankful to my family: Wife Reena, son Anupam and daughter Amrita for their encouragement and understanding.

I am grateful to one of my former students, Dr S Manivannan, who has given the Foreword for the new edition of the text. He is currently Deputy Drugs Controller (India) with vast regulatory experience at national level. This is my privilege and I sincerely thank him.

Hope this new edition of the text would continue to get the patronage from the readers. While every effort has been taken into account to meet the requirement, it may not be able to satisfy all sections due to limitations, as it is not the substitute of the original Acts and Rules. The decision of limiting the text to the level is entirely of mine. I look forward to receiving your critical assessments, feedback and suggestions which would enable me to make it more useful.

Guru Prasad Mohanta
E.mail: gpmohanta@hotmail.com

Preface to the First Edition

"If students do not learn the way we teach, then let us teach the way they learn"

The profession of pharmacy is perhaps the most diversified profession in the world. The persons qualified through a rigorous process of education and training in pharmacy find a wide range of opportunities to build career in: Pharmaceutical industries, health care facilities, contract research organizations, education and research, marketing and regulatory systems to name with. Wherever they may be, they do work in a regulatory system and they need to comply with the regulations.

Hence, the Forensic Pharmacy, literally known as the study of laws and regulations governing the profession of pharmacy, is a part of all pharmacy programmes. Based on the career prospects of pharmacy professionals, the curriculum of almost all universities covers the following laws and regulations: Drugs and Cosmetics Act, Pharmacy Act, Drugs Price Control Order, Narcotic Drugs and Psychotropic Substances Act, Prevention of Cruelty to Animals Act, Patent Act, Drugs and Magic Remedies Act, Medicinal and Toilet Preparations Act, Insecticide Act, and Medical Termination of Pregnancy Act.

As a teacher of pharmacy spanned over more than 25 years, I found that the teaching of forensic pharmacy gets low priority. One of the reasons perhaps is lack of good textbook as most of the textbooks available in the market cover the subjects as narration of the laws and regulations without giving explanations or case studies. The laws are just narrated, not discussed. The students find the available books difficult to follow. In this book, I have made an attempt to bridge this gap and make the forensic pharmacy an interesting subject.

In addition to the laws and regulations mentioned above, the Right to Information Act, the Code of Ethics in Pharmaceutical Marketing, and Pharmaceutical Policy are included as they are relevant in the present context. The textbook is intended for the students and teachers of Bachelor of Pharmacy, Master of Pharmacy and Doctor of Pharmacy programme of Indian Universities. I am sure they would find it useful. The Pharmacy Professionals already in the field too may find this as their companion.

I express my gratitude to the authorities of Annamalai University for permitting me to write this text. I am indebted to Dr P K Manna, Professor of Pharmacy, who has always been my guide and inspiration. His support is gratefully acknowledged. I shall fail in my duty if I do not say a few words of my family members: My wife, Mrs Reena; my son, Anupam, computer engineer; and my daughter, Amrita, doing her schooling. They have spared me to complete the present project of writing this text. Without their help and cooperation, it would have never been possible.

It is my honour that Mr Prafull D Sheth, one of the most respected Pharmacy Professionals in the country, has written foreword of this book introducing it to the students and professionals. He is the Vice-President of International Pharmaceutical Federation (FIP) and Professional Secretary of SEARPharm Forum.

Last but not least, I appreciate the CBS Publishers & Distributors interest for taking up the job of publishing this book.

Though due care has been taken while writing the text, there may be some errors left inadvertently. I do not claim this as perfect and there is always a scope for improvement. I shall appreciate the feedback from the readers for further improvement of the textbook and their contributions will be gratefully acknowledged.

Guru Prasad Mohanta

E.mail: gpmohanta@hotmail.com

Contents

Abbreviations

AICTE	All India Council for Technical Education
AIIMS	All India Institute of Medical Sciences
ANC	Assistant Narcotics Commissioner
API	Active Pharmaceutical Ingredient
ASCI	Advertising Standard Council of India
ASU	Ayurvedic, Siddha and Unani
AYUSH	Ayurveda, Yoga and Naturopathy, Unani, Siddha and Homeopathy
BCS	Biopharmaceutical Classification System
BIS	Bureau of Indian Standards
BMS	Bare Metal Stent
CAG	Comptroller and Auditor General
CAGR	Compound Annual Growth Rate
CDL	Central Drugs Laboratory
CDSCO	Central Drugs Control Organization
CEA	Clinical Establishment Act
CFR	Case Fertility Ratio
CIC	Central Information Commission
CIMS	Current Index of Medical Specialities
CL	Compulsory Licence
CLA	Central Licencing Authority
CLAA	Central License Approving Authority
COPP	Certificate of Pharmaceutical Products
CPCSEA	Committee for the Purpose of Control and Supervision of Experiments on Animals
CRCL	Central Revenue Control Laboratory
CRI	Central Research Institute
CRO	Clinical Research Organization
CSIR	Council of Scientific and Industrial Research
D & C	Drugs and Cosmetics
DCC	Drugs Consultative Committee
DCGI	Drugs Controller General India
DCI	Dental Council of India
DDMAC	Division of Drug Marketing, Advertising and Communication
DEC	Drugs Enquiry Committee

DES	Drug Eluting Stent
DGFT	Directorate General of Foreign Trade
DGHS	Director General Health Services
DHMS	Diploma in Homeopathic Medicine and Surgery
DIPP	Department of Industrial Policy and Promotion
DNC	Deputy Narcotics Commissioner
DNP+	Delhi Network of Positive People
DOO	District Opium Officer
DoP	Department of Pharmaceuticals
DoR	Department of Revenue
DPCO	Drug Price Control Order
DPCRC	Drug Price Control Review Committee
DPEA	Drug Price Equalization Account
DPRC	Drug Price Review Committee
DST	Department of Science and Technology
DTAB	Drugs Technical Advisory Board
DTCA	Direct to Consumer Advertising
EC	Excise Commissioner
EDL	Essential Drugs List
EMR	Exclusive Marketing Rights
ER	Education Regulation
EXIM	Export Import
FIR	First Information Report
FTC	Federal Trade Commission
GATT	General Agreement on Tariff and Trade
GCP	Good Clinical Practice
GMP	Good Manufacturing Practices
GOAW	Government Opium and Alkaloid Works
GOI	Government of India
HAL	Hindusthan Antibiotics Limited
HCV	Hepatitis C Virus
I – MAK	Initiative for Medicine, Access and Knowledge
IAEC	Institutional Animal Ethics Committee
ICMR	Indian Council for Medical Research
IDMA	Indian Drugs Manufacturers Association
IDPL	Indian Drugs and Pharmaceuticals Limited
IEC	International Electro Technical Commission
IFPMA	International Federation of Pharmaceutical Manufacturers and Associations
INP +	Indian Network of People living with HIV
IPA	Indian Pharmaceutical Association

IPAB	Intellectual Property Appellate Board
IPC	Indian Pharmacopoeia Commission
IPG	Indian Pharmaceutical Guide
IPO	Indian Patent Office
IPR	Intellectual Property Rights
ISO	International Organization for Standardization
JAMA	Journal of American Medical Association
LA	Licensing Authority
LVP	Large Volume Parenterals
M	% Margin to retailer
M&TP	Medicinal and Toilet Preparations
MAT	Moving Annual Turnover
MCI	Medical Council of India
MHA	Ministry of Home Affairs
MHRA	Medicines and Health Products Regulatory Authority
MIMS	Monthly Index of Medical Specialities
MNC	Multi-national Companies
MoEF&CC	Ministry of Environment, Forest and Climate Change
MOH&F	Ministry of Health Family Welfare
MQY	Minimum Qualifying Yield
MR	Medical Representative
MRL	Maximum Residual Limit
MSJE	Ministry of Social Justice and Empowerment
MTP	Medical Termination of Pregnancy
NACEN	National Academy of Customs, Excise and Narcotics
NC	Narcotic Commissioner
NCB	Narcotic Control Bureau
NCHRH	National Council for Human Resources in Health
NCI	Nursing Council of India
NDPS	Narcotic Drugs and Psychotropic Substances
NIB	Narcotics Intelligence Bureau
NIPER	National Institute of Pharmaceutical Education and Research
NLEM	National List of Essential Medicines
NOC	No Objection Certificate
NPPA	National Pharmaceutical Pricing Authority
NPPP	National Pharmaceutical Pricing Policy
OPPI	Organization of Pharmaceutical Producers of India
P(c)	Ceiling price of the scheduled formulation
P(s)	Average Price to Retailer for the same strength and dosage of the medicine
P2P	Product to Product

PCI	Pharmacy Council of India
PEPAC	Pesticide Environmental Pollution Advisory Committee
PFA	Prevention of Food Adulteration
Pharm D	Doctor of Pharmacy
PIO	Public Information Officer
PPP	Public—Private Partnership
PRDC	Pharmaceutical Research and Development Committee
PSR	Professional Service Representative
PSUR	Periodic Safety Update Report
PWN	Positive Women's Network
PWR	Preliminary Weighment Register
R & D	Research and Development
RDTL	Regional Drugs Testing Laboratory
RTI	Right to Information
SC	Supreme Court
SIC	State Information Commission
SOP	Standard Operating Procedure
SPCA	Society for Prevention of Cruelty in Animals
TGA	Therapeutics Goods Administration
TKDL	Traditional Knowledge Digital Library
TNC	Trans National Companies
TRIPS	Trade Related Intellectual Property Rights
UCPMP	Uniform Code for Pharmaceutical Marketing Practices
UGC	University Grants Commission
USA	United States of America
USD	United States Dollar
USFDA	United States Food and Drugs Administration
WHO	World Health Organization
WIPO	World Intellectual Property Organization
WPI	Wholesale Price Index
WTO	World Trade Organization

1

Pharmaceutical Scenario and Related Regulations—from Past to the Present

"One of the greatest delusions in the world is the hope that the evils in the world are to be cured by Legislation"

— *Thomas Brackett Reed*

After reading this chapter, you should be able to understand and appreciate:
- Pharmaceutical regulatory systems in three phases: Preindependence, postindependence and liberalized era
- Development and growth of pharmaceutical industries and education over these periods
- Various committee reports and their impact in changing the pharmaceutical scenario

Drugs (or medicines) are special commodities and are perhaps the greatest weapon of the mankind to fight against diseases. They are used for diagnosis, prevention, mitigation or treatment of diseases. They play a crucial role in protecting, maintaining and promoting health of the people. But they are double-edged weapons. If drugs available for use are not of good quality and/or not used appropriately, they often harm the users. Thus, it is essential to ensure that the medicines made available to the people, are of assured quality, purity and strength and are packaged in containers which maintains the potency of the product and labelled with necessary information for proper use of medicines.

In an effort in this direction, government makes legislation to control the manufacture and distribution of medicines to ensure the availability of quality products. Currently, the drugs, medical devices, cosmetics, and medicines of Indian system and homeopathy are regulated. But the genesis of these regulations could be traced back to the pre-independence era. Accordingly the historical account of development of regulations along with changing pharmaceutical scenario is divided into three periods: Preindependent era, postindependent era and postliberalized period.

PREINDEPENDENT ERA

Despite having well-drafted statutes in Britain such as sale of Food and Drugs Act 1875, Food and Drugs (Adulteration) Act 1828, Therapeutics Act 1925, Dangerous Drugs Act 1920, to protect the health of the community, in British India there was no legislation which could directly prevent drug adulteration or assure conformity to proper standard of purity and strength. The drugs were part of other goods and certain provision in Indian Penal Code, Indian Merchandise Marks Act 1889, and Sea Customs Act 1878 were the guiding force. The intentional adulteration or sale of a drug which was not of the nature, quality or substance demanded by the purchaser was punishable under Indian Penal Code. The Indian Merchandise Marks Act provided a check on misbranding, false marketing and also trade description. Goods with false description were prohibited items for importing into India under the Sea Customs

Act. The Cantonment Act 1924 empowered the Cantonment Authority to enter any shop or place and seize any article of medicine which was adulterated or different from what was reported to be. The Opium Act 1878, Poison Act 1919, Dangerous Act 1930 were basically designed to meet excise and custom requirements and to prevent the illicit use of certain dangerous drugs. Thus, these Acts were just to control the manufacture, import and sale of certain drugs while they had no authority on the subject such as adulteration or standard of strength. The overall situation was grave.

Realizing the gravity of situations rising out of rampant availability of adulterated or inferior quality drugs in British India, in March 1927, the council of states recommended the Governor General in the council to urge all provincial governments to take necessary steps to control the indiscriminate use of medicinal drugs and to legislate for standardization of preparations and for the sale of such drugs. But this yielded no action. Being no effective law prevailing, one was free to start a shop and call himself 'chemist' and could deal with deadliest drugs in a way which might well harm the public.

The real pharmaceutical awakening in India came through the Report of the Drugs Enquiry Committee (1931). The Drugs Enquiry Committee (DEC) was constituted in August 1930 under the chairmanship of Col. Ram Nath Chopra, Professor of Pharmacology at School of Tropical Medicine and Hygiene, Calcutta. The establishment of Drugs Enquiry Committee has been the most significant event which laid the foundation of drugs and pharmacy statutes in the country. The main recommendations of the committee include: Enactment of central legislation to control drugs and pharmacy either through a combined legislation or separate Drugs Act and Pharmacy Act; creation of an Advisory Board in drafting rules under the Act to be enacted; establishment of a central laboratory, compilation of Indian Pharmacopoeia, etc.

The British (India) Government did not show any interest on the recommendation of Drugs Enquiry Report for some period. The Anderson Report of 1937 helped raising the awareness and impressed the medical professionals on need of legislations. Dr. Anderson, Secretary of British Medical Association, after visiting India submitted his critical report on pharmacy and drugs control. The medical profession in India was disturbed due to lack of organized or self-contained profession of pharmacy and lack of measure of drugs control. He observed "There is a lack of adequately qualified men among those who take up profession of pharmacy and there is absence of any restrictive laws preventing the practice of pharmacy by unqualified persons. No attempt is made to control the quality of drugs sold, with the result that market in India is flooded with drugs and preparations of impure quality and defective strength. It was represented that the legislation to improve this state of affairs is badly needed and should apply to the whole of India".

Under the pressure from various groups, a piecemeal approach was initiated by the government and Import of Drugs Bill was introduced in Indian Legislative Assembly in October 1937 to regulate the import of drugs and medicines into British India. The bill was finally withdrawn on opposition from professionals.

After 9 years of Drugs Enquiry Committee's recommendations, the Government of India moved the Drugs Bill 1940 before the Legislative Assembly to regulate the import, manufacture, distribution and sale of drugs in British India. The bill received the Governor General's assent in November 1940 leading to enactment of Drugs Act 1940. Following this, Drugs Technical Advisory Board (DTAB) was constituted in 1941 to draft the rules under the Act. The Rules were published as Drug Rules 1945. The Biochemical Laboratory of Calcutta established during 1937 was converted to Central Drugs Laboratory, the apex analytical laboratory under the Act.

The Drugs Act 1940 has been amended on several occasions: 1962 amendment brought the Cosmetics under its purview and thereafter the Act came to be known as Drugs and Cosmetics Act 1940. The statute was further amended in 1964 to widen its scope to bring

Ayurvedic (including Siddha) and Unani drugs under its domain.

The Drugs Enquiry Committee (Chopra Committee) recommended the necessity of minimum qualification for registration as pharmacists and it suggested that post-matriculation two years Diploma Course in Pharmacy as the minimum qualification. It has also recommended starting degree courses in Pharmaceutical Chemistry in different universities and provision for registration of such qualified persons.

Pharmacy Profession at Britain and India

In England, apothecaries separated from grocers during seventeenth century and later known as 'pharmacy' and 'chemists and druggists'. They formally organized themselves into the Pharmaceutical Society of Great Britain in 1841 and this society established a school of pharmacy in 1842. The Pharmacy Act 1852 authorized the society's council to set up a register of chemists and druggists, off associates and students and to examine persons for regis-tration. The titles 'pharmaceutical chemists', 'chemists and druggists' were protected only under the Pharmacy Act 1868. Subse-quently Poison and Pharmacy Act 1908 was introduced to control the profession of pharmacy to some extent.

On the contrary, the situation of pharmacy practice in India was in apathetic state. There was no legal restriction. Some fringe restrictive provisions were available in local Municipal Acts. There was no formal educa-tion or training was required for dispensing of medicines and was largely responsibility of compounders. However, the first attempt was made by the British government to provide formal education initiating a chemists and druggists' class in 1870s at Madras Medical College. Unfortunately the pro-gramme was not popular but continued to exist. There were sharp differences in pharmaceutical services within British India: British and native troops had the benefit of trained apothecaries and hospital assistants, there were drug houses in metropolitan and big cities run by European Pharmacists, but the general sectors of societies had to depend largely on the ill-trained and ill-qualified compounders. The compounders were the pharmacists of the less privileged common people.

In 1943, the Government of British India appointed a Committee called Health Survey and Development Committee under the chairmanship of Sir Joshep Bhore, to make a broad survey of the existing position of health conditions and health organizations in British India and recommendations for future developments. The report of this committee was widely regarded as Blueprint of Health Services for Independent India as country was fast approaching towards achieving cherished goal of independence from British Empire.

POSTINDEPENDENT ERA

The industrial policy of independent India was aimed to build a diversified, relatively balanced, self-reliant economy in which growth would be accompanied by a modi-cum of distributive justice, i.e. socialism. The government played a critical role in building core industries, boosting agricultural growth to achieve self-reliance in food production, creating diversified research and develop-ment infrastructure, training skilled and scientific personnel and building public distribution system.

At the time of independence, the drug supply situation in the country was marked by a preponderance of mainly transnational companies (TNC) running a small number of plants which only imported and formulated a limited range of medicines. The healthcare infrastructure was poor and modern healthcare coverage was confined to a less than one-tenth of population, mainly in bigger cities and towns. There was a little or no control over the quality of drugs, price tended to be high and ungoverned, and profiteering was rampant. Misprescription was widespread; so too arbitrary choice of drugs for patients by dispensing chemists who were usually untrained but were called poor man's doctor.

There were no standard dosage, no effective labelling regulation, and no control on the kind or quality of information to be provided with medicinal formulations.

The Government of India set up the Pharmaceutical Enquiry Committee in 1953 under the chairmanship of Major General S. L. Bhatia to study the working of existing pharmaceutical concerns with reference to demand for drugs produced and their essentiality; the quality of drugs; the cost of productions; the efficiency of the process employed; and to recommend steps for encouraging the manufacture of important drugs which are imported into the country. The committee observed that the then pharmaceutical industries in the country could be considered to be non-existent compared to the situation in the USA and the UK. But the tempo of development of pharmaceutical industries was maintained. The export market was developed for glandular and alkaloids. This happy position did not last long. The products from better established and well-known pharmaceutical producers in countries soon replaced the Indian products. Even within the country the domestic companies were facing severe competition from foreign products or producers. The committee suggested the manufacturing of bulk drugs from the basic materials not only for India but also to cater the market of other countries.

The global pharmaceutical boom during 1950s and 1960s, when many new discoveries and inventions had taken place, had a direct bearing in Pharmaceutical scenario in the country. The Transnational Companies (TNCs) promoted their products through aggressive promotional techniques. One classic example was the promotion of extremely toxic antibiotic, chloramphenicol (though meant for typhoid fever), as common cure for a variety of infections including cough and common cold. This sort of unethical drug promotion led to resistance to the drug among the typhoid bacteria and eventually the drug became ineffective. When typhoid fever broke out in South India in 1960s, the chloramphenicol was found to be useless because of resistance.

Against this backdrop the Government of India took measures to create alternate source of drug supply and introduce systems for regulating industries. The following measures were initiated:

- The Drug (Display of Price) Order was passed in 1962 and the Drugs Price Control Order (DPCO) was issued in 1963 covering a small number of products under the Defence of India Act. The DPCO was subsequently modified in several occasions.

- Setting up of public sector pharmaceutical manufacturing units to manufacture new drugs needed for the treatment of infectious diseases especially penicillin and streptomycin. The private sectors particularly foreign companies were reluctant to manufacture such drugs. The Government of India set up in 1954 Hindusthan Antibiotics Limited (HAL) at Pimpri for manufacture of antibiotics and Indian Drugs and Pharmaceuticals Limited (IDPL) in 1961 with two units: one at Hyderabad for the production of synthetic drugs and the other at Rishikesh for the production of antibiotics. These industries were developed with an objective of making the country self-reliant in drugs and pharmaceuticals, to free the country from foreign exploitation and to produce cheaper medicines in adequate quantity for the benefit of the people. However, the production commenced only in 1968 and in 1955 at IDPL and HAL respectively.

- Changed the Intellectual Property Rights (IPR) system radically through Indian Patent Act 1970 looking at national interest. The new law disallowed product patents completely in food and health related sector. The process patent was only recognised for pharmaceuticals, which was limited to between five and seven years. The law also provided provision of compulsory licensing system for health-related items. The Patent Act revised in 2005 and reintroduced the product patent system in pharmaceuticals as a part of international obligation in post-liberalised period.

- Created a basic regulatory system for testing quality of drugs. The registration of drugs through drugs controller of India's office (central government) and control over all other aspects of medicines including manufacturing, sale and quality were vested on state government.

There were major developments in late 1960s and early 1970s: the then Prime Minister, Smt. Indira Gandhi, nationalising the major private commercial banks and strengthening antimonopoly and protectionist measures. A vigorous public sector and growing of wholly owned Indian private companies emerged.

Despite the production of about ₹ 370 crore worth of pharmaceuticals during 1973, it was estimated that modern drugs were accessible to only 20% of the population. Large-scale expansion of drug industries envisaged during fifth five year plan period with a view to ensuring the regulated and rapid growth of drug manufacture. With this background in mind, the Government of India appointed a committee under the chairmanship of Jaisukhlal Hathi, a respected politician, in 1974 to go into various facets of the drug industries with a view to promote Indian and small scale pharmaceutical industries, improve technological developments, take effective quality control measures, reduce price of medicines, and provide essential drugs throughout the country. The Hathi Committee report, which was submitted in 1975, was widely acclaimed as one of the best policy documents ever produced in the country. But the report was more in favour of industrial pharmaceutical policy rather than of health concern. One of the major concerns of the committee was dependence of the drug industries on import.

Important Recommendations of Hathi Committee Report

- A clear distinction should be made between the public, wholly owned Indian sectors on the one hand and the foreign sectors on the other.
- Some product lines should be reserved for public sectors.
- The indigenous drug industry should be encouraged through the phased imposition of bans on the import of bulk drugs.
- The state should take complete responsibility for supporting research to develop new drugs, especially for tropical diseases.
- Foreign companies should reduce their equity in pharmaceutical companies to 40% forthwith and gradually to 26%. To ensure that this actually dilutes foreign control, the government should purchase their shares either directly or through public sector undertakings.
- Foreign companies using imported bulk drugs should start manufacturing from the basic stage within a period of three years.
- An effective system of monitoring should be evolved to check compliance.
- Foreign companies should not be allowed to operate in small scale sector.
- Within one year foreign firms should switch over 50% of their production to manufacturing bulk drugs and formulations.
- There should be gradual changeover from brand names to generic names.
- Future steps towards a national drug formulary, better prescription practices and monitoring of drug abuse should be planned.

Between mid 1970s and late 1980s, there were many attempts of cooperation between pharmaceutical industries and public R&D laboratories. The prominent R&D organizations: National Chemical Laboratory, Pune; Central Drug Research Institute, Lucknow; and Regional Research Laboratory, Hyderabad (now known as Indian Institute of Chemical Technology) developed several cost effective, energy efficient processes and some new products which could compete internationally with dominant manufacturers' or original innovator's products. Dissemination of technology was relatively rapid and widespread. This helped in developing drugs from the basic stages and reducing the prices of final products. For instance, in 1993, the price of ranitidine in India was 16.58 times lower than the price at which Glaxo was selling in the UK.

Indian companies and laboratories became sufficiently strong and equipped to produce the same molecules by different and cost effective method of synthesis. The Patent Act 1970 encouraged such innovations. The country has greatly benefited from this generic drugs that were made available plenty.

Based on Hathi Committee report, though many recommendations were diluted, the first Drug Policy was drawn up in 1978. As a follow up of this, the DPCO 1970 was modified introducing Drug Price Equalization Fund and a system of monitoring the production of bulk drugs. These provisions are regulated by the Ministry of Chemicals and Fertilisers and the Bureau of Industrial Costs and Prices of Ministry of Industries. The Drug Policy 1978 was a licensing and pricing policy without overt linkages with the Health Policy of the country. The policy was not implemented with a strong political will. Though the public sector was projected as a key driver of drug industry, this never happened. In fact, within a few years the public sectors got progressively weaker.

Between 1947 and 1969, the drug industry was dominated by multinational companies (MNCs). In late 1950s and early 1960s, the establishment of public sector initiated drug production in organized sector. In 1970 Indian owned companies had 10 to 20% share of total drug market while MNCs accounting for the remaining 80–90%. By 1980, Indian and MNCs had approximately equal shares and by 1993, the share of Indian firms had grown to 61%.

POSTLIBERALIZED PERIOD

The year 1990–1991 is considered to be the cut-off year for liberalization in the country. Contrary to the common perception to liberalization for it being against the "aam aadmi", there has been a hefty increase in free economic environment in social sectors such as education, health, rural development and food. The developments occurred in post-liberalized period are discussed under the following headings:

Policy

The signing of new International Trade Agreement under the Uruguay Round of the General Agreement on Tariffs and Trade (GATT) in December 1993 brought a new paradigm in Indian scenario drifting from socialism to capitalism where market forces would decide what is essential and what is not.

With this backdrop the Drug Policy 1994 was introduced. The policy outlines 'the measures for rationalisation, quality control and growth of drugs and pharmaceutical industries in India. Besides these, it proposed to ensure abundant availability of essential and life saving and prophylactic medicines of good quality, at reasonable prices. The Drugs Price Control Order (DPCO) was issued in 1995 to regulate the prices of medicines. However, with successive orders, the number of drugs under DPCO is limited to 74 as on July 2006 with decreasing number from 347 in DPCO 1979 to 142 in DPCO 1987 and 76 under DPCO 1995. In order to give further teeth to DPCO, the National Pharmaceutical Pricing Authority (NPPA) is created in 1997. The NPPA is an independent body of experts under the Ministry of Chemicals and Fertilisers, Department of Pharmaceuticals, is assigned the task of price fixation or revision and other related matters such as monitoring of the prices of decontrolled drugs and formulations. With the Supreme Court's intervention the Government of India brought a revised DPCO 2013 paving a way to regulate the prices of all medicines under National List of Essential Medicines. However, the DPCO 2013 significantly differ from DPCO 1995 at least on two aspects: All medicines including coronary stents are now under price capping and price capping is not based on manufacturing cost. The readers can find more details in the chapter: Drug Price Control order.

Then the new policy 'Pharmaceutical Policy 2002' was announced but could not be implemented because of protests from several corners and high court judgement. This policy further proposed price deregulation to bring down the number of drugs under DPCO is just to 35 from 74. The rationale behind this liberalization was that completion stabilises price of consumer products where consumers have a direct choice. But the medicines are different commodities where real consumers have no choice.

The new draft policy was then released in 2006 "National Pharmaceutical Policy 2006". The Sandhu Committee and Pronab Sen Committee's report on access and affordability of medicines to the vulnerable and poorer segments of the population were the part of the draft policy. This too could not be materialised.

Thus the policy of 1994 is in existence.

The Government of India, instead of concentrating on Pharmaceutical Policy, has notified National Pharmaceutical Pricing Policy 2012 (NPPP 2012) on July 2012. The NPPP is the extension of Drugs Policy of 1994. The objective of the policy is to place a regulatory framework for pricing of drugs to ensure availability of required medicines— "essential medicines"—at reasonable prices and at the same time providing sufficient opportunity for innovation and competition to support the growth of industry, thereby meeting the goals of employment and shared economic well-being for all. The outcome of NPPP is the DPCO 2013 which currently regulates the prices of all medicines listed in NLEM 2015.

In September 2014, the Indian Government launched the "Make in India" campaign, with the objective of making India a global manufacturing hub; thus, bringing foreign technology and capital into the country. In 2017, the draft pharmaceutical policy is announced inviting stakeholders' comments before finalizing the long pending holistic pharmaceutical policy.

Infrastructure and Administration

The Government of India established a separate 'Department of Pharmaceuticals' under the Ministry of Chemicals and Fertilisers to look after the following divisions: Pharmaceutical Industries, Public Sector Pharmaceutical Industries, National Institute of Pharmaceutical Education and Research (NIPER), Research and Development and National Pharmaceutical Pricing Authority (NPPA). The department is headed by a secretary and assisted by two joint secretaries, one economic adviser, and one Deputy Director General.

The Central Drugs Standard Control Organization (CDSCO) has shifted its operation from the Nirman Bhawan to a newly build palatial FDA Bhawan. The then newly appointed Drugs Controller General India (DCGI) initiated several steps such as improving the manpower through recruiting drugs inspectors and other staff, promoting the present staff to various levels and promising e-governance like online submission of all forms and applications, digitalised interactive portals, online approvals with digital signature, nearly paperless office, etc. The CDSCO has been strengthened over the years with more number of employment of regulatory officers.

Over the years, CDSCO has changed its role too. Initially, it was perceived just as regulator. Its website now projects its vision "To Protect and Promote Public Health in India" and mission as "To safeguard and enhance the public health by assuring safety, efficacy and quality of drugs, cosmetics and medical devices".

Schedule M is made mandatory for all manufacturing companies with effect from 1st July 2005 which further ensures that India produces quality medicines. The Government now proposes to upgrade the Schedule M to be on par with WHO GMP. The Schedule M (III) for Medical Devices too made mandatory.

Against the backdrop of campaign that India has a significant spurious drugs market, the Government of India constituted an expert committee under the chairmanship of Dr R A Mashelkar, Director General of

Council of Scientific and Industrial Research in January 2003. The committee was assigned to undertake comprehensive review of drug regulatory issues including the problems of spurious drugs and to evaluate the extent of problem of spurious drugs and measures required to tackle the problem effectively. Some of its recommendations are made into effect later.

The Government too made some proactive steps to curb the menace of spurious drugs. It has introduced a handsome reward scheme for whistle blowers to encourage good intentioned people (informers) who provide specific information to the designated authorities leading to the seizure of spurious, adulterated, misbranded and not of standard quality drugs, cosmetics and medical devices in 2009. It seems to be giving encouraging result.

Contrary to the public perception and sensational headlines in newspapers about the quality of medicines produced in India, the latest report of GOI, the biggest drug quality survey result, pegs the percentage of substandard drugs produced and sold in India at 3.5%. This figure is much lower than the proportion of 'Not of Standard Quality' medicines elsewhere in the world. [National Drug Survey 2014–2016 Report].

The GOI has also brought the new National Intellectual Rights Policy in May 2016 reinforcing the strengths of IPR to acquire both economic and social benefits on a bigger and higher scale. It proposes to have a vibrant IP ecosystem.

There is also a move to bring all activities under one umbrella. Currently the Department of Pharmaceuticals of the Ministry of Chemicals and Fertilisers looks into pharmaceutical policy and price regulations including the growth of pharmaceutical industries. On the other hand, the Ministry of Health and Family Welfare is entrusted with the task of ensuring quality of medicines, clinical research, and activities related to approval of new drugs, manufacturing, distribution and sale of medicines. This move would help in harmonization of the work of CDSCO and Department of Pharmaceuticals.

Legislations

Based on several recommendations beginning from the Hathi Committee Report to Mashelkar Committee Report, the Government of India proposed to have Central Drugs Authority with a power of regulating all aspects related to Drugs and Cosmetics leaving just regulating sales to the state governments. Accordingly Drugs and Cosmetics (Amendment) Bill 2007 was introduced to the Parliament. But it could not get through as was rejected by the Parliamentary Panel. This left the dream of having a strong drugs controlling authority in the country though government continues pursuing the agenda.

Based on Mashelkar Committee report on spurious drugs, the Government of India through Drugs and Cosmetics (Amendment) Act 2008 enhanced the penalties for various offences relating to spurious drugs and made such offences as cognizable and non-bailable. This overcomes the previous difficulties the prosecution authorities used to face as the offences were non-cognizable and bailable besides meagre punishments.

Keeping the tune of commitments to the World Trade Organization (WTO), the Government of India first promulgated an ordinance on December 26, 2004 and then subsequently passing Patent (Amendment) Act 2005. The Act received the Presidential Assent on 4th April 2005 making the country as TRIPS agreement compliant. The country comes under the banner of product patent for not only medicines but also for agriculture and softwares despite the powerful protest from various quarters including International NGOs, individuals, public concerned with public health. The impact of this product patent on Indian economy, growth of pharmaceutical industries and public health is yet to be seen.

As biologicals constitute a sizeable proportions of medicinal products and they differ from usual chemical-based pharmaceuticals, the Department of Biotechnology proposed to establish National Biotechnology Regulatory Board to regulate the development of drugs and vaccines from natural sources such as humans, animals or microorganisms. If this happens, the regulatory mechanism will shift from Ministry of Health

(CDSCO) to Ministry of Science and Technology (Department of Biotechnology).

The medical devices are different from drugs. There have been long standing demand to have separate authority, or at least have separate set of rules for medical devices. In this direction, the government has notified the Medical Device Rules 2017 but would be effective from 01st January 2018. The following medical devices are notified as drugs to have effective control under Drugs and Cosmetics Rules: Cardiac stents, drug eluting stents, catheters, intra-ocular lenses, IV cannulae, bone cements, heart valves, scalp vein set, orthopaedic implants, and internal prosthetic replacements in 2005. Often, it is said "A country has standard for condoms but not for medical devices". In fact, a separate standard and regulations are necessary. The new rule is now notified.

With increased focus on clinical research in India, the Government of India initiated regulatory measures to ensure that the rights of research participants are protected. Accordingly, the Schedule Y is amended in 2005 to include mandatory Good Clinical Practice (GCP) compliance for carrying out clinical research. With reports of exploitation of innocent people participating in the clinical research, the Supreme Court intervened. Subsequently, the schedule Y was further amended making mandatory provision for registration of ethics committee, compensation payment in case of injury. Other measures like liberalizing the requirement of study site and limiting the number of trials per investigator are likely to boost the clinical research industry.

Pharmacovigilance is made mandatory. The guidance document for adoption by pharmaceutical industries is issued.

Education

There are dramatic improvements in education sectors in postliberalized period. The potential growth of pharmaceutical industries both in manufacturing sectors as well as in research led to the growth of pharmaceutical education in the country. But the growth is not proportionate to the requirements leaving many institutions striving to get students to sustain. They are not proportionately located and most of the institutions are located in southern part of the country.

The first National Institute called "National Institute of Pharmaceutical Education and Research" at Mohali is established under an Act of Parliament as Institute of National Importance on 26th June 1998. At present there are seven NIPERs located at: Mohali, Ahmedabad, Hyderabad, Kolkata, Hajipur, Guwahati and Raebareli. Four more NIPERs are under process of being established: Madurai (approved in 2012), one each at Chhattisgarh, Maharashtra and Rajasthan (announced during budget of 2015–2016).

The Pharmacy Council of India too introduced new Education Regulation to introduce six years Doctor of Pharmacy (Pharm. D.) and three years Post Baccalaureate Pharm. D. programme in 2008. The Annamalai University is the first institute in the country to start the Pharm. D. programmes with support from University Grants Commission. Pharm. D. is also notified as registrable qualification for pharmacists. Pharm. D. programmes are launched online with the programmes of the United States of America.

There are 968 approved pharmacy colleges offering degree courses in the country as on May 2014 (http://pib.nic.in/newsite/erelease.aspx?relid=107825). In spite of having large number of institutions, there is no clarity and confusion still prevailing. The debate continues on the multi-control of Pharmaceutical Education by three statutory bodies: Pharmacy Council of India (PCI), All India Council for Technical Education (AICTE) and University Grants Commission (UGC). The Pharm. D. programme is also brought under the regulatory purview of AICTE with effect from 2018-2019 academic session.

In order to strengthen the pharmaceutical education and practice of pharmacy, a series of regulations were framed with the initiative of PCI. They are: Minimum Qualification for Teachers in Pharmacy Institutions Regulations, 2014; Master of Pharmacy (M. Pharm.) Course Regulations 2014; Bachelor of Pharmacy (B. Pharm.) Course Regulations, 2014; and Pharmacy Practice Regulations, 2015.

Industries

The Indian pharmaceutical industries have made significant progress over the years and more so during the postliberalized period.

There are more than 10500 pharmaceutical industries in the country of which majority are in small sector. About 300–400 units are categorized as medium and large ones. These industries are not equally distributed throughout the country. While five states: Maharastra (29.7%), Gujarat (14.4%), West Bengal (7.2%), Andhra Pradesh (6.9%) and Tamil Nadu (5.4%) account for about two-third of total number of manufacturers and another 22 States and Union Territories account for only little over one-third of total number of pharmaceutical manufacturers [2008–2009 Annual Report of Department of Pharmaceuticals]. This is on line with industrial development clusters developed by the respective states.

The Indian pharmaceutical industry has grown from a mere USD 0.3 billion turnover in 1980 to about USD 19 billion in 2008. The country now ranks 3rd in terms of volume of production (10% of global share) and 14th largest by value (1.5%). One reason for lower value share is the lower cost of drugs in India ranging from 5% to 50% less as compared to developed countries. Indian pharma industry growth has been fuelled by exports and its products are exported to more than 200 countries with a sizeable share in the advanced regulated markets of the US and Western Europe. Indian pharma industry employs over 42 lakhs directly and indirectly. 40% of the world's bulk drug requirement is met by India. (Third Round up, Department of Pharmaceuticals, July 2009).

The Indian Pharmaceutical Companies have been currently growing at a compound annual growth rate (CAGR) of approximately 10% for the period 2010–11 to 2014–15. The growth rate has come down from 14.36% in 2010–11 to 8.68% in 2014–15 [Draft Pharmaceutical Policy 2017]. The growth of pharmaceutical industries could not be sustained due to several reasons: Non-adherence to quality standards and norms; growing competition from other countries; dependence on imports of API and other starting materials; lack of R&D and discovery of new formulations. Even the domestic compulsion of price capping of all essential medicines too contributed the slowdown the economic growth of pharmaceutical industries. The USFDA has issued several warning letters and import alerts to Indian companies. As on end of 2015, 42 Indian facilities of 28 pharmaceutical companies were under import alert. The tough completion from even our neighboring countries: Vietnam, Sri Lanka, Korea, Bangladesh posing a threat to generic market. The most of the APIs are now imported and the overdependence on one or two countries is a serious concern for drug security. In fact, during 1954 to 1966, India was able to produce most of APIs and intermediate products making India sustainable. The R&D spending is so low that not able to show any visible results in terms of drug discovery.

In spite of the current slowdown, the prospects looks to be optimistic. The government's efforts

Total domestic Indian market in crore (Indian Rupees)	November 2004	2005	2006	2007	2008
	33036	35764	42355	47596	52491

The export growth is above 17%:

Export Figure in crore (Indian Rupees)	2002–2003	2003–2004	2004–2005	2005–2006	2006–2007	2007–2008	2008–2009 (up to September 2009)
	12826	15213 (17.38%)	17857 (24.41%)	22216 (21.06%)	26895 (14.37%)	30759 (18.61%)	18021.16

(*Source:* Annual Report, Department of Pharmaceuticals, 2008–2009).

to making business easier in the country and completion of all the initiated projects would likely boost the growth. Glaxosmithkline Pharmaceuticals, Shantha Biotechnics, Cipla Biotec and Aurobindo Pharma are some of the companies which completed their projects during the period [Annual report 2016–2017, Department of Pharmaceuticals]. The increasing healthcare spending, changing demographic trends with increasing elderly persons, increasing disposable income and increasing emergence of lifestyle diseases would likely to contribute the domestic growth.

In addition to the manufacturing activity, India becomes the favourite destination for clinical research. The multinational pharmaceutical companies are looking towards India for outsourcing data for new drugs approval mostly because of low cost and likely credible data. This has brought increased growth of Clinical Research Organizations (CROs) in the country. The Indian CRO market is likely boom further after a brief slowdown.

Indian Pharmaceutical Industry at a Glance

- India has the largest number of USFDA approved manufacturing facilities (262). Its 253 plants are approved by European Directorate for the Quality of Medicines (EDQM) and has 1300 WHO GMP compliant units [Draft Pharmaceutical Policy 2017].
- Indian pharma sector is largely fuelled exports and is the third largest foreign exchange earner for India. It exports to more than 200 countries, often called the 'Pharmacy of the World'.
- Compound annual growth rate for the last five years was 8.8% [Annual Report 2016–2017, Department of Pharmaceuticals].
- Currently, India's share of Abbreviated New Drug Approvals (ANDA) is 31.8%.
- Position of Indian pharmaceutical industries': 3rd in terms of volume, 14th in terms of value, 4th in terms of generic production, and 17th in terms of export value [Indian Pharma Sector Dissected, Choice, June 6, 2017).

- Sun Pharmaceutical Industries Limited is the biggest pharmaceutical company in the country.

Like international players the Indian pharmaceutical companies too strategically acquired several firms to enter new markets and consolidate their positions. Indian firms made 18 international acquisitions between January 2004 and October 2005, including Matrix Labs' acquisition of Belgium's Docpharma for USD 263 million in June 2005; Dr Reddy's acquisition of Roche's API business for USD 59.6 million; Ranbaxy's acquisition of a 40% stake in Japan's Nihon Pharmaceutical Industry; and Sun Pharma's completion of its purchase of ICN Hungary for an undisclosed sum. In 2006, Ranbaxy acquired a South African generics company, Be-Tabs, apart from Ethimed (Belgium), Therapia (Romania) and Mundogen (Spain). In 2006, Dr Reddy bought out Germany's fourth-largest generics company, Betapharm Arzneimittel, from UK-based 3i for USD 573.6 million, which was the biggest acquisition seen in the sector until then. Nicholas Piramal's acquisition of Avecia Custom Drug Synthesis of the UK for USD 16.7 million in 2005 and Jubilant Organosys acquired Hollister-Stier Laboratories (US) in May 2007. Wockhardt acquired the Wallis Laboratory (1997) and CP Pharmaceuticals (2003) based in the UK and Esparma, Germany, in 2004 for its biopharmaceutical work.

At the same time there are disturbing trends too. The Indian companies are purchased by multinational foreign companies. Acquisition of a 50% stake in Ranbaxy by Daiichi Sankyo makes Ranbaxy Japanese Company. Similarly companies such as Piramal Healthcare, Santha Biotech and Dabur Pharma are acquired by Abott Lab. (USA), Sanofi Pasteur SA (USA) and Fresenius Kabi AG (Germany) respectively. There are apprehensions that this would result in foreign multinational companies gaining market supremacy. Fortunately, the Sun Pharmaceutical Industries Limited acquired back the Ranbaxy from Japanese making Sun Pharma, the biggest Indian Pharma. The deal was completed in 2015.

Top 10 Acquisitions in India's Pharmaceutical Sector

Company acquiring	Company merged	Year and deal
Sun Pharma	Ranbaxy	2015: USD 4 billion
Abbott (US)	Formulation Unit of Pirmal Healthcare	2010: USD 3.72 billion
Daiichi (Japan)	Ranbaxy	2008: USD 4.6 billion
Lupin	Gavis (US)	2015: USD 880 million
Lupin	Biocom (Russia)	2015
Sun Pharma	Taro (Israel)	2007: USD 454 million
Dr Reddy's	UCB in India (Belgium)	2016: USD 128.38 million
Dr Reddy's	Betapharm (Germany)	2006: Euro 480 million
Torrent Pharma	Elder Pharma	2014: USD 324 million
Cipla	InvaGen and Exelan (US)	2016: USD 550 million

Merger and acquisition may help improving the capital, productivity and innovation, there are apprehension that this may adversely affect the access to medicines.

The growth and competency of Indian pharmaceutical industries over the last decade or so became the worrisome for multinational foreign companies. One or other way, the multinational foreign companies have been trying to trouble or halt the growth of Indian companies by widening the definition of counterfeit medicines (there is no such definition in Indian Legislation) and Indian generic supply have been termed counterfeit and seized at different ports and airports of European Union while they are exported to third world countries. The Government of India lodged a protest to WTO on this. The products are genuine products manufactured under a license valid both in the country of origin and destination country. They are seized on the ground that they infringed on Intellectual Property Rights or violated the patent rights (2010).

There is another malicious campaign that the most of the fake or spurious drugs originate from India. This is not true. Here is a classic example where foreign made but Indian Label fake medicines circulating (See Box). Even to counter the move of this malicious campaign, the Government of India conducted a countrywide survey on spurious medicines (2014–2016) and reported that the prevalence of not of standard quality medicines in domestic market is less than 3.5%. But the report of the study would be how effective in increasing the global trust is yet to be seen. Even inside the country, it is hard to trust the result when there have been frequent report of fake and substandard and recycling of expired drugs appearing in daily newspapers.

Fake Drugs from China - India lodges Protest

http://timesofindia.indiatimes.com/Govt-protests-fake-India-tag-on-China-drugs/articleshow/4643585.cms

Times of India, 12 Jun 2009, 0509 hrs IST, TNN New Delhi: India has asked the Chinese government to take action against bootleggers who are making fake drugs and shipping them abroad with 'Made in India' tags as a tactic to cover the origin. The commerce department has lodged a complaint with the Chinese embassy here and the Indian embassy in Beijing has been asked to push for action against the impostors.

The Indian action comes after Nigeria's pharma regulator reported the detention of a large consignment of fake drugs for treating malaria. The consignment carried 'Made in India' labels but was produced in China. A laboratory test of the consignment of Maloxine and Amalar tablets proved these were fake. Had the drugs flowed into the market, over 600,000 lives would have been affected. After getting information from Nigerian authorities, the Indian high commissioner in Nigeria indicated that the consignment containing drugs were produced, packed and shipped from China. Fake Chinese drugs with 'Made in India' tag hurts reputation of Indian pharmaceuticals industry and is expected to give rise to more trouble for genuine Indian consignments to Africa and elsewhere transiting through Europe.

The government is making efforts at brand promotion of Indian pharmaceuticals and generic drugs in Africa. An Indian delegation recently met African health ministers and officials to assure them that genuine Indian generic pharma was as safe as patented versions and was available at more reasonable prices.

The African ministers were also informed that the Indian government had launched a massive offensive against manufacture and sale of spurious medicines. Drug Controller General of India regularly conducts on-the-spot inspections and lift samples at random. A study of samples of drugs tested all over the country in the last 4–5 years revealed that about 0.3% to 0.4% of around 40,000 samples fell within the category of spurious drugs.

Drugs and Cosmetics Act

"The *National Human Rights Commission* (NHRC) has described the manufacture, distribution and sale of unsafe drugs and medical devices as a violation of human rights."

— www.drugscontrol.org

After reading this chapter, you should be able to understand and appreciate:
- Need of drugs control mechanism
- Regulation relating to import and export, manufacture, labelling and packaging, sale of medicine of allopathic, homeopathic and Ayurvedic, siddha and unani systems and cosmetics.
- Regulation relating to medical device.
- Regulation relating to quality of medicines and cosmetics
- Administrative procedure for implementing the regulations
- Regulatory Authorities of other countries.

Drugs or medicines (often used inter-changeably) are part of our lives. They not only save lives and promote health, but also prevent epidemics and diseases. They have been recognised as the greatest weapon of mankind to fight diseases and deaths. But they need to be safe, effective, and of good quality and used appropriately. This in turn requires that their development, production, importation, exportation and subsequent distribution must be regulated to ensure that they meet the prescribed standard. With advancement of science and technology, many new and sophisticated medicinal products have been introduced into the market for the patient care. But at the same time, circulation of toxic, substandard, and counterfeit drugs on the national and international market has increased. The use of toxic, substandard and counterfeit medicines is not only a waste of money, but

may also threaten the health and lives of those who take them. The issue of safety, efficacy, and quality can be effectively controlled or redressed through effective drug regulation.

Legal structures form the foundation of drug regulation. The drug laws provide basis for drug regulation. Throughout the world the drug legislation exists. Drug regulation comprises all measures: Legal, administrative and technical—which the government takes to ensure the safety, efficacy and quality of medicines or similar products, besides ensuring appropriate product information.

The genesis of drug control in India could be traced back to the preindependence era. The council of states adopted a resolution in 1927 to initiate immediate measures to control the indiscriminate use of drugs and to legislate for standardization of the pre-parations and for sale of such drugs. In persuasion of this resolution and in response to the public opinion against the defective drugs, the then Government of India in 1930 appointed a committee known as Drugs Enquiry Committee. The mandate of the committee was to enquire the extent to which drugs of impure quality or defective strength were being imported, manufactured, or sold in India; and to recommend steps for controlling such import, manufacture and sale in public interest. This committee was also known as Chopra Committee as Col. R. N. Chopra was the Chairman. One of the recommendations of the committee was to make a Central Legislation to control drugs. In response to this recommendation, the Government of India passed the Drugs Act in 1940 to regulate the import, manufacture, distribution and sale of drugs. The rules under the Act were framed in 1945 to give effect to the provision of the Act. It came into force from 1st of April 1947.

The Drugs Act 1940 was a colonial legislation designed to protect the opportunistic rights of foreign traders who were controlling the import and distribution of drugs in India. The Drugs Act was first amended in 1955 in which central government was empowered to frame rules under the Act in respect of control over manufacture and sale of drugs. Prior this amendment the state governments had power to frame rules. In subsequent

amendment in 1962 "cosmetics" were brought under control of the statute and consequently the name of the Act was changed from the Drugs Act to Drugs and Cosmetics Act. The Ayurvedic (including Siddha) and Unani drugs were brought under the statute with Drugs and Cosmetics (Amendment) Act 1964. Similarly comprehensive provisions were introduced in 1964 in the Drugs and Cosmetics Rules for exercising control over Homeopathic Medicines. Separate regulations for medical devices also introduced. The Act has undergone several amendments since 1940 and the salient features of these amendments are given in a tabular form.

The Drugs and Cosmetics Act is a life-saving statute. It regulates the import, manufacture, distribution and sale; and standards of drugs and cosmetics. The **Act is administered by the Ministry of Health and Welfare at National level and Department of Health at State level.** However, it does not regulate the possession of drugs or the use of drugs by any person or by medical practitioner. It does not control the practice of medicine too. There are two organizations with clear-cut responsibilities have control over drugs and cosmetics: Central Drug Standard Control Organization (CDSCO) headed by Drugs Controller (General) India; and State Drug Control Organization in each state has often different name: Directorate of Drugs Control [West Bengal], Food and Drug

Country	Legislation	Regulating agency
USA	Food, Drugs and Cosmetics Act	Food and Drug Administration (FDA)
Canada	Food and Drug Act and Regulations	Health Canada
Australia	Therapeutics Goods Act	Therapeutics Goods Administration (TGA)
Thailand	Drug Control Act 1967	Food and Drug Administration (FDA)
Malaysia	Poison Ordinance and Control of Drug and Cosmetic Regulations	National Pharmaceutical Control Bureau
South Africa	Medicines and Related Substances Control Act 1965	Medicines Control Council in South Africa
India	Drugs and Cosmetics Act 1940 and Drugs and Cosmetics Rules 1945	Central Drug Standard Control Organization
UK	Medicines Act 1968	Medicines and Health Products Regulatory Agency (MHRA)
Japan	Pharmaceutical Affairs Law	Organization of Pharmaceutical and Food Safety Bureau (PFSB) and Pharmaceuticals and Medical Devices Agency (PMDA)

Administration [Maharashtra]. The primary responsibility of central government with respect to drugs control is on imported and new drugs while responsibility of manufacture, sale and distribution lies with the state government.

The provisions of this Act are in addition to Drugs and Psychotropic Substances

Milestone in Drugs Legislation in India	
Committee/Legislation	Main features
Drugs Enquiry Committee (Chopra Committee) 1930	Recommended to make central legislation to control drugs and pharmacy.
Drugs Act 1940	To regulate the import, manufacture, distribution and sale of drugs.
Health Survey and Development Committee 1943	Recommended the establishment of All India Pharmaceutical and Provincial Pharmacy Councils, setting up of Central Drugs Laboratory; and operation and rigid enforcement of Drugs Act throughout the country.
Drug Rules 1945	To give effects to the provision of Drugs Act.
Pharmaceutical Enquiry Committee with Major General S L Bhatia as Chairman 1953–1954	Recommended for enforcing quality control measures by amending Drugs Act.
Drugs (Amendment) Act 1955	The central government was empowered to frame rules under the Act in respect of control over manufacture and sale of drugs (earlier it was with respective state governments)
Health Survey and Planning Committee under the Chairmanship of Dr. A. Lakshmanswami Mudaliar 1959–1961	Recommended the necessity to bring drugs prepared according to indigenous system of medicine under the purview of Drugs Act.
Drugs (Amendment) Act 1960	The central government was empowered to appoint government analyst and drugs inspector as well. The central government assumed statutory powers to give directions to the states to carrying into execution of any provision of the Act or Rules.
Drugs and Equipments Standard Committee (Naskar Committee) 1962–1965	To assess *inter alia* the extent of spurious drugs moving in the country and the steps that should be taken to augment Drug Control Administration and its enforcement.
Drugs (Amendment) Act 1962	Cosmetics were brought under control.The statute known as Drugs and Cosmetics Act.
Drugs and Cosmetics (Amendment) Act 1964	Ayurvedic (including Siddha) and Unani drugs were brought under the purview of statute.
Borkar Committee 1964–1966	To study the set up of State Drugs Control Administration, Inspectorate Staff, and Drug Testing facilities.
Purabi Mukopadhay Committee 1966	To study the set up of Drugs Control Administration in the light of Naskar Committee and Borkar Committee reports.
Drugs and Cosmetics (Amendment) Act 1972	Extended to the State of Jammu and Kashmir.
Hathi Committee 1974–1975	To enquire into the progress made by drug industry and recommend measures for effective quality control of drugs.
Drugs and Cosmetics (Amendment) Act 1982	Devices were considered as drugs.The central government was empowered to prohibit import or manufacture and sale of drugs and cosmetics in public interest. Ayurvedic, Siddha and Unani systems were considered as three different systems (earlier Siddha was part of Ayurveda).

(Contd...)

(Contd...)

Committee/Legislation	Main features
Task Force on Drug Control 1982	To study the existing status of drugs control enforcement and recommend suitable measures for its improvements.
Drugs and Cosmetics (Amendment) Act 1986	To give effect of Consumer Protection Act.
Director General Health Services (DGHS) combat Committee 2001	Suggested certain remedial measures needed to be taken to the menace of spurious drugs.
Mashelkar Committee 2003	Recommended the restructuring of the CDSCO into a strong Central Drug Authority. Taking over of manufacturing license from state regulation to central authority.
Drugs and Cosmetics (Amendment) Bill 2007	Proposed establishment of Central Drug Authority in which Controller (India) will be Secretary and Chief Executive Officer of the CDA. The Bill could not get through.
Drugs and Cosmetics (Amendment) Act 2008	Revised Penalty for dealing with spurious and adulterated drugs.
PN Tandon Committee (2009)	To study the growing menace of spurious drugs, medical devices and plight of diagnostic centers in the country and to suggest ways and means to tackle these issues.
Drugs Bill 2013 [It did not get through]	Proposed to have Centralized Licensing for Certain Categories of Drugs
Drugs and Cosmetics (Fourth Amendment) Rules 2013	Schedule H1 introduced
Professor Ranjit Roy Chaudhury Expert Committee Report 2013 and Subsequent Amendment of Drug and Cosmetic Rules	Scheduled Y amended introducing features like registration of Ethics Committee, Payment of Compensation
Drugs and Cosmetics (First Amendment) Rules 2013	Introducing the concept of Pharmacovigilance and PSUR made mandatory
Drugs and Cosmetics (Third Amendment) Rules 2015	Prohibiting the advertisement of Drugs in Schedule H, H1 and X
Professor Kokate Committee Report 2016	On Fixed Dose Combinations
Drugs and Cosmetics (Amendment) Rule 2016	Mandating all manufacturers and importers for setting up a pharmacovigilance system managed by qualified and trained personnel within their company
Medical Devices Rules 2017	Separate regulation for Medical Devices, effective from 01.01.2018
Drugs and Cosmetics (Ninth Amendment) Rules, 2017	Biopharmaceutical Classification System introduced making mandatory data of Bioequivalency for oral dosage forms of Category II and Category IV drugs (low solubility and high permeability; low solubility and low permeability)

Act 1985 and any other law for the time being in force. The Government proposes to deal with situations like: Prescribing unnecessary medicines, taking presents from the pharmaceutical companies, accepting their hospitality and conducting clinical trials without following prescribed norms by treating them as offences. Some of the issues are addresses by other Departments or Ministries. The Department of Pharmaceuticals, Ministry of Chemicals and Fertilizers, deal with Pharmaceutical Policy, Price Control of Medicines and Pharmaceutical Industries.

The Drugs and Cosmetics Act and Rules have the following schedules

Schedule to the Act	Explanation
First schedule	List of books on Ayurvedic, Siddha and Unani system of medicines.
Second schedule	Standards to be complied by imported and manufactured drugs for sale, sold, stocked or exhibited for sale or distributed.

Schedule to Rules	Explanation
A	Proforma for application for license, issue and renewal of licenses, sending memorandum and certificate of test or analysis.
B	Fees for test or analysis by Central Drugs Laboratory or the Government Analyst.
C	List of biological and special products.
C (1)	List of special products.
D	List of drugs exempted from the provisions of import drugs.
E(1)	List of poisonous substances under the Ayurvedic (including Siddha) and Unani. Systems of Medicine.
F	Space, equipment and supplies required for a blood bank.
F(I)	Provisions applicable to the production of vaccines, sera and diagnostic antigens.
F(II)	Standards for surgical dressings.
F(III)	Standards for umbilical tapes.
FF	Standards for ophthalmic preparations.
G	List of drugs that are required to be used only under medical supervision and are to be labelled accordingly.
H	List of prescription drugs.
H1	List of high-ended antibiotics, anti-TB and other drugs. This requires special labelling and selling condition. A move to restrict the access of antibiotics to the common public as a measure to combat antibiotic resistance.
J	Diseases and ailments which a drug may not purport to prevent or cure or make claims to prevent or cure.
K	Drugs exempted from certain provisions relating to manufacture, sale and distribution of drugs.
M	Good Manufacturing Practices (GMP) and requirements of premises, plant and equipment.
M-I	GMP for homeopathic medicines.
M-II	GMP for cosmetics.
M-III	GMP for Medical Devices (This is now replaced and made as Quality Management System for Medical Devices and in vitro diagnostics under Medical Device Rules 2017)
N	List of minimum equipment for efficient running of a pharmacy.
O	Standards for disinfectant fluids.
P	Life period of drugs.
P-I	Pack sizes of drugs.
Q	List of dyes, colours and pigments permitted to be used in cosmetics and soaps as amended by Bureau of Indian Standards (BIS).
R	Standards for condoms.
R-I	Standards for certain medical devices as laid down by BIS.
S	Standards for cosmetics.
T	GMP for Ayurvedic, Siddha and Unani medicines.
U	Particulars to be shown in manufacturing records of products, records of raw materials, and analytical records.
U(1)	Particulars to be shown in the manufacturing records and records of raw materials with respect to cosmetics.
V	Standards for patent and proprietary medicines.
W	Drugs which should be marketed under generic names only.
X	List of drugs whose import, manufacture, sale, labelling and packaging are governed by special provisions.
Y	Requirements and guidelines on clinical trials.

Schedule A (various forms)

Form no.	Details
1	Memorandum to the Central Drugs Laboratory (Sending sample by the court to CDL)
2	Certificate of test or analysis by the Central Drugs Laboratory
8	Application for license to import drugs (excluding those specified in Schedule X)
8 A	Application for license to import drugs specified in Schedule X
9	Form of undertaking to accompany an application for an import license
10	License to import drugs (excluding those specified in Schedule X)
10 A	License to import drugs specified in Schedule X
11	License to import drugs for the purposes of examination, test or analysis
11 A	License to import drugs by a Government Hospital or Autonomous Medical Institution for the treatment of patients
12	Application for license to import drugs for purpose of examination, test or analysis
12 A	Application for the issue of a permit to import small quantities of drugs for personal use
12 AA	Application for license to import small quantities of new drugs by a Government Hospital or Autonomous Medical Institution for the treatment of patients
12 B	Permit for the import of small quantities of drugs for personal use
13	Certificate of test or analysis by Government Analyst (Drugs and Cosmetics)
13 A	Certificates of tests or analysis by Government Analyst (ASU Medicines)
14 A	Application from a purchaser for test or analysis of a drug (Drugs and Cosmetics)
14 B	Certificate of test or analysis by Government Analyst (Drugs and Cosmetics)
15	Order not to dispose of the stock in possession
16	Receipt for stock of drugs or cosmetics for record, register, document or material object seized
17	Intimation to person from whom sample is taken
17 A	Receipt for samples of drugs or cosmetics taken where fair price tendered is refused
18	Memorandum to Government Analyst [samples sent by drugs inspector]
18 A	Memorandum to Government Analyst samples sent by drugs inspector for ASU medicines
19	Application for grant or renewal of a license to sell, stock or exhibit or offer for sale, or distribute drugs other than those specified in Schedule X
19 A	Application for the grant or renewal of a restricted license to sell, stock or exhibit or offer for sale, or distribute drugs by retail by dealers who do not engage the services of a registered pharmacist
19 AA	Application for grant or renewal of a license to sell, stock or exhibit or offer for sale by wholesale, or distribute drugs from a motor vehicle
19 B	Application for license to sell, stock or exhibit or offer for sale, or distribute Homoeopathic medicines
19 C	Application for grant or renewal of a license to sell, stock, exhibit or offer for sale, or distribute drugs specified in Schedule X
20	License to sell, stock or exhibit or offer for sale, or distribute drugs by retail other than those specified in Schedules C, C (1) and X
20 A	Restricted License to sell, stock or exhibit or offer for sale, or distribute drugs by retail other than those specified in Schedules C, C (1) and X for dealers who do not engage the services of a registered pharmacist
20 B	License to sell, stock or exhibit or offer for sale, or distribute by wholesale, drugs other than those specified in Schedules C, C (1) and X

(Contd...)

(Contd...)

Form no.	Details
20 BB	License to sell, stock or exhibit or offer for sale by wholesale, or distribute drugs other than those specified in Schedule C and Schedule C (1) to the Drugs and Cosmetics Rules, 1945 from a motor vehicle
20 C	License to sell, stock or exhibit or offer for sale, or distribute Homoeopathic medicines by retail
20 D	License to sell, stock or exhibit or offer for sale, or distribute Homoeopathic medicines by wholesale
20 E	Certificate of renewal of license to sell, stock or exhibit or offer for sale, or distribute Homoeopathic medicines
20 F	License to sell, stock or exhibit for sale or distribute by retail drugs specified in Schedule X
20 G	License to sell, stock or exhibit or offer for sale, or distribute by wholesale drugs specified in Schedule X
21	License to sell, stock or exhibit or offer for sale, or distribute by retail drugs specified in Schedules C and C (1) [excluding those specified in Schedule X]
21 A	License to sell, stock or exhibit or offer for sale, or distribute by retail drugs specified in Schedule C (1) [excluding those specified in Schedule X] for dealers who do not engage the services of a registered pharmacist
21 B	License to sell, stock or exhibit or offer for sale, or distribute by wholesale drugs specified in Schedules C and C (1) [excluding those specified in Schedule X]
21 BB	License to sell by wholesale or to distribute drugs specified in Schedule C and Schedule C (1) to the Drugs and Cosmetics Rules, 1945 from a motor vehicle.
21 C	Certificate of renewal of license to sell, stock or exhibit or offer for sale, or distribute drugs
21 CC	Certificate of renewal of license to sell, stock or exhibit or offer for sale by wholesale, or distribute drugs from a motor vehicle
24	Application for the grant of or renewal of a license to manufacture for sale or for distribution of drugs other than those specified in Schedules C and C (1) and X
24 A	Application for grant or renewal of a loan license to manufacture for sale or for distribution of drugs other than those specified in Schedules C and C (1) and X
24 B	Application for grant or renewal of license to repack for sale or distribution of drugs, being drugs other than those specified in Schedules C and C (1) [excluding those specified in Schedule X]
24 C	Application for the grant or renewal of a license to manufacture for sale or for distribution of homoeopathic medicines or a license to manufacture potentised preparations from back potencies by licensees holding license in Form 20-C
24 D	Application for the grant/renewal of a license to manufacture for sale of Ayurvedic/ Siddha or Unani drugs
24 E	Application for grant or renewal of a loan license to manufacture for sale Ayurvedic (including Siddha) or Unani Drugs
24 F	Application for the grant or renewal of a license to manufacture for sale or for distribution of drugs specified in Schedule X and not specified in Schedules C and C (1)
25	License to manufacture for sale or for distribution of drugs other than those specified in Schedules C and C (1) and X
25 A	Loan license to manufacture for sale or for distribution of drugs other than those specified in Schedules C and C (1) and X

(Contd...)

(Contd...)

Form no.	Details
25 B	License to repack for sale or distribution of drugs being drugs other than those specified in Schedules C and C (1) [excluding those specified in Schedule X]
25 C	License to manufacture for sale or for distribution of Homoeopathic medicines
25 D	License to manufacture for sale of Ayurvedic (including Siddha) or Unani drugs
25 E	Loan License to manufacture for sale Ayurvedic (including Siddha) or Unani Drugs
25 F	License to manufacture for sale or for distribution of drugs specified in Schedule X and not specified in Schedules C and C (1)
26	Certificate of renewal of license to manufacture for sale of drugs other than those specified in Schedule X
26 A	Certificate of renewal of loan license to manufacture for sale of drugs other than those specified in Schedule X
26 B	Certificate of renewal of license to repack for sale or distribution of drugs being drugs other than those specified in Schedules C and C (1) [excluding those specified in Schedule X]
26 C	Certificate of renewal of license to manufacture for sale of Homoeopathic medicines
26 D	Certificate of renewal of license to manufacture for sale of Ayurvedic/Siddha or Unani drugs
26 E	Certificate of renewal of loan license to manufacture for sale of Ayurvedic/Siddha or Unani Drugs
26 E1	Certificate of Good Manufacturing Practices (GMP) to manufacture of Ayurveda, Siddha or Unani Drugs
26 F	Certificate of renewal of license to manufacture for sale of drugs specified in Schedule X
26 G	Certificate of renewal of license to operate a Blood Bank for processing of whole human blood and/or for preparation for sale or distribution of its component
26 H	Certificate of renewal of license to manufacture for sale of Large Volume Parenterals/Sera and Vaccines specified in Schedules C and C(1) excluding those specified in Schedule X
26 I	Certificate of renewal of license for manufacture of blood product
27	Application for grant or renewal of a [license to manufacture for sale or for distribution] of drugs specified in Schedules C and C (1) [excluding those specified in Schedule XB and Schedule X]
27 A	Application for grant or renewal of a loan [license to manufacture for sale or for distribution of] drugs specified in Schedules C and C (1) [excluding those specified in Schedule XB and Schedule X]
27 B	Application for grant or renewal of a license to manufacture for sale or for distribution of drugs specified in Schedules C, C (1) and X
27 C	Application for grant/renewal of license for the operation of a Blood Bank for processing of whole blood and/or preparation of Blood Components
27 D	Application for grant or renewal of a license to manufacture for sale or for distribution of Large Volume parenterals/Sera and Vaccines excluding those specified in Schedule X
27 E	Application for grant/renewal of license to manufacture blood products for sale of distribution
28	License to manufacture for sale or for distribution of drugs specified in Schedules C and C (1) [excluding those specified in Schedule X]
28 A	Loan [License to manufacture for sale or for distribution of] drugs specified in Schedules C and C (1) [excluding those specified in Schedule X]
28 B	License to manufacture for sale or for distribution of drugs specified in Schedules C, CI and X

(Contd...)

(Contd...)

Form no.	Details
28 C	License to operate a Blood Bank for collection, storage and processing of whole human blood and/or its components for sale or distribution
28 D	License to manufacture for sale or for distribution of Large Volume Parenterals/Sera and Vaccines specified in Schedules C and C (1) excluding those specified in Schedule X
28 E	License to manufacture and store blood products for sale or distribution
29	License to manufacture drugs for purposes of examination, test or analysis
30	Application for license to manufacture drugs for purposes of examination, test or analysis
31	Application for grant or renewal of a license to manufacture cosmetics for sale or for distribution
31 A	Application for grant or renewal of loan license to manufacture cosmetics for sale or for distribution
32	License to manufacture cosmetics for sale or for distribution
32 A	Loan license to manufacture cosmetics for sale or for distribution
33	Certificate of renewal of license to manufacture cosmetics for sale
33 A	Certificate of renewal of loan license to manufacture cosmetic for sale
34	Certificate of test or analysis of cosmetic by the Central Drugs Laboratory or the Government Analyst
35	Form in which the Inspection Book shall be maintained
36	Application for grant or renewal of approval for carrying out tests on drugs/cosmetics or raw materials used in the manufacture thereof on behalf of licensees for manufacture for sale of drugs/cosmetics
37	Approval for carrying out tests on drugs/cosmetics and raw materials used in their manufacture on behalf of licensees for manufacture for sale of drugs/cosmetics
38	Certificate of renewal of approval for carrying out tests on drugs/cosmetics and raw materials used in the manufacture thereof on behalf of licensees for manufacture for sale of drugs/cosmetics
39	Report of test or analysis by approved institution
40	Application for issue of Registration Certificate for import of drugs into India
41	Registration Certificate to be issued for import of drugs into India
44	Application for grant of permission of import or manufacture a New Drug or to undertake clinical trial
45	Permission to import Finished Formulation of the New Drug
45 A	Permission to import raw material (new bulk drug substance)
46	Permission/Approval for manufacture of new drug formulation
46 A	Permission/Approval for manufacture of raw material (new bulk drug substance)
47	Application for grant or renewal of approval for carrying out tests on Ayurvedic, Siddha and Unani drugs or raw materials used in the manufacture thereof on behalf of licensees for manufacture for sale of Ayurvedic, Siddha and Unani drugs
48	Approval for carrying out tests or analysis on Ayurvedic, Siddha and Unani drugs or raw materials used in the manufacture thereof on behalf of licensees for manufacture for sale of Ayurvedic, Siddha and Unani drugs
49	Certificate of renewal for carrying out tests or analysis on Ayurvedic, Siddha or Unani drugs or raw materials used in the manufacture thereof on behalf of licensees for manufacture for sale of Ayurvedic, Siddha or Unani drugs
50	Report of test analysis by approved Laboratory

IMPORT OF DRUGS

Drugs may be imported into India under the authority of license excepting those whose import is prohibited. The Drugs Controller General (India) is the Licensing Authority for granting import licenses. He may delegate the powers of signing licenses to his officers. The CDSCO has initiated the process of inspecting manufacturing sites abroad as large number of bulk drugs are imported.

Drugs Permitted to be Imported

- Drugs of standard quality.
- Patent or proprietary medicines on the condition that the composition is declared on the label and these conform to the standards of quality, purity and strength.
- Approved new drugs.
- Drugs (not approved) for experiment, test, research or clinical trials under a test license.
- Drugs for personal use in small quantity under an import permit.

Procedure for Import

Application with prescribed fees by the importer in the prescribed form seeking license or permit to import along with the relevant following documents:

- Undertaking by the manufacturer abroad that he has complied with the requirements of the Drugs and Cosmetics Rules to ensure that drugs to be exported to India by him conform to standards of strengths, quality and purity.
- Copy of the prescription of the registered medical practitioner (no fees required).

↓

License or permit for import is issued in the prescribed form which is valid up to 31st December of the year.

↓

Importer places the order for import and the consignment arrived at seaport or airport

(Seaport: Chennai, Kolkata, Mumbai, Cochin, Nhava Sheva, Kandla, Inland Container Depots at Tugla and Patparganj in Delhi, Tuticorin (Tamil Nadu), Marmugao port in Goa and Visakhapatnam in Andhra Pradesh; Rail: Ferozpur Cantonment and Amritsar in frontier with Pakistan and Ranaghat, Bongaon and Mohiassan in frontier with Bangladesh)

↓

Release of imported drugs or returned back to the country of origin or destroyed.

Other conditions and release of imported drugs on arrival:

- Import of biological and special products (Schedule C and C(1)): License does not restrict the quantity of drugs to be imported. The label of the containers of the drugs is required to bear the import license number. The importer needs to comply with the storage condition in drug stocking premises.
- Import of psychotropic drugs (Schedule X): Importer has to maintain detailed records of the stock imported, sold and the balance in hand.
- Import for examination, test or analysis: The drugs cannot be sold and are to be used for clinical trials or tests or research.
- Import of new drugs: The importer has to apply DCGI giving all documents of safety, efficacy, standards, testing methods and status of new drug in the country of manufacturer and other countries. On approval for the new drug, the importer has to follow the process of import.
- Import of fixed dose combination drugs: The applicant has to submit the data and information as specified in Schedule Y. The Licensing Authority after being satisfied that the fixed dose combination if approved to be manufactured shall be effective and safe for use in the country, issues permission. When it is felt that the data generated on the fixed dose combination is inadequate, the Licensing

Authority informs in writing that the conditions need to be satisfied before issuing approval.

- Import of drugs for personal use:
  - As a part of bonafide baggage—the drugs are intended for exclusive personal use of the passenger. If required it needs to be declared to the custom authorities. The quantity of any single drug does not exceed 100 average doses (The Licensing Authority can sanction the import of larger quantity in an exceptional case).
  - Not forming part of personal baggage— a permit from Licensing Authority is essential for which one has to apply. The applicant has to apply to the Assistant Drugs Controller/Technical Officer/ Drugs Inspector of the respective port offices of CDSCO in prescribed format along with the prescription clearly mentioning the name, quantity and duration of medication.

- A drug manufacturer holding the manufacturing license for biological and special products need not obtain import license for importing bulk drugs needed for his manufacture.

- Before any drug is released for entry into the country, bills of entry (through a clearing agent), protocols of test and analysis of manufacturer, sample of the label, sample of drug or any other information are submitted by the importer to the collector of customs at the point of entry. Once the office of customs collector passes the bill of entry to the Assistant Drugs Controller or the Technical Officer of CDSCO, the documents are examined.

- Samples of the drugs are drawn for test and the consignment is released only when the test report declares the drugs are of standard quality. The sample is either tested in a local private laboratory or is sent to Central Drugs Laboratory, Kolkata (for antibiotics, corticosteroids, and chemotherapeutic agents), the Central Research Institute, Kasauli (for Sera and Vaccines), the Central Indian Pharmacopoeial Laboratory, Ghaziabad (for Condoms), the Indian Veterinary Research Institute, Izzatnagar (for veterinary biological products) or Central Drug Testing Laboratories of Mumbai and Chennai. As the testing in government laboratory takes time, consignments can be released on a Letter of Guarantee, but the importer cannot sell or use such drugs. When the test result shows that the drugs do not conform to the required standard, they may be either sent back to the country of origin or destroyed.

- An importer has to comply with other Acts: Sea Customs Act, the Import and Export trade (Control) Regulation and the Indian Customs Tariff Regulations.

- If the drug is in transit through India to a foreign country, these legal requirements are not applicable.

Refusal of License

The Licensing Authority may refuse to grant license if he is satisfied that:

- The applicant has not complied with the provision of Act or Rules.
- The applicant has been convicted under Dangerous Drugs Act or Narcotic and Psychotropic Substances Act or Rules.
- The applicant's license has been previously suspended or cancelled.

The applicant aggrieved by the decision of the Licensing Authority may appeal to the central government within 30 days of the receipt of the order. The central government may take the final decision after giving the appellant an opportunity for making a presentation and any enquiry as required.

Cancellation /Suspension of License

If the manufacturer or licensee fails to comply with any condition of license, the Licensing Authority may cancel or suspend the license after giving an opportunity to licensee to make representation. The aggrieved licensee has an opportunity to appeal.

Prohibited to be Imported

- Drug which is not of standard quality.
- Misbranded, spurious or adulterated drug.

- Drug for which import license is prescribed, otherwise without a license.
- Patent and proprietary medicines whose true formula or list of ingredients with quantity is not displayed on the label or container.
- Drug which purports or claims to cure or mitigate any such disease or ailment specified Schedule J.
- Drugs whose manufacture, sale or distribution is prohibited in the country of origin. (But can be imported for examination, test or analysis.)
- Drugs not labelled and packed in the prescribed manner.
- Unapproved new drugs.
- Biological and other special products specified in Schedule C or C (1) whose potency is lost or acquired toxicity (after expiry date).
- Drug whose import is prohibited by the rule.

MANUFACTURE OF DRUGS

The following classes of drugs are prohibited to be manufactured:

- Substandard, misbranded, adulterated or spurious drugs;

- Patent or proprietary medicine unless true formula or list of ingredients including quantities used is displayed on the label;
- Drug which purports or claims to prevent, cure or mitigate any disease or ailment described in Schedule J.

However, prohibition is not applicable for manufacturing of small quantities of any drug for the purpose of examination, test or analysis.

Manufacturing of drugs can be undertaken only under a manufacturing license. The state Drugs Controller is the Licensing Authority. There are six different types of license for manufacture of drugs.

- License to manufacture drugs other than those specified in Schedule C, C(1) and X. These drugs are liquid orals, tablets and ointments, and are not psychotropic substances.
- License to manufacture Schedule X drugs. These are psychotropic drugs for oral administration.
- License to operate blood bank or process whole human blood for components or manufacture blood products.
- License to manufacture Large Volume Parenterals (LVP), sera or vaccines. The LVP means sterile solutions intended for

Schedule D (List of drugs exempted from the provisions of import drugs)	
Class of drugs	*Extent and conditions of exemption*
Substances not intended for medical use.	Import permissible if imported in bulk and the importer certifies that the substance is for non-medical use. If not in bulk, then each container must indicate that it is not for medicinal use.
Substances included in Schedules C and C (1) required for manufacturing purposes but not intended for medical use in the form in which they are imported.	No license is necessary if the importer holds a license for manufacture of Schedule C and C (1) drugs.
Substances used as articles of food as well as drugs: Condensed or powdered milk whether pure, skimmed or malted, fortified with vitamins and minerals; farex, oats, lactose and all other cereal preparations fortified with vitamins (excepting those for parenteral use); virol, bovril, chicken essence and all other predigested foods; ginger, pepper, cumin, cinnamon and other similar spices and condiments if they are not labelled to have in conformity of official standards as prescribed under the Act and Rules.	No regulation.

Offences and punishments relating to import of drugs

Nature of offence	Punishment for the first offence	Punishment for the subsequent offences
Import of adulterated or spurious drug	Imprisonment up to 3 years and fine up to ₹ 5000	Imprisonment up to 5 years or with fine up to ₹ 10000 or with both.
Import of any drug which has been prohibited to be imported	Imprisonment up to 6 months or with fine up to ₹ 500 or both	Imprisonment up to 1 year or with fine up to ₹ 1000 or with both
Import of any drug which has been banned in public interest	Imprisonment up to 3 years or with fine up to ₹ 5000 or with both	Imprisonment up to 5 years or with fine up to ₹ 10000 or with both

parenteral administration with a volume of 100 ml or more and are for single use. It covers anti-coagulant solutions.

- License to manufacture Schedule C and C (1) drugs (excluding Schedule X drugs, whole human blood or blood products, large volume parenterals, sera and vaccines). These are injections and oral vitamins, antibiotics, corticosteroids, fish liver oils, and other thermolabile drugs.
- License to manufacture Schedule C, C (1), and X drugs.

Besides these, there are provisions for license to manufacture drugs for examinations, test or analysis; manufacture of new drugs; loan license and repacking license.

The manufacturer needs to satisfy the following pre-requisite conditions to be eligible for grant of a license.

1. Employ competent technical staff under whose active direction and personal supervision manufacturing would take place.
2. Have good manufacturing practices facilities (Schedule M).
3. Maintain hygienic conditions and adequate premises for the manufacture.
4. Maintain necessary equipment and appliances required for the manufacture of drugs.
5. Have independent drug testing laboratory to test raw materials and every batch of drugs manufactured. The qualification required for head of the testing unit:
   - degree in medicine; or
   - degree in science; or
   - degree in pharmacy; or
   - degree in pharmaceutical chemistry with adequate experience in testing of drugs (no period of experience specified).
6. Have adequate storage arrangements for manufactured drugs.
7. Have evidence and data for justifying manufacturing of patent and proprietary medicines:
   - contains ingredients in therapeutic or prophylactic quantities;
   - vehicles, excipients, additives, pharmaceutical aids are safe for use;
   - the product is stable; and
   - contain such ingredients and in quantities which are therapeutically justifiable.

Licensing Procedure

Application to the State Drugs Controller (Drug Licensing Authority) on fulfilling the prerequisite conditions

↓

Inspection of the premises, facilities for manufacture, testing facilities by Drugs Inspector (Joint inspection by State and Central Drugs Inspectors for manufacturing of LVP, sera, vaccines, operating blood bank, processing of whole human blood, manufacturing blood products)

↓

Granting of manufacturing license in the prescribed format (License issued by State Drugs Controller is to be approved by Central License Approving Authority, Drugs Controller General, India)

The rejection of application for grant of license is to be communicated to the applicant giving reasons for rejection and the conditions which must be satisfied before a license can be granted. The copy of the inspection report is also to be supplied. If within six months of rejection, the applicant fulfils the conditions and applies for inspection, then after the inspection by the authority concerned may grant a license.

Checklist for application for manufacturing license to manufacture pharmaceutical products

(*Source:* Pharma Web, January–February–March 2009)

- Application in Form 24, 27 and 36, duly filled and signed by the applicant.
- Original challan for ₹ 7500/- being the license fees remitted under correct heads of account.
- Courts fees stamp to the value of ₹ 2/- fixed on each application.
- Xerox copies of partnership deed/ attested copies of memorandum and articles of association.
- Plan of the manufacturing premises showing the various sections and measurements and duly signed by the applicant and by a licensed surveyor.
- Xerox copy of rent agreement deed, rent receipt, lease deed.
- List of machineries/plants/equipment provided for the manufacture of drugs and for the analysis of raw materials/ finished products with xerox copies of purchase invoices.
- Xerox copies of educational qualification certificate and previous experience certificate in respect of manufacturing and analytical chemists.
- Full time employee declaration of manufacturing chemists and analytical chemists.
- Letter of undertaking for the analysis of raw materials and finished products.
- Other declaration letter.
- Specimen labels in triplicate.
- Therapeutic justification, method of analysis.
- List of drugs to be permitted to manufacture in quadruplicate.

- Original licenses in Form 25 and 28.
- Latest renewal certificate.
- Dissolution deed.
- Original list of drugs permitted to be manufactured under licenses in Form 25/28.
- Director's/Partner's/Proprietor's address proof, specimen signature and photograph with attestation.
- Address proof and photograph of chemists.
- Copy of latest property tax receipt.

For 25A and 28A, the following additional documents are to be submitted:

- Copy of wholesale license.
- Consent letter from manufacturer where they believe to have the loan license.

[*Note:* Extra fees need to be paid for more than 10 products under each category (tablets, capsules, liquid orals, external preparations, injectables)]

Qualification and Training of Competent Technical Staff

Manufacturing of drugs specified in Schedule C, C(1) and X/Schedule C and C (1) drugs (excluding Schedule X drugs, whole human blood or blood products, large volume parenterals, sera and vaccines)/large volume parenterals, vaccines, sera:

- Graduate in Pharmacy or Pharmaceutical Chemistry of a recognized university having at least 18 months practical experience after graduation in the manufacture of relevant drugs. The period of experience is relaxed by six months if the person has undergone training of manufacturing of relevant category of drugs for a period of six months during university programme; or
- Graduate in Science of a recognized university and studied Chemistry or Microbiology as a principal subject and having at least three years experience in the manufacture of relevant category of drugs after graduation; or
- Graduate in Medicine of a recognized university and having at least three years

experience in the manufacture and pharmacological testing of biological products after graduation; or

- Graduate in Chemical Engineering of a recognized university having at least three years practical experience in the manufacture of relevant categories of drugs after graduation; or
- Holding any foreign qualification comparable in quality and content of training as described above and is permitted to work as competent technical staff by the central government.

For Veterinary Medicines (specified in Schedule C and C1): Graduate in Veterinary Science, general Science, Medicine or Pharmacy from a recognized university with at least three years experience in the manufacture of biological products.

Conditions of license: The licensee will:

a. Maintain the building and different premises for manufacture, processing, packing, and labelling in good condition. Maintain good water supply and disposal of waste. Make arrangements to look after the health, clothing, and sanitation of workers. Ensure medical services and sanitation in the manufacturing premises.

b. Maintain GMP requirements as laid down in Schedule M.

c. Maintain Master Formula Records and Batch Manufacturing Records.

d. Keep inventory of raw materials , arrange for good manufacturing operations. Maintain reprocessing and recovery, distribution, and complaint and adverse reaction records.

e. Ensure the functioning of Quality Control System as laid down in Schedule M for testing every batch of drug manufactured in the premises.

f. Maintain the record of drug manufacture and drug testing in the prescribed proforma (Schedule U).

g. Allow the Drugs Inspector to inspect the plant, premises, process of manufacture, testing, records, registers, and permit him to draw samples.

h. Maintain reference samples from each batch of drug manufactured.

i. Maintain an inspection book to enable the Drugs Inspector to record his observation.

Manufacture of LVPs, sera, vaccines, processing of whole human blood, manufacture of blood products: These operations require the licensing system by both state and central drug authorities. It is a two-tier control system to bring more rigidity and stricter discipline in the system or process. The application for manufacture has to be made to the State Licensing Authority in triplicate giving the details of premises, list of equipment, names of expert with qualification and experience and also those in charge of testing. The State Licensing Authority arranges inspection of plant and premises by State Drugs Inspector, either alone or with expert. On satisfaction based on inspection report, the State Licensing Authority forwards his recommendation along with the application to the zonal office of CDSCO. Zonal office after scrutiny of the papers arranges for inspection by Central Drugs Inspector either alone or with expert. After the second inspection, the inspection report and recommendation of the zonal office is sent to Central License Approving Authority (CLAA). There is a provision of joint inspection and this can be done at any stage. When the license is granted, the CLAA after approval keeps one copy, sends a copy to the applicant and the third copy to State Licensing Authority.

Manufacture for examination, test or analysis: The drug(s) are not only used for the benefits of human beings or animals, but also used for experimental purposes. The license from the State Licensing Authority is necessary to manufacture drug(s) to be used for examination, test or analysis. The application is to be signed by the head of the institution or the director of the manufacturing firm. The license will permit manufacturing as well as testing of the drug. This drug cannot be sold for use by the patient. The licensee is required to keep the record of quantity of drug manufactured and the person to whom such drug is supplied. In case, the drug is a new drug, not so far approved for use, it is necessary that the applicant submits no objection certificate from the Drugs Controller General (India).

Manufacture of new drugs: The manufacturer is required to obtain approval of the new drug from DCG(I). The applicant has to submit the details described in Schedule Y including the results of clinical trials and approval details of DCG(I) to the State Licensing Authority for obtaining approval (not license). The new bulk drug (Active Pharmaceutical Ingredient) can be sold only to those manufacturers who have permission to either to use the drug for development purpose, clinical trial, or bioequivalence study or to manufacture the formulation. For manufacturing of formulation separate approval is necessary from licensing authority.

Manufacture of fixed dose combinations: The applicant has to submit the data and information as specified in Schedule Y. The Licensing Authority, after being satisfied that the fixed dose combination if approved to be manufactured shall be effective and safe for use in the country, issues permission. When it is felt that the data generated on the fixed dose combination is inadequate, the Licensing Authority informs in writing that the conditions need to be satisfied before issuing approval. Fixed dose combinations of two or more drugs, individually approved for certain claims, which are now proposed to be combined for the first time or the ratio of ingredients of approved combination is proposed to be changed, for use with new indication, new form including sustained release dosage forms are treated as new drugs.

The DCGI in 2007 ordered the withdrawal of 294 irrational fixed dose combinations. The DCGI is of the opinion that the State Licensing Authority should stop issuing new license or renewal of the existing license for manufacture of fixed dose combinations. The license to manufacture requires the approval of Central Licensing Authority. Later, based on the report of the Professor Kokate Committee, the Government has issued order banning of 344 FDCs. The matter is now pending at SC as Government filed appeal against the Delhi High Court's order quashing the ban notification. The DCGI has issued order with respect to FDCs which the Kokate Committee has approved as rational. The NOC by the DCGI would be issued within 30 days of application for clearance, This NOC is required for the state licensing to issue manufacturing license for FDCs. Every FDC manufacturer needs to comply with submission of periodic safety update report (PSUR). Failure to submit PSUR is the contravention of rules.

Loan License: A loan licensing system is available for manufacturing of drugs. Under this provision, a person can get drugs manufactured from manufacturing premises which is licensed for manufacturing. The loan license is issued for both biological and non-biological products. Loan license is not issued for Schedule X drugs. The licensee has to comply with all conditions of manufacture and testing. The licensing authority needs to be satisfied himself before issuing license that the manufacturing unit has adequate equipment, staff, capacity to manufacture and facilities for testing to undertake the manufacture on behalf of the applicant for a loan licensee.

Repacking of Drugs

Though there is no need to comply with usual conditions specified for manufacturing drugs, a license is required for repacking. Repacking means making small packs from large containers for household use. The repacking license is not issued for biological products specified in Schedule C and C (1) and drugs specified in Schedule X.

Conditions for issuing or renewing of license: The following must be complied.

- The repacking operation is to be carried out under hygienic conditions and under the supervision of a competent person (a registered pharmacist; person holding Diploma in Pharmacy; a person passed Intermediate examination with Chemistry as one of the principal subjects, or an equivalent examination recognized by the Licensing Authority; a person passed in matriculation examination and has not less than four years practical experience in the manufacture, dispensing or repacking of drugs);

- The factory premise complies with GMP (Schedule M) and
- There is adequate arrangement in the premises for carrying out tests for strength, quality and purity of the drugs at a

testing unit which is separate from the repacking unit.

Any change in the competent staff named in the license needs to be informed forthwith to the Licensing Authority. For repacking of additional items, it is necessary that the licensee applies for endorsement of such items. In addition to other requirements of labelling, the label of repacked products must contain the name and address of the licensee and the Rpg. Lic. No.

Offences and Punishments relating to manufacture of drugs

Nature of offence	Punishment
*Manufacture of any adulterated or spurious drug or any drug which when used by any person is likely to cause his death or likely to cause harm on his body which is treated as grievous hurt.	Imprisonment for not less than 10 years which may extend to a term of life and fine of not less than ₹ 10,00,000/- or three times the value of drugs confiscated.
Manufacture of any adulterated drug.	Imprisonment for not less than 3 years extendable to 5 years with a fine of not less than ₹ 1,00,000/- or three times the value of drugs confiscated, whichever is more. The court may reduce both the minimum punishments citing adequate and special reasons.
Manufacture without a valid license	Do
Manufacture of spurious drug.	Imprisonment for not less than 7 years extendable to life imprisonment with a fine of not less than ₹ 3,00,000/- or three times the value of confiscated products, whichever is more. (Court may impose a sentence of imprisonment of less than 7 years but not less than 3 years and fine of less than ₹ 1,00,000).
Manufacture of any drug in contravention of any provision of act or rules other than mentioned above.	Imprisonment of not less than 1 year extendable to 2 years and with fine of not less than ₹ 20,000/-.
Non-disclosure of the name of the manufacturer or non-disclosure of the place where drugs are manufactured or kept.	Imprisonment up to 1 year or with fine not less than ₹ 20,000/- or with both.
Non-maintenance of registers and documents and non-disclosure of the information relating to them.	Imprisonment extendable to 1 year or with fine of not less than ₹ 20,000/- or both.
Manufacture of any drug which has been banned under public interest.	Imprisonment up to 3 years and with fine up to ₹ 5,000/-
Use of any report of a test or analysis by the Central Drugs Laboratory or by a Government Analyst or any abstract from such report for the purpose of advertising any drug.	Fine up to ₹ 5000/-.

* The amount recovered or realised from convictions, is to be paid to the relative of the person who had died due to the use of such products: (spouse, minor legitimate son, unmarried legitimate daughter, widow mother, parent of minor victim, person wholly dependent on the earning of the deceased person).

Offences relating to manufacture of spurious and adulterated is cognizable and non-bailable offences. Provision of fast track court to deal with cases relating to spurious drugs is also made.

The manufacturing Licence for drugs and cosmetics remains valid if licence holder continues paying the retention fees before the expiry of a period every succeeding five years. Before issuing licence, there will be joint inspection of State and Central Drugs Inspectors to ensure the compliance. The premises need to be inspected at least once in three years or as required based on risk assessment. For this too there will be joint inspection.

Whistle Blower Policy on Dealing with Spurious Drugs (2009):

The spurious drugs not only affect the health of the citizens, but also affect the prestige of India's pharmaceutical trade. Hence a whistle blower policy is announced by the Health Ministry in 2009. The policy intends to handsomely reward both the public and the officials who provide information about and help seizure of spurious, adulterated, misbranded drugs, cosmetics and medical devices.

The reward of a maximum of 20% of the total cost of a consignment seized will be payable to the informer which should not exceed ₹ 25 lakh in each case. In case of government officials or officials of CDSCO, the reward would not exceed ₹ 5 lakh for one case and a maximum of ₹ 30 lakh in his or her entire service.

LABELLING AND PACKAGING OF DRUGS

The labels on drugs package are essential for identifying the product and ensuring the proper use of medicines. The containers of drugs should have labels giving all particulars which would comply with legal requirements and help in identifying the product and its use.

The following particulars need to be either printed or written in indelible ink and appear in a conspicuous manner on the label of the innermost containers and every other package:

1. **Name of the drug:** Proper name of the drug should be in a more conspicuous manner than the trade name (if any). The trade name should be shown immediately after or under the proper name. When drug is included in official pharmacopoeias the name should be followed by IP or NFI to express its quality of Pharmacopoeial standard. For other drugs, the international non-proprietary name suggested by WHO should be used.

2. **Net contents:** Weight, measure, volume, number of units of contents, number of units of activity, as expressed in metric system.

3. **Strength of the product:**
   Oral liquids:
   - Contents per single dose being indicated in 5 milliliters;
   - When dose is less than 5 milliliters, it is in terms of 1 milliliter or its fraction;
   - If dose is more than 5 milliliter, then in terms of single dose.

   Liquid injections:
   - In terms of 1 milliliter or percentage by volume or per dose in single dose container;
   - If product is in ampoule, the composition may be shown on the label or wrapper affixed to any package in which ampoule is issued for sale.

   Solids for injections:
   - In terms of units or weight per milligram or gram. Tablets/Capsules/other single dosage form;
   - In terms of contents in each unit of tablet/capsule, etc.

   Other products:
   - In terms of percentage by weight or volume or in terms of unitage per gram or milliliter.

   The expression of contents is not applicable for products described in pharmacopoeias or national formulary.

4. **Name of the manufacturer and the address where the drug has been manufactured:** If the drug is supplied in small container like ampoule, it is sufficient if the name of the manufacturer and its principal manufacturing place is shown.

5. **The Batch or Lot Number** expressed as "Batch" or "B No" or "Lot No" or "Lot".

6. **The Manufacturing License Number** expressed as "Manufacturing License Number" or "Mfg. Lic. No." or "M.L.".

7. **Import License Number** for imported drugs.

8. **Date of Manufacture and Date of Expiry.**

9. **Alcohol Content:** If the alcohol content is not less than 3 percent by volume, it needs to be expressed on the label.

   Special requirements: This is in addition to the labelling requirements described earlier.

10. **Free sample distribution to medical profession:** "Physician's sample–Not to be sold".

11. **For drugs like narcotic drugs, analgesics, hypnotics, sedatives, tranquilizers, corticosteroids, hormones, hypoglycemics, anti-microbials, anti-epileptics, anti-depressants, anti-coagulants, anti-cancer and all other drugs belonging to Schedule G, H and X:** A conspicuous red vertical line on the left side running throughout the body of the label which shall not be less than 1 mm width and without disturbing the other details.

   But this clause is not applicable to:

   - Preparations intended for animal treatment;
   - Preparations intended for external use;
   - Ophthalmic preparations and ear drops; and
   - Sterile preparations such as sutures, surgical dressings, and preparations intended for parenteral use.

12. **Schedule G drug for internal use:** "Caution: It is dangerous to take this preparation except under medical supervision".

13. **Schedule H drug for internal use:** R_X on the left top corner of the label with the words "Schedule H drug –

    Warning: To be sold by retail on the prescription of a Registered Medical Practitioner only".

Schedule H1: R_X in red in the left top corner with the box warning with red border:

"Schedule H1 Drug—Warning:

- It is dangerous to take this preparation except in accordance with the medical advice
- Not to be sold by retail without the prescription of a Registered Medical Practitioner."

14. **Drug belongs to Schedule H and also to Schedule X:** Symbol N R_X in red on the left top corner of the label and also with the words:

    "Schedule H drug –

    Warning: To be sold by retail on the prescription of a Registered Medical Practitioner only".

15. **Schedule X drug for internal use:** Symbol X R_X in red on the left top corner of the label and with the words:

    "Schedule X drug –

    Warning: To be sold by retail on the prescription of a Registered Medical Practitioner only".

16. **Contraceptives:**

    Mechanical contraceptives like condoms:

    - Manufacturer's name and address and trade name of the condom(if any);
    - Batch number;
    - Date of expiry (month and year); The shelf life would not be more than 36 months.
    - The words " For single use only".

    Locally used contraceptives like cream, jelly or foam tablets:

    - All requirements mentioned under mechanical contraceptive;
    - The date of manufacture;
    - The date of expiry;
    - Storage condition.

    Oral pills:

    - The date of manufacture only.

17. **External application products:** FOR EXTERNAL USE ONLY in capital letters.

18. **Drug for animal treatment:** Not for Human Use: For animal treatment only. In addition, the label should show the head of a domestic animal.

19. **Drug containing Industrial Methylated Spirit:** For external use only.

20. **Unsterilized surgical ligature or suture:** In red ink.

    Non-sterile surgical ligature (suture): Not to be used for operations upon the human body unless efficiently sterilized.

21. **Patent and proprietary medicine:** The true formula or the list of ingredients to be disclosed on the label.

22. **The label of the container of a drug shall not give any idea that**
    - It may prevent or cure the disease or ailment specified in Schedule J;
    - It may procure miscarriage in women.

23. **Biological products (Schedule C):** Should also comply with other requirements specified in Schedule F.

24. Ophthalmic preparations:
(a) **Ophthalmic solutions and suspensions:**
    - On the container:
      - The statement "Use the solution within one month after opening the container";
      - Name and concentration of preservative, if any;
      - The words NOT FOR INJECTION
    - On the container or carton or package leaflet:
      - Special instruction regarding storage, where applicable;
      - A cautionary legend reading as

    "Warning (i) if irritation persists or increases, discontinue the use and consult physician; (ii) Do not touch the dropper tip or other dispensing tip to any surface since this may contaminate solutions"

(b) **Ophthalmic ointments:**
    - Special instructions regarding storage as required.
    - A cautionary legend reading:

    "Warning: If irritation persists or increases, discontinue the use and consult physician"

25. **Disinfectants:** For Black and White Fluids:
    - Name of the product;
    - The name and full address of the manufacturer;
    - Grade, type and RW coefficient of the product;
    - Date of manufacture;
    - Quantity present in the container;
    - Indications and mode of use;
    - The date up to which the product can be used.

Packing of drugs: Pack size of certain drugs are specified in Schedule P(1). Unless covered in Schedule P(1), they should:
- Tablets/Capsules: When the number is less than 10, they should be in integral number. For numbers above 10, pack size should contain multiple of 5.
- Oral liquids: 30 ml (paediatrics)/60 ml/100 ml/200 ml/450 ml;
- Paediatric oral drops: 5 ml/10 ml/15 ml;
- Eye drop/Nasal drop/Ear drop: 3 ml/5 ml/10 ml;
- Eye ointment: 3 g/5 g/10 g;
- Schedule X drugs: Packing not exceeding 100 unit doses in case of tablets or capsules; 300 ml in case of oral liquids; 5 ml in case of injections. This rule is not applicable if supplies are made directly to the hospitals/dispensaries and are not supplied to a retail dealer or to a Registered Medical Practitioner.

These provisions of rule are not applicable to:
- Imported formulations in finished form;
- Preparations for veterinary use;
- Preparations for export;
- Vitamins/tonics/cough preparations/antacids/laxatives in liquid oral forms, unit dose including applicaps;
- Pack size meant for retail sale to hospitals, Registered Medical Practitioners, nursing homes;
- Physician samples;
- Pack size of large volume intravenous fluids.

The GoI notified, on 23 July 2017, an amendment to Legal Metrology (LM) Act 2009 to be effective from 01 January 2018. The new rule regulates the content of labels of all pre-packaged goods sold in India. All pre-packaged commodities should carry declaration and particulars as prescribed under LM Rules. The drugs that are covered under DPCO 2013 are exempted from this provision. The LM rule requires the following to be mentioned on the label:

- Maximum retail price;
- Common or Generic Name;
- Month and Year in which commodity manufactured;
- Name, address, telephone number, e-mail address of the person who can be or office to which be contacted in case of consumer complaint;
- Actual corporate name and complete address of domestic manufacturer or importer or packer;
- Declaration.

Some of these details are required under Drugs Rule also.

DISTRIBUTION AND SALE OF DRUGS

Sale of drugs is permitted by a dealer who has obtained a license. Sale of medicine is under the control of state government and the state drugs controller is the licensing authority. The applicant intends to open a shop for sale of medicines needs to apply to the state licensing authority with supporting evidence that he has required premises, competent person for sale of medicines, and proper storage facilities. The premise of the person is inspected by the drug inspector and the license is issued on the basis of this report.

In granting a license the authority may consider the number of licenses granted in the locality during one year immediately preceding (restricted license—sale does not require the supervision of a qualified person); the average number of licenses granted during the period three years immediately preceding and the occupation, trade or business carried out by the applicant during this period.

A sale license remains valid if the licence holder continues paying the retention fees before the expiry of a period of every succeeding five years. This brought a big relief to all wholesalers and retailers.

There are four types of drug trade(sale):

1. Retail sale.
2. Wholesale.
3. Sale by retail (grocer chemist) and itinerant vendors.
4. Wholesale from a motor vehicle.

General Conditions of License

- Records and registers are to be maintained by the dealer to prove that the drugs have been purchased from licensed manufacturer/dealer and they are sold as per the conditions laid down. The dealer should be able to prove that the stock of drugs in hand is correct on the basis of purchase and sale records.
- The dealer has adequate space and necessary cold storage facility.
- The dealer is not engaged in stocking and sale of spurious and adulterated drugs or drugs like Physician's sample, or those bearing mark like "Hospital Supply".
- The wholesale dealer or retailer engages the service of a qualified person to supervise the sale operation.
- Expired drugs are to be kept separately marked " Not for Sale".

Retail Sale License

There are three types of License:

- Retail sale of non-biological drugs (other than those included in Schedule C and C(1));
- Retail sale of biological and special products;
- Retail sale of psychotropic drugs (Schedule X)

There are three types of retail units:

- **Drug Store:** This does not require the service of registered pharmacist. Sells only such drugs whose sale does not require any technical supervision.

- **Chemists and Druggists:** These require the service of a registered pharmacist and sell all types of drugs except those which are to be compounded.
- **Pharmacy, Pharmacist, Dispensing Chemist, Pharmaceutical Chemist:** These require the services of a registered pharmacist and maintain a pharmacy with space and equipment as per Schedule N and dispense drugs including the drugs which have to be compounded.
- Space requirement: 15 square meter.

Other Conditions

- Purchase records are to be maintained by the retail chemist: the date of purchase; the name and address of the supplier with license number; the name of the drug, the quantity and batch number; the name of the manufacturer.
- Supply records to be maintained either in a register or cash memo: serial number of entry; the date of supply; name and address of prescriber; the name and address of the patient (or name and address of the animal owner); the name of drug or preparation and quantity; the manufacturer, batch number and expiry date in case of Schedule C and H drugs; the signature of registered pharmacist or under whose supervision medicine supplied. These records are not necessary if drug is supplied against the prescription under the Employees' State Insurance Scheme or sale of drugs other than those specified in Schedule C and H, if supplied in the original unopened container.
- If drug is compounded, sale record is to be maintained in a prescription register.
- For Schedule X drugs, the prescription has to be in duplicate and a copy is to be retained by the chemist: the record of sale is to be maintained in a bound and serially registered bound register. Date of transaction; quantity received and name and address of the supplier including quantity received; name of the drug; quantity supplied; manufacturer's name; batch number; the name and address of the patient or purchaser; reference number of the prescription against which supplies were made; bill number; signature of the person under whose supervision the drugs were supplied.
- The medicines for the treatment of animals need to be kept in a cupboard or drawer reserved solely for storage of veterinary medicines and should be labelled with the words "Not for human use—for treatment of animals only".
- The Schedule X drugs are required to be kept under lock and key in cupboard or drawer reserved for the purpose and only the responsible person should have access.
- Dispensing of Schedule H and X: The prescription must not be dispensed more than once unless prescriber intended; at the time of dispensing this must be recorded above the signature of the prescriber—the name and address of the seller and the date on which dispensed.
- Schedule H1 drugs: Sale is to be recorded in a separate register at the time of the supply giving the name and address of the prescriber, the name of the patient, the name of the drug and the quantity supplied and such records shall be maintained for three years and be open for inspection.
- A retail chemist has to supply the Schedule H or X drugs given by name in the prescription and he cannot give any substitute.

The entry in the carbon copy of the cash or credit memo is usually acceptable. However, the licensing authority may require the entries be made in register if the carbon copy entries are not legible.

The medicines supplied on the prescription (ready for use should have the following particulars: the name and address of the supplier; the name of the patient and the quantity of the medicine; the number representing serial number of the entry in the prescription register; the dose, if the medicine is for internal use; the words 'For External use only' shall be printed on the label if the medicine is for external application.

Wholesale License

Like retail, there are three types of license.

- Space requirement: Not less than 10 sq m.
- Sale operation should be in charge of registered pharmacist/matriculation with four years of experience in dealing with drugs/recognized university degree with one year experience dealing with drugs.
- Maintains purchase records.
- Maintains sales records: The date of sale; the name and address of licensee to whom sold and his license number; the name and address of authority, institution, or registered medical practitioner if the medicines are sold to government, institution or registered medical practitioner; the name of the drug, quantity and the batch number; the name of the manufacturer; and the signature of the competent person under whose supervision the sale was effected. The carbon copy of the cash or credit memos need to be preserved for three years from the date of sale.
- Can sell to hospitals, medical institutions and registered medical practitioners and such records have to be maintained.

In the internet age and opportunities of home delivery of every commodities, the on-line business of or sale of medicines is not an exception. Though not legal, it has been in operation. The GoI now proposes to allow on-line pharmacy operation and brought a draft in June 2017 called "Drugs (Sale and Distribution Rules) 2017. It proposes to have legal operation of e-pharmacy. A strict enforcement of law is necessary to prevent illegal sale and to protect the public health.

SALE LICENCE CONDITIONS

[http://www.drugscontrol.tn.gov.in/guidelines_procedures_grant_renewal_retail_wholesale_licences_allopathic_drugs.html accessed on 22.10.2017]:

Licensing Authority

The Assistant Director of Drugs Control of Concerned zone

Documents to be Submitted

- Covering letter addressed to the Assistant Director of Drugs Control of **Concerned zone** along with Rs. 2/- court fee stamp for each licence.
- **Form 19** duly filled and signed by the applicant. **Form 19**—One number for each form of Licence, as applicable
- Authorization letter, in case of application signed by the authorized signatory in stamp paper/Board resolution.
- **Declaration form** duly filled and signed by the applicant and pharmacist/competent person.
- Fees of Rs. 1500/- for each form of licence.
- Premises details
  - Ownership document of the premises
  - Plan of the premises
  - Rental agreement of the premises, if applicable
- Pharmacist/competent person's details
  - Pharmacy council registration certificate/ Education qualification certificate
  - Experience certificate of competent person
  - Declaration of pharmacist/ competent person
- Applicant details
  - Document relating to constitution of concerned firm/Company/LLP and others
  - Passport size photos—3 of each and every applicant
  - Address/ID proof of the applicant
  - Legal tenancy affidavit
- Storage Accommodation details
  - Purchase bills of A/C and refrigerator along with working condition/ installation certificate

In case of change of premises and change in constitution.

Enclose Original Licence

Documents related to change in constitution like sale deed, Dissolution/Reconstitution deed, Amalgamation court order if it is Private Limited Company with board resolution and any other document.

Any other documents/particulars which are related to the above mentioned documents to verify the correctness of the particulars submitted by the applicant, if required.

Space Requirements

Minimum area required for
- Retail – 10 sq m
- Wholesale – 10 sq m
- Retail and Wholesale – 15 sq m
- Storage facilities racks, Refrigerator and A/C has to be provided.

Procedure Followed

The applicant has to submit the required statutory application in prescribed Form, Fees along with documents to the concerned Assistant Director of Drugs Control.

After the receipt of application, the Licencing authority will scrutinize the application file within 3 working days.
- If the file is in complete shape, it will be forwarded to the Drugs Inspector for inspection.
- If the file is incomplete, the required particulars/documents will be called from the applicant by the Licensing authority within 7 working days. And after the receipt of required particulars, the file will be forwarded to the Drugs Inspector for inspection.

The Drugs Inspector will inspect the premises and resubmit the file with Inspection Report within 7 working days.

After the receipt of the file with Inspection Report from the Drugs Inspector, the Licencing authority will scrutinize the file,
- If the file is in complete shape, the License will be issued within 7 working days.
- If the recommendation of Drugs Inspector is for rejection, the Licensing authority will take necessary follow-up action for rejection within 7 working days.

Overall Processing Time

- In case of grant of licence: 30 days
- In case of renewal of licence: 60 days

Restricted License to sale drugs by retail (grocer chemist) and itinerant vendors (travelling salesman):
- For sale of common household remedies in unopened container.
- Injections are not permitted.
- Drugs to be sold do not require any supervision by registered pharmacist (not containing drugs given Schedule G, H and X).
- Village with less than 1000 population does not need license under this category.

Sale by wholesale or distribution from a motor vehicle:

Two types of license:
- For drugs other than those specified in Schedule C and C(1).
- For drugs specified in Schedule C and C(1).
- A license is not required where public carrier or a hired vehicle is used for transportation or distribution of drug.

Offences and punishments related to sale of medicines (see box):

If on test any sample drawn from the dealer fails, the dealer can be prosecuted by the drugs inspector. In such situation the dealer needs to prove that the drugs were purchased from licensed dealers (purchase vouchers) and that the drug in the container while in his possession was in the same state as he had purchased and not tempered with. If these two facts are established, the dealer may not be treated as guilty and the liability shifts to manufacturer.

In case of cancellation or suspension of license, the dealer can appeal to the state government against the order.

Sale License for Pharmacies Attached to Private Hospitals (Kerala High Court) (Pharmabiz. Dated April 14, 2010)

The Kerala High Court came out with a significant judgement last month making it mandatory for all pharmacies attached to private hospitals in the state to obtain a drug license for running these stores. The court verdict is an affirmation of the state government order issued to the private hospitals in this connection two decades ago. The state branch of IDMA and Qualified Medical Practitioners Association had then moved the High Court challenging the state government order. The High Court upheld the directive of the state government. The doctors associations then filed a suit against the order in the Supreme Court but the apex court had asked the state HC to hear the case once again. Now the High Court order is final and binding on the state government. As per the provisions of the Drugs and Cosmetics Act, a drug license is required to run a pharmacy store whether it is owned by a hospital or an individual with a pharmacy registration. It is rather shocking to learn that pharmacies in private hospitals in a state with a high literacy rate were being run without a drug license and pharmacist for so many years. This would also mean that these hospital medical stores were not subjected to any checks by the state drug control department with regard to quality, price and ethics.

The Drugs Control Department had issued a directive to all the private hospitals in the State to obtain the license before July 31 following a High Court directive. However, the private hospitals have approached the Supreme Court against the High Court ruling and a verdict from the apex court is awaited.

Offences and punishments relating to sale of medicines

Offences	Punishments
*Sale or distribution of adulterated or spurious drug or any drug which when used by any person is likely to cause his death or likely to cause harm on his body (grievous hurt).	Imprisonment for not less than 10 years which may extend to a term of life and fine of not less than ₹ 10,00,000/- or three times the value of drugs confiscated.
Sale or distribution of any adulterated drug	Imprisonment for not less than 3 years extendable to 5 years with a fine of not less than ₹ 1,00,000/- or three times the value of drugs confiscated, whichever is more. The court may reduce both the minimum punishments citing adequate and special reasons.
Sale of drugs without a valid license	Do
Sale or distribution of any spurious drug	Imprisonment for not less than 7 years extendable to life imprisonment with a fine of not less than ₹ 3,00,000/- or three times the value of confiscated products, whichever is more. (Court may impose a sentence of imprisonment of less than 7 years but not less than 3 years and fine of less than ₹ 1,00,000.)

* The amount recovered or realised from convictions, is to be paid to the relative of the person who had died due to the use of such products (spouse, minor legitimate son, unmarried legitimate daughter, widow mother, parent of minor victim, person wholly dependent on the earning of the deceased person).

Offences relating to sale of spurious and adulterated are cognizable and non-bailable offences. Provision of fast track court to deal with cases relating to spurious drugs is also made.

Classes or list of medicines exempted from sale license (Schedule K)

Class of drugs	Remarks
Drugs (coming under the definition of drugs) not intended for medicinal use	No sale license subject to the condition that the drug is not sold for medicinal use or for the use in the manufacture of medicines and that each container is labelled conspicuously with the words "Not for medicinal use".

(Contd...)

(Contd...)

Class of drugs	Remarks
Quinine and other anti-malarial drugs	No sale license for persons selling the drugs by retail under arrangements made by the state government for sale and distribution of drugs.
Drugs supplied by registered medical practitioner to his own patient or any drug specified in Schedule C supplied by registered medical practitioner at the request of such practitioner if it is especially prepared with reference to the condition and for use of an individual patient provided the registered medical practitioner is not (a) keeping an open shop or (b) selling across the counter or (c) engaged in importation, manufacture, distribution or sale of drugs in India.	No sale license subject to the conditions: 1. The drugs shall be purchased only from a licensed dealer or manufacturer, and maintains records of such purchases showing the names and quantity of such drugs including batch number, manufacturer, etc. (Such records are subjected to inspection and samples may be drawn). 2. In case of medicines containing a substance specified in Schedule G, H or X, the following additional conditions are to be complied: • The medicines shall be labelled with the name and address of the registered medical practitioner by whom it is supplied. • If the medicine is for external application, it shall be labelled with the words "For External Use only", or if it for internal use, then with the dose. • Register to be maintained giving details such name and quantity of medicine, name of the patient, etc. • Entry in the register shall be given a number and that number should be entered on the label of the container. • The register and the prescriptions any need to be preserved for not less than two years from the date of prescription. 3. The drugs shall be stored under proper storage condition as directed on the label.
Drugs supplied by a hospital or dispensary maintained or supported by government or local body.	No sale license is required subject to the following conditions: • The dispensing and supply of drugs shall be carried out by or under the supervision of a qualified person (registered pharmacist). • The premises where drugs are supplied or stocked are open for inspection and sampling of drugs. • Drugs stored under proper storage condition. • Purchased from licensed dealer or manufacturer or transferred from hospital store.
Whole human blood/components stored for transfusion by first referral units, community health centre, primary health centre and hospital.	No license to operate blood bank.
Substances used as food and drugs: • All condensed or powdered milk whether pure, skimmed or malted, fortified with vitamins and minerals or otherwise. • Farex, oats, and all other similar cereal preparations whether fortified with vitamins and minerals or otherwise. • Virol, bovril, chicken essence and all other similar pre-digested foods.	No sale license.

(Contd...)

(Contd...)

Class of drugs	Remarks
• Ginger, pepper, cumin, cinnamon and all other similar spices and condiments unless they specially labelled as conforming to the standards in the Indian Pharmacopoeia or the official pharmacopoeia of drug standards prescribed in Drugs and Cosmetics Act and the Rules.	
Substances intended to be used for destruction of vermin or insects which cause disease in human beings or animals (insecticides and disinfectants).	No sale license subject to the condition that no keeping stock of materials after expiry dates. If kept, should be labelled with 'Not for sale.'
Household Remedies: • Aspirin tablets. • Paracetamol tablets. • Analgesic Balms. • Gripe water for use of infants. • Inhalers containing drugs for treatment of cold and nasal congestion. • Syrups, lozenges, pills and tablets for cough. • Liniments for external use. • Skin ointments and ointments for burns • Absorbent cotton wool, bandages, absorbent gauze, and adhesive plaster. • Castor oil, liquid paraffin and epsom salt. • Eucalyptus oil. • Tincture iodine, compound benzoin Tincture and mercuchrome solution in containers not exceeding 100 ml. • Tablets of quinine sulphate. • Tablets of iodochlorohydroxy quinoline 250 mg.	No sale license subject to the conditions: • The drugs are sold only in village having population of not more than one thousand persons and where there is no licensed dealer. • The drugs do not contain any substance specified in Schedule G, H or X. • The drugs are sold in the original unopened container of the licensed manufacturer. • No need of a competent person (if sold in village having population of not more than one thousand persons and where there is no licensed dealer).
Mechanical contraceptives like condoms.	No sale license subject to the condition that no keeping stock of materials after expiry dates. If kept, should be labelled with 'Not for sale'.
Vaginal contraceptive pessaries containing nonoxynol.	No sale license subject to the condition that no keeping stock of materials after expiry dates. If kept should be labelled with 'Not for sale'.
Chemical contraceptive having the following composition per tablet: • DL-Norgestrel – 0.3 mg Ethinyloestradiol – 0.03 mg • Levonorgestrel – 0. 15 mg • Centchroman – 0.15 mg • Desogestrel – 0.150 mg Ethinyloestradiol – 0.030 mg • Levonorgestrel – 0.1 mg Ethinyloestradiol – 0.02 mg	No sale license is required.
Ophthalmic ointments of tetracycline group of drugs.	Persons authorized by the government to sell under National Trachoma Control Programme do not require license.

(Contd...)

(Contd...)

Class of drugs	Remarks
Radiopharmaceuticals.	Sale provision of the Drugs and Cosmetics Act not applicable.
Tablets of chloroquine salts.	No sale license if selling in strip pack under Commercial Distribution Scheme of National Malaria Eradication Programme and duly labelled as "National Malaria Eradication Programme, Ministry of Health and Family Welfare, Government of India"
Sales from restaurant cars of trains and from coastal ships of household remedies which do not require the supervision of qualified person for their sale.	No sale license if • Records of purchase and sale are maintained and subjected to inspection. • Place where such drugs are stocked is subject to inspection and sampling.
Drugs supplied by multipurpose workers attached to primary health centres/sub centres; community health volunteers under rural health scheme; nurses, auxiliary nurses, mid-wives and lady health visitors attached to the Urban Family Welfare Centres/Primary Health Centres/Sub centres; Anganwadi Workers.	No sale license if drugs are supplied under health or family welfare programme of central or state government.
Preparations applied to the human body for the purpose of repelling insects like mosquitoes.	No sale license subject to the conditions that such product has been manufactured under valid drug manufacturing license.
Medicated dressings and bandages for first aid	No sale license subject to the conditions that such product has been manufactured under valid drug manufacturing license.
ORS	No sale license subject to the conditions that such product has been manufactured under valid drug manufacturing license.
Morphine tablets	No sale license if • Supplied by state government approved palliative care centre to terminally ill cancer patients. • To be kept under custody of medical officer in charge. • Subjected to inspection and sampling.
Homeopathic hair oils having active ingredients up to 3X potency only	No sale licence if manufactured under licence and sold in original container.
Custom made device	No sale licence if device is made in accordance with qualified medical practitioner's prescription only
Zinc sulphate tablets and oral solutions having 10 mg and 20 mg elemental zinc	No sale license if manufactured under licence.

EXPORT OF DRUGS

India is the 3rd largest producer of drugs in the world and exports drugs to over 200 countries which include both regulated and unregulated markets. The quality of drugs to be exported is equally controlled as products meant for domestic use (even more stringently). The drugs to be exported to be labelled based on the specific requirements of the importing country.

In addition, the following particulars must appear on the label of the innermost container and also outer coverings:

• Name of the drug;
• Name and address of the manufacturer;
• The manufacturing license number;
• The batch or lot number;
• The date of expiry.

As some of the importing countries do not require the label to contain all the above particulars including the name and address of manufacturer, the label of the container should bear a code number as approved by DCGI. As some of the exporters/manufacturers/merchant exporters are trying to export the drug formulations manufactured under neutral code of actual manufacturer mentioning their name 'manufacturer' or 'manufactured by' or 'the manufacturer', this would lead to confusion and will be treated as spurious drugs. Hence, the DCGI has instructed the state drug controllers and port and zonal officers to ensure that all the exporters/merchant exporters should mention their name and address with their status as 'Manufacturer', 'Manufactured by' and 'The Manufacturer'—Manufactured under neutral code of actual manufacturer on the label of export of drug formulations.

However, sera and vaccines for human use, all veterinary biological products, blood products, Schedule X preparations (psychotropic substances) and narcotic drugs cannot have any code number and needs to have name and address of manufacturer on the label.

Now some of the importing countries insist on WHO certification for Good Manufacturing Practices for accepting products. The WHO has a scheme of certification of pharmaceutical products (COPP) for pharmaceuticals moving in international commerce. After joint inspection by drug inspectors of central and state government to verify that the unit has complied with WHO GMP requirements, the COPP certificate is issued by the state licensing authority. The scheme of issuing COPP by State Dru Regulating Authority is scrapped and the responsibility is taken over by Central Authority (DCGI). From October 1, 2009, CDSCO will issue the COPP certificate after inspecting the manufacturing facility by CDSCO officials. The order of DCGI is stayed by the Madras High Court.

Drugs for export must carry barcode to put an end to allegations overseas that some local firms shipout counterfeit medicines. The Directorate General of Foreign Trade (DGFT) made it mandatory for all pharmaceutical exporters to send their shipments under a trace and track system of surveillance to prevent spurious drug manufacturers in countries like China to pass off their medications as Indian products. This is operative from 1st July, 2011.

Domestic drug companies engaged in contract manufacturing of medicines meant for export markets will have to furnish validation certificates to prove the authenticity of the importing firms. All contract manufacturers exporting medicines using neutral code (which do not mention the name of the manufacturing or marketing firm) will have to present certificates from the regulators of the importing country to prove the genuine nature of the importing firm. In other words, the foreign regulator will have to endorse the product name and marketing registration these companies have obtained from the regulator.

DCGI Directs SLAs, Port Officers to Act Against Exporters Breaching Labelling Rules (Pharmabiz Dated 25 October 2009)

Mumbai, 25 Oct: The Drugs Controller General of India (DCGI) Dr Surinder Singh has asked all state drug controllers, port and zonal officers to initiate action against the exporters and merchant exporters who violate the labelling provisions and put only neutral code on the labels of their products in violation of the Drugs and Cosmetics Act. In a directive to the state drug controllers and all port and zonal officers, the DCGI has said it has been brought to the notice of this Directorate that some of the exporters/manufacturers/merchant exporters are trying to export the drug formulations manufactured under neutral code of actual manufacturer mentioning their name as 'manufacturer' or 'manufactured by' or 'the manufacturer'. "This Directorate may like to inform you that such type of labelling amounts to contravention of provisions of the Drugs and Cosmetics Rules and would be covered under the definition of Spurious Drugs'," he said. The DCGI has asked the state drug controllers and port and zonal officers to ensure that all the exporters/merchant exporters should mention their name and address with their status as 'Manufacturer', 'Manufactured by' and 'The Manufacturer'—manufactured under neutral code of actual manufacturer on the label of export of drug formulations. As per Rule 94 of the Drugs and Cosmetics Rules, the exemption is given to the manufacturer to mention neutral code issued by state licensing authority in place of name and address of the manufacturer on the label to meet the requirement of exporting country. The DCGI's action in this regard comes in the wake of complaints against several exporting companies. Some of the com-panies against whom complaints have been received by the DCGI office included M/s. Promed Exports Pvt Ltd, New Delhi, M/s. Protech Biosystems Pvt Ltd, Haryana, M/s Hindustan Syringes and Medical Devices Ltd, Haryana and M/s. Harsoria Healthcare Pvt Ltd, Haryana.

ADMINISTRATION OF ACT

The central and state governments enforce the provision of the Drugs and Cosmetics Act through implementation of Drugs and Cosmetics Rules. In order to enforce the Act, there are provisions of statutory bodies; central and state drugs control authorities; and analytical laboratories. The regulatory system for health care products is given Table 2.1.

Table 2.1: Regulatory system for health care products

Ministry of Health and Family Welfare	Ministry of Chemicals and Fertilizers	Ministry of Commerce	Ministry of Science and Technology	Ministry of Environment
Directorate General of Health Services (DGHS) Indian Council of Medical Research (ICMR)	Department of Pharmaceuticals	Patent office	Department of Biotechnology (DBT)	Environmental clearance for manufacturing
Central Drugs Standard Control Organization (CDSCO) headed by Drug Controller General of India, DCGI (I) + Statutory Committees + Advisory Committees + State Licensing Authorities	National Pharmaceutical Pricing Authority (NPPA): Drugs (Prices Control) Order (DPCO) 2013	Controller General of Patents	Council of Scientific and Industrial Research (CSIR) Laboratories	

Statutory committees: DCC and DTAB
- **Advisory committees:**
  - Subject Expert Committees (SEC) advise on approvals of clinical trials, drugs and medical devices.
  - New Drug Advisory Committee (NDAC) and Investigational New Drugs Committee (INDC) provide recommendations on approval of clinical trials.
  - The Indian Council of Medical Research (ICMR) provides assistance in evaluation of Phase I clinical trials.
- **For biologicals:** Department of Biotechnology (DBT) supports in identifying, formulating, implementing and monitoring of various activities related to biotechnology, e.g. through Division of Biologicals and the Cellular Biology-Based Therapeutic Drug Evaluation Committee (CBBTDEC).
- For medical devices (except investigational ones): Medical Devices Advisory Committee (MDAC) advises on review and approval of products and clinical trials

Source: Medicine Regulation—Regulatory System in India, WHO Drug Information Vol. 31, No. 3, 2017

Statutory Bodies

The two statutory bodies are formed under the act for advising governments on different matters relating control of drugs and cosmetics.

Drugs Technical Advisory Board (DTAB): DTAB is constituted by the central government under the act to advise the central and state governments on technical matters arising out of the administration of the act. No rule can be made by the central government without consulting DTAB.

The Director General of Health Services is the *ex-officio* chairman and the Drugs Controller General (India) is the member secretary. It is composed of the following 18 experts:

I. Ex-officio members:

- The Director General of Health Services;
- The Drugs Controller General (India);
- The Director of Central Drugs Laboratory, Kolkata;
- The Director of Central Research Institute, Kasauli;
- The Director of Indian Veterinary Research Institute, Izatnagar;
- The President of Medical Council of India;
- The President of Pharmacy Council of India;
- The Director of Central Drugs Research Institute, Lucknow.

II. Nominated Members:

- Two persons nominated by the central government from among the persons in charge of drugs control of the states;
- One person nominated by the central government from the pharmaceutical industry;
- Two government analysts nominated by the central government.

III. Elected Members:

- One person elected by the Executive Members of the Pharmacy Council of India from among the teachers in pharmacy or pharmaceutical chemistry or pharmacognosy of an Indian university or affiliating college;
- One person elected by the Executive Members of the Medical Council of India from among the teachers in medicine or therapeutics of an Indian university or affiliating college;
- One pharmacologist elected by the Governing Body of the Indian Council of Medical Research;
- One person elected by the Central Council of Indian Medical Association;
- One person elected by the Council of Indian Pharmaceutical Association.

The nominated and elected members of the board hold office for three years but are eligible for nomination or election. The persons who are nominated or elected by virtue of their position can hold office as long as they continue in their position.

The board, with approval of central government, regulates its own procedure and conducts all business. It may appoint sub-committees for a period not exceeding three years.

Drugs Consultative Committee (DCC)

The DCC is the statutory advisory committee constituted by the central government to advise the DTAB, central government and state governments on any matter tending to secure of uniform administration of the Act throughout the country. The Drugs Controller General (India) is the chairman of the DCC. It consists of two representatives of central government nominated by the central government and one representative of each state government (usually Drugs Controler of the state) nominated by the concerned state government. DCC meets as and when required by the central government.

Drugs Control Authorities

There are two drugs control authorities with clear cut responsibilities functioning under the Act. The first one at National Level called Central Drugs Standard Control Organization of Government of India and is headed by the Drugs Controller General (India). The second one is at each state level: State Drugs Control organization and is responsible for exercising control over manufacturing, sale or distribution of drugs and cosmetics within its territory. Refer to the box on the next page.

Central Drug Standard Control Organization (CDSCO): The CDSCO is the part of the Directorate General of Health services in the Ministry of Health and Family Welfare, Government of India. The CDSCO is staffed with DCGI as head and other staff like Deputy Drugs Controllers, Assistant Drugs Controllers, and Technical Officers. The headquarter is located in New Delhi (FDA Bhawan). The CDSCO has six zonal offices: At Mumbai (West zone), Kolkata (East zone), Chennai (South zone), Ghaziabad (North zone), Hyderabad (Hyderabad zone), and Ahmedabad (Ahmedabad zone). The zonal offices work in collaboration with state drugs control department to enforce regulations over manufacture of drugs. There are five sub-zonal offices: Baddi, Bangalore, Jammu & Kashmir, Goa and Indore. It has 13 port offices and 8 laboratories under its domain.

State Drug Control Organization

In the states and union territories, state drugs control department is functioning. The state drugs control department is also known as Food and Drugs Administration in some states like Gujarat and Maharashtra.

Drugs Controller General of India

- Head of CDSCO;
- Central License Approving Authority (CLAA);
- Central Licensing Authority (CLA);
- Chairman of DCC;
- Secretary of DTAB;

Qualification of Licensing Authority and Controlling Authority

- Graduate in Pharmacy or Pharmaceutical Chemistry or Medicine with specialization Clinical Pharmacology or Microbiology from Indian University; and
- Experience in manufacturing or testing of drugs or enforcement of the Drugs and Cosmetics Act for a minimum period of five years.

(MD Pharmacology is acceptable qualification to satisfy the requirement—specialization in Clinical Pharmacology. Super-speciality is not contemplated.)

However, the academic qualification would not apply to those inspectors and government analysts who were holding these positions as on 12 April, 1989.

At state level the licensing authority and controlling authority are the same.

Drugs Control Administration	
Functions of Central Government (CDSCO) http://cdsco.nic.in/writereaddata/Pr.pdf accessed on 22.10.2017	Functions of State Government (State Drugs Control Department) http://cdsco.nic.in/writereaddata/statefunction.pdf accessed on 22.10.2017
• Approval of new drugs and clinical trials • Import Registration and Licensing • License approving of Blood Banks, LVPs, Vaccines, r-DNA products and some medical devices (CLAA Scheme) • Amendment to D & C Act and Rules • Banning of drugs and cosmetics • Grant of test license, personal license, NOCs for export • Testing of new drugs • Oversight and market surveillance through Inspectorate of Centre over and above the State Authority	• Licensing of manufacturing site for drugs including API and finished formulation • Licensing of establishment for sale or distribution of drugs • Approval of drug testing laboratories • Monitoring of quality of drugs and cosmetics marketed in the country • Investigation and prosecution in respect of contravention of legal provision • Recall of sub-standard drugs

Drugs Controller (India) Recruitment Rule 2011

The Drugs Controller (India) is required to be appointed only by deputation including short-term contract. The maximum age limit at the closing date of application is not exceeding 56 years. The period of deputation including the period of deputation held earlier shall ordinarily not exceed 5 years.

Essential Educational Qualification and Experience:

- Graduate Degree in Pharmacy or Pharmaceutical Chemistry or in Medicine with specialization in Pharmacology or Microbiology from a recognised university established in India by law;
- Postgraduate Degree in Pharmacy/ Pharmaceutical Chemistry/Biochemistry/ Chemistry/Microbiology/Pharmacology from a recognized university or equivalent; and
- 15 years experience in manufacture or testing of drugs in a concern of repute or enforcement of provision of Drugs and Cosmetics Act and the Rules.

Desirable Educational Qualification and Experience:

- Two years experience in dealing with problems connected with drug standardization and control and import and export of drugs and/or administration of the Drugs and Cosmetics Act and the Rules;
- Ph. D. in Pharmaceutical Sciences.

Disqualification: The following persons are disqualified:

- Who has entered into or contracted a marriage with a person having spouse living;
- Who, having a spouse living, has entered into or contracted a marriage with any person.

However, the Central Government has the power to exempt any person from the operation of the rule, if such a marriage is permissible under personal law to such person and other party to the marriage.

Drugs Inspector

The Drugs Inspectors are appointed by both central and state government. The central inspectors are under the control of DCGI and the state inspectors work under the controlling authority (drugs controller).

Qualification

- Degree in Pharmacy or Pharmaceutical Sciences, or Medicine with specialization in clinical pharmacology or microbiology from an Indian University.
- For inspection of manufacturing of Schedule C drugs: The inspector should have at least 18 months experience in manufacturing of at least one drug specified in Schedule C; or have at least 18 months experience in testing of at least one substance specified in Schedule C; or have at least three years of experience in inspecting firms involve in manufac-turing of drugs specified in Schedule C.

The educational qualification is not applicable for inspectors already appointed on or before 18 October 1993.

Now, there is a move to expand the qualification further to have inspectors from all related scientific discipline as therapeutic sciences has developed extensively comprising products of biotechnology, genetic engineering, medical devices, gene therapy etc.

Now, there is a move to expand the qualification further to have inspectors from all related scientific discipline as therapeutic sciences has developed extensively comprising products of biotechnology, genetic engineering, medical devices, gene therapy, etc.

Power of Inspectors

1. To inspect:
   a. the premises where drugs and cosmetics are manufactured and means employed for standardising and testing drug or cosmetic.
   b. the premises where drug or cosmetic is sold, stocked or exhibited or offered for sale or distributed.

2. To take samples of any drug or cosmetic:

a. which is being manufactured or being sold or is stocked or exhibited or offered for sale, or is being distributed.

b. from any person who is in the course of conveying, delivering or preparing to deliver drug or cosmetic to a purchaser or consignee.

3. At all reasonable time:

a. search any person who is believed to have committed an offence relating to drug or cosmetic.

b. enter or search any place where believed to have committed an offence.

c. stop and search any vehicle or vessel or other conveyance believed to have been used committing an offence.

d. order the person, possessing the drug or cosmetics in respect of which offence has been committed, not to dispose for a period not exceeding 20 days and if required seize the stock.

e. examine any record, register, document or any other material object and seize them if it is believed that they provide evidence.

f. require the person to produce record, register or other document relating to manufacture, distribution, stocking, exhibition for sale, offer for sale or distribution of any drug or cosmetic believed to have involved in offence.

g. exercise such other powers necessary for carrying out the provision of act and the rules.

The code of criminal procedure is to be followed to any search or seizure operation. Every record, register or other documents seized need to be returned within a period of 20 days after making copies or extracting.

Any person wilfully obstructs an inspector in exercise of powers or refuse to produce any record, register or other document as required is punishable with imprisonment extending to 3 years or fine or with both.

Duties of Inspectors for Inspecting Premises for Sale

- To inspect all premises licensed for sale within its jurisdiction for at least once in three years;
- To satisfy himself that the conditions of the licenses are observed;
- To procure and send for analysis of any suspected samples contravening the provision of the Act;
- To investigate any complaint made to him in writing;
- To institute prosecution in case of breach of Act;
- To maintain record of all inspections, sampling, seizure of stocks, etc. and inform the controlling authority;
- To make such enquiries and inspections to detect the sale contravening the provision of Act;
- To detain imported packages if suspected to contravene the Act, if authorized by the state government.

Duties of Inspectors for Inspecting Premises for Manufacturing

- To inspect all manufacturing premises at least once in a year to satisfy himself that the conditions of the license and provisions of the Act are observed;
- Schedule C and C(1) drugs: To inspect the plant and process of manufacture, standardization and method of testing, the methods and place of storage, technical qualification of staff employed, and details of location, construction, and administration of the establishment which is likely to affect the quality of product;
- To submit the report forthwith to the controlling authority giving details of conditions observed or not observed;
- To take samples manufactured in the premises and send them for test or analysis;
- To institute prosecution in case of breach of Act and Rules.

Procedure for Inspectors

- An inspector will not disclose the information acquired by him during course of his duties without written sanction of his superior officer and except for the official purpose or required by court of law.

- When he believes that stocks of drugs/ cosmetics in possession of a person are prohibited from manufacturing and sale, he should issue an order in the prescribed form (Form 15) to the individual not to dispose of stock for a specified period. The person in possession of such drug/ cosmetics should not dispose off or sale such stock. If it is ascertained that the materials concerned does not contravene the provision of the Act and Rules, he should revoke his order forthwith. Similarly if the alleged contravention is due to defect and he is satisfied that the defect is remedied, he should revoke the order forthwith.

- When the stock of drugs/cosmetics, records, registers, documents or materials are seized; he should issue a receipt in prescribed form (Form 16). After seizing he should inform the judicial magistrate as soon as possible and take his orders to take custody of such materials.

- He should return the seized documents after making copies or extracts within 20 days of such seizure.

Taking samples:

- While taking samples for test or analysis, he should give intimation in writing in Form 17, offer a fair price and ask for written acknowledgement for payment. When price tendered is refused, he should tender a receipt for taking samples in Form 17A.

- He should divide the samples into four portions in the presence of the person concerned unless he wilfully absents, seal and suitably mark and permit the person to add his seal and mark. If sampling is from the manufacturing units, the sample should be divided into three portions.

- Where the sample is of small volume, instead of dividing them, four or three such containers are to be taken.

- He should restore one portion of the sample or one such container to the person concerned and dispose of the remaining as follows: One portion to send government analyst, one to keep with himself for producing before the court if required, and one to send to the manufacturer.

- He should send the samples to the government analyst by registered post or deliver by hand in a sealed packed enclosed together with memorandum in Form 18 with the outer cover addressed to the government analyst. A copy of the memorandum and specimen impression of the seal used to seal the packet should be sent to the government analyst separately by registered post or by hand.

- Disposal of confiscated drugs: If the drugs are of standard quality, he should report the same to the court and disposes them by giving the stock to hospital or dispensary maintained or supported by the government or charitable institutions as ordered by the court. If they are not of standard quality, he should supervise the destruction of such materials in the presence of such authority as specified by the court.

Analytical Laboratories

Central Drugs Laboratory (CDL): The CDL is a statutory laboratory established by the central government under the Act at Kolkata in 1947 (The Biochemical Standardization Laboratory established during 1937 was converted as CDL) and it functions under the control of a director.

The functions of the laboratory include:

I. Statutory Functions

a. Analytical quality control of majority of the imported Drug available in Indian market.

b. Analytical quality control of drug and cosmetics manufactured within the country on behalf of the Central and State Drug Controller Administrations.

c. Acting as an Appellate authority in matters of disputes relating to quality of Drug.

II. Other Functions

a. Collection, storage and distribution of International Standard, International Reference Preparations of Drug and Pharmaceutical Substances.

b. Preparation of National Reference Standards and maintenance of such standards. Maintenance of microbial cultures useful in drug analysis Distribution of Standards and Cultures to State Quality Control Laboratories and drug manufacturing establishments.

c. Training of Drug Analysts deputed by State Drug Control Laboratories and other institutions.

d. Training of World Health Organization fellows from abroad on modern methods of drug analysis.

e. To advise the Central Drug Control Administration in respect of quality and toxicity of drug awaiting license.

f. To work out analytical specifications for preparation of Monographs for the Indian Pharmacopoeia and the Homoeopathic Pharmacopoeia of India.

g. To undertake analytical research on standardisation and methodology of drug and cosmetics.

h. Analysis of cosmetics received as survey samples from Central Drug Standard Control Organisation.

i. Quick analysis of life-saving drug on an all-India basis received under National Survey of Quality of Essential Drug Programme from Zonal Offices of Central Drug Standard Control Organisation.

In addition to the above functions, the Central Drug Laboratory also actively collaborates with the World Health Organisation in the preparation of International Standards and Specifications for International Pharmacopoeia. It also undertakes collaborative study on behalf of the Indian Pharmacopoeia Committee. The senior officers of the Laboratory have been

Classes of drugs	Institute or Laboratory
Sera, solutions of serum proteins intended for injection, vaccines, toxins, antigens, anti-toxins, sterilized surgical ligature and sterilized surgical suture, bacteriophase	Central Research Institute (CRI), Kasauli.
Oral polio vaccine	1. CRI 2. Pasteur Institute of India, Conoor. 3. Enterovirus Research Centre (ICMR), Haffkine Institute Campus, Mumbai. 4. The National Institute of Biologicals, Noida.
Anti-sera, vaccines, toxoids, and diagnostic antigens for veterinary use	1. Indian Veterinary Research Institute, Izatnagar. 2. Indian Veterinary Research Institute, Mukteshwar.
Condom	Central Indian Pharmacopoeia Laboratory, Ghaziabad (currently known as Indian Pharmacopoeia Commission)
VDRL Antigen	Laboratory of Serologist and Chemical Examineer, Kolkata
Intra uterine devices and falope rings	Central Drug Testing Laboratory, Thane
Homeopathic medicines	Homeopathic Pharmacopoeia Laboratory, Ghaziabad
Blood grouping reagents and, Hepatitis B surface antigens and Hepatitis C virus	National Institute of Biologicals, Noida
Human blood or blood products including components, to test for freedom of HIV antibodies	1. National Institute for Communicable Disease, Department of Microbiology, Delhi. 2. National Institute of Virology, Pune 3. Centre of Advanced Research in Virology, Christian Medical College, Vellore.

appointed as Government Analysts on the behalf of most of the States of the Union for analysis of drug samples.

It tests the sample sent by CDSCO, Central Drug Inspectors, and custom authorities and courts. It tests all antibiotics, steroids, vitamins, chemotherapeutic substances, and phytopharmaceuticals and cosmetics. The functions of the CDL in respect of certain classes of drugs entrusted to the following other laboratories or institutes:

There are other Central Laboratories: Central Drug Testing Laboratory, Chennai; Central Drug Testing Laboratory, Mumbai; Regional Drugs Testing Laboratory (RDTL), Guwahati; and Regional Drugs Testing Laboratory (RDTL), Chandigarh.

Sending of Samples to Central Drugs Laboratory: The samples for test or analysis should be sent by registered post in a sealed packet along with a covering letter (memorandum in Form 1) in an outer cover addressed to the Director. The packet as well as outer cover should be marked with a distinguish number.

A copy of the memorandum in Form 1 and a specimen impression of the seal used should be sent separately by registered post to the Director.

Procedure to be followed by CDL

- On receipt of the packet, it will be opened only by authorised officer who should record the condition of the seal on the packet.

- After test or analysis, CDL supplies the results with full protocols of the test applied to the sender in prescribed format (Form 2).

- Certificates of the test results should be signed by the Director or any other officer authorised by central government.

Indian Pharmacopoeia Commission (IPC)

Indian Pharmacopoeia Commission is an Autonomous Institution under the Ministry of Health and Family Welfare, Govt. of India dedicated for setting of standards for drugs, pharmaceuticals and healthcare

devices/ technologies, etc. besides providing Reference Substances and Training. Its functions are:

a. To develop comprehensive monographs for drugs to be included in the Indian Pharmacopoeia, including active pharmaceutical ingredients, excipients and dosage forms as well as medical devices, and to keep them updated by revision on a regular basis.

b. To accord priority to monographs of drugs included in the national Essential Drugs List and their dosage forms.

c. To prepare monographs for products that have normally been in the market for not less than 2 years except for certain special categories of new drugs like antiretrovirals, antituberculosis and anticancer drugs and their formulations introduced more recently, which may be accorded priority attention.

d. To give special attention to the methods of manufacture used by the indigenous industry in selecting the pharmacopoeia tests for monitoring the toxic impurities of the concerned drug.

e. To take note of the different levels of sophistication in analytical testing/ instrumentation available while framing the monographs.

f. To accelerate the process of preparation, certification and distribution of IP Reference Substances, including the related substances, impurities and degradation products required.

g. To collaborate with pharmacopoeias like the Ph Eur, BP, USP, JP and International Pharmacopoeia with a view to harmonizing with global standards.

h. To organize educational programs and research activities for spreading and establishing awareness on the need and scope of quality standards for drugs and related articles/materials.

Government Analyst: The central government and state governments appoint government analysts, by notification in the official gazette, in respect of drug(s) or cosmetics. The person having financial interest in the import, manufacture or sale of drugs cannot be appointed as government analysts.

Qualifications: The person must be one of the following:

- Graduate in Medicine or Science or Pharmacy or Pharmaceutical Chemistry of a recognised University and has not less than five years postgraduate experience in testing of drugs in a laboratory under the control of (i) a government analyst or (ii) head of the institution or approved testing laboratory; or has completed two years training on testing of drugs including items of Schedule C in Central Drugs Laboratory;

- Postgraduate in Medicine or Science or Pharmacy or Pharmaceutical Chemistry of a recognised University or Associate Diploma of Institution of Chemists (India) obtained by passing examination with 'Analysis of Drugs and Pharmaceuticals' as one of the subjects and has at least three years experience in testing of drugs in a laboratory under the control of (i) a government analyst or (ii) head of institution or approved testing labora-tory; or has completed two years training on testing of drugs including items of Schedule C in Central Drugs Laboratory.

For examination of items in Schedule C:

- The Government Analysts appointed under the above two categories and have degree in Medicine, Physiology, Phar-macology, Microbiology, Pharmacy should have experience or training in testing of these items in an approved institution or laboratory for a period of not less than six months;

- The Government Analysts appointed under the above two categories but not having degree in the above subjects should have experience or training in testing of Schedule C items for a period of not less than three years in an approved institution or laboratory or have completed two years training on testing of drugs in CDL.

For examination of antisera, toxoid, vaccines and diagnostics antigens for veterinary use, the following qualifications are necessary:

- The person needs to be graduate in Veterinary Sciences, or General Science, or Medicine or Pharmacy with not less than five years experience in the standardisation of biological products. OR

- The persons with a postgraduate degree in Veterinary Science, or General Science, or Medicine, or Pharmacy or Pharma-ceutical Chemistry with an experience of at least three years in the standardisation of biological products.

Duties of Government Analyst

- To analyse or test samples of drugs or cosmetics samples sent by drugs inspectors or any person or recognised consumer association or other authorities.

- To submit reports relating analytical and research work to the government with a view to their publication at government's discretion.

Procedure for Government Analyst

- On receipt of the sample, Government Analyst needs to compare the seals on the packet or on portion of the sample or container with the specimen impression received separately from the sender of the sample.

- Then to note down the condition of the seals on the packet or on the portion of the sample or container.

- On completion of analysis, to supply a report in triplicate to the Drugs Inspector in prescribed form (Form 13) along with the full protocol of the tests or analysis used.

- On completion of analysis, to supply a report to the person who has sent the sample in prescribed form (Form 14B).

Protocol for Test or Analysis

1. Pharmacopoeial Drugs: Pharmacopoeial Methods.

2. Patent or Proprietary Medicines:
   a. Any available Pharmacopoeial Method.
   b. Modified Pharmacopoeial Method.
   c. Method of analysis described in standard books or journals (if no pharmacopoeial method available).
3. Drugs for which no available method: The method developed by government analyst.

Drugs and Cosmetics (Amendment Bill) 2007 (The Bill could not get through as Parliamentary Panel rejected)

- Propose to create an independent central drugs authority (CDA) with headquarter at Delhi;
- CDA would appoint Drugs Controller (India) who would be the secretary of CDA.

- DTAB would be replaced by CDA.
- Centralized licensing procedure for manufacturing of drugs and cosmetics.

The Parliamentary panel (standing committee on health and family welfare) has rejected the proposal for a new central drug authority and instead recommended setting up of a central drug administration as an independent body under the ministry with headquarter in Delhi and its zonal and sub-zonal offices at state level, by strengthening, modernizing and restructuring the CDSCO. (Pharmabiz dated 23.10.2008)

HOMEOPATHIC MEDICINES

The homeopathy was brought to India as early as 1810 from the West by travellers,

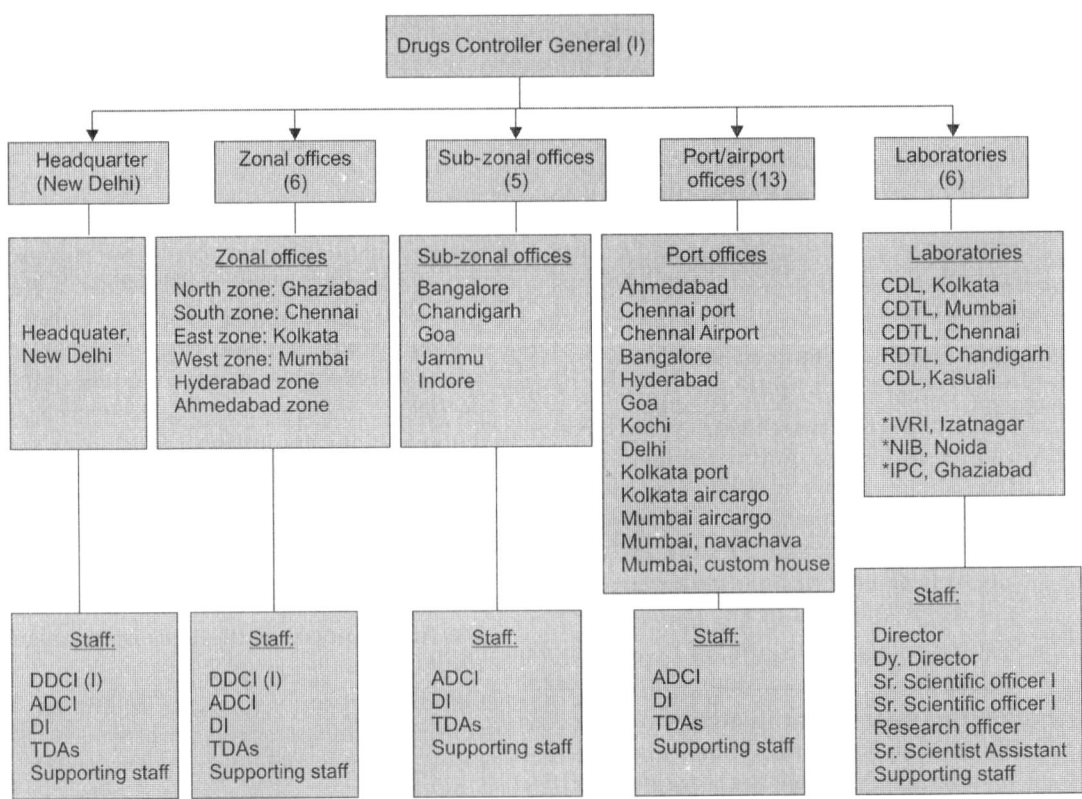

Abbreviations CID & CO-central drug standard control organisation; CDL-central drug laboratories; CDTL-central drug testing laboratories; RDTL-regional drug testing laboratories, IVRI-Indian Veterinary Research Institute: NIB-National institute of Biologiostic; IIPC-Indian Pharmacoposts commission; DDC(I)-Deputy Drugs controller (I); AIDC (I)- Assistant drugs controller; DIs Drugs inspectors; TDAs- Technical data associates

Organisation chart central drugs standard control organisation missionaries, and military personnel. However, the official patronage started when a visiting Romanian person Dr John Martin Honiberger cured Maharaja Ranjit Singh of Lahore suffering from paralysis of vocal cords with swelling of feet in 1839. Soon he was recognized as Chief Physician of the Royal Court. Later on the science and practice of homeopathy flourished in West Bengal especially in Calcutta (now Kolkata). Now homeopathy is one of the recognized medical systems in the country. The homeopathic medicines were kept out of purview of Drugs and Cosmetics Act and the Rules up to 1963. In 1964 the comprehensive provisions were made in the statute for bringing the homeopathic medicines within the scope of drugs control.

Combinations of homeopathic medicines are treated as homeopathic medicines but the injection form of any drug is not recognized as homeopathic medicine.

Standards of Homeopathic Medicines

Current edition of Homeopathic Pharmacopoeia of India is the official books of standards. If the homeopathic medicine is not described in the current edition of Homeopathic Pharmacopoeia of India, then standards given in the current edition of Homeopathic Pharmacopoeia of the USA, the UK or Germany are acceptable. When the homeopathic medicines do not find the standards in any of the above pharmacopoeias, the standards would be the formula or list of ingredients displayed on the label.

Import: It is not necessary to have any license for importing homeopathic medicines into India but the importer has to comply with the following conditions:

- The imported medicines are packed and labelled in conformity with the rules;
- They conform to the standards prescribed.

In case of new homeopathic medicines, approval from Drugs Controller General (India) is necessary.

New homeopathic medicine means:

- The homeopathic medicines not specified in recognized pharmacopeias.

- The homeopathic medicines not recognized in authoritative homeopathic literatures.
- Combination of homeopathic medicines when one or more medicines belong to either of the above categories.

During import, the bill of entry is referred by the Collector of Customs to the Assistant Drugs Controller (India) at the port of entry for examination of import documents and sampling before clearance.

Manufacturing: Manufacturing of homeopathic medicines are required to be carried out under a license issued by State Drugs Control Authority. The conditions for manufacturing license:

- The manufacturing is required to be carried out under the supervision of at least one whole time employed technical person:
  - A graduate in science with chemistry as one of the subjects with three years experience in manufacturing of homeopathic medicines.
  - A graduate in pharmacy with 18 months of experience in manufacturing of homeopathic medicines.
  - A recognized qualification such as Diploma in Homeopathic Medicine and Surgery (DHMS), Bachelor of Homeopathic Medicine and Surgery, etc. (under Schedule II and Schedule III of Homeopathy Central Council Act 1973 with 18 months of experience in manufacturing of Homeopathic medicines.)
- Comply with requirements and conditions specified in Schedule M-I (Good Manufacturing Practices).
- Comply with the prescribed standards and packed and labelled properly.
- If mother tincture is manufactured, the total solids and content should be determined. No colour should be added to mother tincture.
- The premises must be distinct and separate from the premises used for residential purposes.

- They are not manufactured simultaneously with medicines of the other systems.
- Availability of proper storage.

A separate license is necessary for each manufacturing premise. All records of manufacturing should be kept for a period of five years. Other conditions and procedures are similar to allopathic medicines. The license is valid till the 31st December of the year.

New homeopathic medicines manufacturing license can be issued only after the approval of Drugs Controller General (India).

Sale: A sale license is necessary. There are two types of sale license: Retail sale and wholesale. Drugs controller of the state is the licensing authority.

Conditions to be complied for sale license:

- Sale premises should be maintained under clean condition.
- Sale is required to be conducted under the supervision of a competent person to deal with homeopathic medicines.
- For retail dealer the person is to be approved by the licensing authority. However, no approval is necessary if Registered Homeopathic Medical Practitioner practices and deals with homeopathic medicines.
- Purchase and sale records of medicines containing alcohol should be maintained. However, there is no necessity for keeping sale record for potentized preparations in containers of 30 ml or lower capacity and in respect of mother tinctures made up in quantities up to 60 ml.

Labelling and Packing: The following particulars must be printed or written in indelible ink in conspicuous manner on the label:

- "Homeopathic Medicine"
- The name of the medicine:
  - Name as described in recognized Pharmacopoeias;
  - Drugs not described in homeopathic pharmacopoeia—the name describe the real nature of the drug.

- Potency of the homeopathic medicine: Either in decimal, centesimal or millisimal system (give a note of these units). In case of combination of medicines, name of each ingredient with its potency and proportions.
- Name and address of the manufacturer have to be given, if sold in the original containers. If not sold in the original containers, the name and address of the seller have to be given.
- Alcohol content: In terms of percentage by volume of ethyl alcohol. However, alcohol content need not be mentioned on the label if the total content of the container is 30 ml or less.
- Homeopathic mother tincture: Additional requirements include:
  - "Batch No."/"Batch"/"Lot Number", etc.
  - "Manufacturing License Number"/ "Mfg. Lic. No./, "ML", etc.

The single ingredient homeopathic medicine cannot have proprietary name on its label. Homeopathic medicines containing more than 12%v/v ethyl alcohol cannot be packed and sold in packing or bottles of more than 30 ml unless they are meant for hospitals/ dispensary in packing of not more than 100 ml.

COSMETICS

In the original statute "Drugs Act 1940" cosmetics were not controlled, but later when reports of ill effects of using harmful cosmetics especially skin diseases started appearing, the need of controlling the operation of cosmetics was felt. Consequently the statute was renamed "Drugs and Cosmetics Act" in 1962 with "Drugs Amendment Act 1962". Thus cosmetics were brought under the control of Drugs and Cosmetics Act.

Import of Cosmetics: Though import of cosmetics is regulated under the rules, an import license is not necessary. However, the following provisions are applicable for importation:

1. Cosmetics must be registered with the licensing authority.

2. Consignment of cosmetics sought to be imported must be accompanied by an invoice giving details of name and quantities, name and address of manufacturer.

3. A declaration signed by the importer is to be submitted that the cosmetics are not under prohibited category to the custom collector.

4. Samples of cosmetics can be withdrawn and sent for analysis. If the sample fails the test, import is not permitted.

5. An undertaking or self-declaration that the cosmetics have not been tested on animals.

6. The free sale certificate from the responsible person like National Regulatory Authority or Competent Association or Organization is necessary in addition to certification by manufacturer.

The drugs control officer at the point of entry finds or suspects defects in the cosmetics, he sends the sample to the designated laboratory for performing tests. The consignment of such cosmetics can be detained till the test result report is received. If the importer gives an undertaking not to dispose off the consignment without the consent of the collector of customs, the latter may handover/permit the importer to take away the cosmetics. The importer is required to return the consignment within 10 days of receipt of the notice from the collector of customs.

If the test report confirms the contravention of the Act or Rule, the collector of customs communicates the report forthwith to the importer. The importer is required to either send back the cosmetics to the exporter country or handover them to the central government for destruction within 2 months of receiving communication from the collector of customs.

If the importer makes a representation within 30 days of receipt of test report, the collector of customs may forward the representation with a fresh sample of cosmetics to the Drugs Controller General India (DCGI). The orders of the DCGI would be final. However, he may obtain the report of Central Drugs Laboratory (CDL).

Cosmetics Prohibited to be Imported

- Cosmetics not of standard quality
- Misbranded or spurious cosmetics
- Cosmetics containing mercury compounds
- Cosmetics containing hexachlorophene. Soaps may contain hexachlorophene not exceeding 1% w/w is permitted if appropriately labelled that not meant for babies.
- Cosmetics containing lead or arsenic compounds (used for colouring)
- Cosmetics tested on animals
- Cosmetics intended for use in the area of eye, level of mercury is exceeding seventy parts per million (0.007%) as preservative.
- Other cosmetics containing unintentional mercury exceeding 1 parts per million.
- Any other cosmetic which is prohibited.

The cosmetics imported for manufacture and export by units situated in "special economic zones" are exempted from the provisions of import license, import registration, import through notified ports. These cosmetics are not to be divided for sale in the country. However, such products are permitted for sale in India, if they meet the requirements of standard, procedure for import and registration.

Import for Personal Use

Small quantities of cosmetics which are otherwise prohibited (spurious, misbranded and cosmetics not complied with the standard) can be imported for personal use. The cosmetics should form part of the passenger's baggage and intended for bonafide use of the passenger. This may be declared as directed by the custom authorities.

Import Routes

By Rail: Ferozpur Cantonment and Amritsar Railway Station across the frontier with Pakistan; Ranaghat, Bongaon and Mohiassan Railway Station across the frontier with Bangladesh; Raxual across the frontier with Nepal.

By Road: Raxual across the frontier with Birganj of Nepal.

By Sea: Chennai, Kolkata, Mumbai, Cochin, Nharva sheva and Kandla.

By Air: Chennai, Kolkata, Mumbai, Delhi, Ahmedabad and Hyderabad.

Manufacture: The cosmetics manufacture is permitted under a license from state drugs controller. The original license or renewed license (including loan license) is valid for a period of five years unless sooner suspended or cancelled. The misbranded or adulterated cosmetics (and all other prohibited products like cosmetics containing colours other than prescribed) are prohibited from manufacture. The conditions of the license are:

- Manufacturing is conducted under the direction of a competent technical staff.
- Manufacturing complies with good manufacturing practices (Schedule M-II).
- Records of manufacturing and testing are maintained as specified in Schedule U (1).
- The records are to be maintained for a period of three years.
- Manufacturer should have own testing facility or make arrangement with other laboratories to test raw materials and finished cosmetic products.
- No animal testing is permitted.
- Mercury content should not exceed 70 parts per million where it is used as preservative (products used near eyes) and in other situation it should not exceed 1 part per million.

Competent Technical Staff (Qualification)

- Holds an approved Diploma in Pharmacy; or
- Is a registered pharmacist; or
- Passed the Intermediate Examination with Chemistry as one of the subjects or any other recognized equivalent examination.

The manufacturing under loan license is also permitted and the conditions of the license are similar to license for regular manufacturing.

Packaging and labelling: The outer and inner label should give the: Name of the cosmetics; and name and complete address of manufacturer. The outer label should show:

- The net content [weight for solids and semi-solids, fluid measures for liquids]. This is exempted for a package of perfume, toilet water, etc. when net content does not exceed 60 ml and 30 g for a package of solid or semi-solid.
- Distinctive Batch Number. [Not applicable to cosmetics containing 10 g or less for solids and semi-solids; 25 ml or less if in liquid state.] For soaps, instead of batch number, the month and year of manufacture is recommended.
- Manufacturing License Number.

The inner label should contain instruction for safe use, precautions (or any warning for the consumers) and contents of hazardous chemicals. When the package has only one label, it should contain all relevant information required to be shown on both the inner and outer labels.

Special Instruction Labels

Hair dyes containing dyes, colours and pigments [to be written in English and local language]:

"**Caution:** This product contains ingredients which may cause skin irritation in certain cases and so a preliminary test according to the accompanying direction should first be made. This product should not be used for dyeing the eye-lashes or eye-brows; as such a use may cause blindness".

The package should have instruction in English and local language for carrying out the test.

"This preparation may cause serious inflammation of the skin in some cases and so a preliminary test should always be carried out to determine whether or not special sensitivity exists. To make the test, cleanse a small area of skin behind the ear or upon the inner surface of the forearm, using either soap and water or alcohol. Apply a small quantity of the hair dye as prepared for use to the area and allow it to dry. After twenty-four hours, wash the area gently with soap and water. If no irritation or inflammation is apparent, it may be assumed that no hypersensitivity to the dye exists. The test should, however, be carried out before each and every application. This preparation should on no account be used for dyeing eye-brows or eye-lashes as severe inflammation of the eye or even blindness may result."

Toothpaste Containing Fluorides

- Fluoride content in ppm on the tube and carton. [Fluoride content should not exceed 1000 ppm].
- Date of Expiry both on the tube and carton.

Sale: The sale of cosmetics does not require a license but they should have manufactured under a license if manufactured in India. They are freely sold.

Kerala DC seizes stocks of Fair and Lovely Products [Pharmabiz. Dated May 12, 2012)

The seizure of several products was done after a state wide raid in the premises of wholesaler and stockists. It was alleged that the manufacturer has given misleading claims on the container and outer cartoons. The seized products were produced before the Chief Judicial Magistrate of the respective area.

Fair and Lovely (Ayurvedic Care) was manufactured under a cosmetics licence. The inner tube and outer cartoon of the label indicated that the product contained 'Kumkumadi Tailam", an Ayurvedic pre-paration. This is a case of misbranded cosmetics. [Misbranding—it bears a state-ment which is false or misleading; or not labelled in prescribed manner.

Other products were also seized during the raid.

Standards of Cosmetics

1. The cosmetics must use the dyes, colour and pigments from the specified list of Bureau of Indian Standard (BIS) and Schedule Q. The permitted synthetic organic colours and natural organic colours should not be more than:
   - 2 parts per million of arsenic calculated as arsenic trioxide;
   - 20 parts per million lead.
   - 100 parts per million of heavy metals other than lead calculated as the total respective metals.
2. As specified by BIS and given in Schedule S.
3. Fluoride content in toothpaste should not be more than 1000 ppm.

Delhi Metropolitan Court Convicts Spurious Cosmetics Maker for Rigorous Imprisonment (Pharmabiz, 6/5/10)

Chennai, 5 May: The Delhi Metropolitan Magistrate Vishal Singh, has sentenced a person for one year rigorous imprisonment for manufacturing a cosmetic product secretly in his house without a license. The case was filed in 1987. Besides, the jail term, the punishment involves a fine of ₹ 20,000 or another period of 10 months of simple imprisonment. PK Jaggi, Assistant Drug Controller of Delhi, told this reporter that the person was manufacturing spurious cosmetic item of Fair and Lovely face cream, in his home in Delhi. He said, PK Gupta, drug inspector of the department during his investigation in 1987 had found the illegal activity of the convict and he sought the help of police to conduct a raid of his house. Following the raid, Mohan Lal was apprehended with spurious products. Later the drug inspector Gupta filed the case with the Metropolitan Magistrate court, and the accused was facing trial till date. The accused in the case has been pleading for leniency for his old age and family responsibility. The court has sentenced the convict for a period of one year rigorous imprisonment under Section 27 A (i) of Drugs and Cosmetics Act, 1940. He is further sentenced for a period of six months rigorous imprisonment for the offence under Section 27 A (ii) of the D and C Act. Both the sentences should run concurrently, the court said.

Cosmetics for which BIS has Specified Standards

If the cosmetic is listed in Schedule S of the Act, then it must conform to the relevant quality parameters as prescribed by the relevant product standard issued by Bureau of Indian Standards (BIS). If not, then manufacturers have to comply with their own in-house specifications. Safety and microbiological quality of the cosmetic product are dictated by the relevant BIS standards. The BIS has specified standards for: Skin powders, tooth powder, toothpaste, skin creams, hair oils, soap-based shampoo, detergent-based shampoo, hair creams, liquid oxidation hair dyes, cologne, nail polish (nail enamel), after shave lotion, pomades and brilliantines, depliatories chemical, shaving creams, cosmetic pencils, lipstick, toilet soap, liquid toilet soap, baby toilet soap, shaving soap, transparent toilet soap, lipsalve, powdered hair dye, liquid bindi, kum kum powder, and heena powder. *No standard is specified for quality of gudakhu. Hence penalty prescribed for infringement of standard quality of gudakhu could not be applied.*

MEDICAL DEVICES

It was often commented that there is no control or standard for medical devices but we do have standards for condoms. Of late, government notified 22 items as drugs for regulating under Drugs and Cosmetics Act and the Rules. Schedule M-III was notified as GMP for Medical Devices. In other parts of the world, there has been separate regulations for medical devices which are different from regulations controlling drugs. Finally, the Government has notified the Medical Device Rules on 01st January 2017 to be effective from 01st January 2018. The rules are simplified and less cumbersome compared to rules applicable for drugs. The rules are customized to meet the need of medical devices. The salient point of the rule are mentioned here.

Various Forms Under Medical Devices Rules

Form number	Details
MD – 1	Application for grant of Certificate of Registration of a Notified Body
MD – 2	Certificate of Registration for a Notified Body
MD – 3	Application for Grant of Licence to Manufacture for Sale and Distribution of Class A or Class B Medical Device
MD – 4	Application for Grant of Loan Licence to Manufacture for Sale or for Distribution of Class A or Class B Medical Device
MD – 5	Licence to Manufacture for Sale or for Distribution of Class A or Class B Medical Device
MD – 6	Loan Licence to Manufacture for Sale or for Distribution of Class A or Class B Medical Device
MD – 7	Application for Grant of Licence to Manufacture for Sale or for Distribution of Class C or Class D Medical Device
MD – 8	Application for Grant of Loan Licence to Manufacture for Sale or for Distribution of Class C or Class D Medical Device
MD – 9	Licence to Manufacture for Sale or for Distribution of Class C or Class D Medical Device
MD – 10	Loan Licence to Manufacture for Sale or for Distribution of Class C or Class D Medical Device
MD – 11	Form in which the Audit or Inspection Book shall be maintained
MD – 12	Application for licence to manufacture medical device for purpose of clinical investigations, test, evaluation, examination, demonstration or training
MD – 13	Licence to Manufacture Medical Devices for the Purposes of Clinical Investigations or Test or Evaluation or Demonstration or Training
MD – 14	Application for issue of import licence to import Medical Device
MD – 15	Licence to Import Medical Device

MD – 16	Application for Licence to Import Medical Devices for the Purposes of Clinical Investigations or Test or Evaluation or Demonstration or Training	MD – 29	Permission to Import or Manufacture new *in vitro* diagnostic Medical Device
MD – 17	Licence to Import Medical Devices for the Purposes of Clinical Investigations or Test or Evaluation or Demonstration or Training	MD – 30	Memorandum to the Central Medical Device Testing Laboratory
		MD – 31	Certificate of test or evaluation by the Central Medical Device Testing Laboratory
MD - 18	Application for licence to import investigational medical devices for the purposes by a government hospital or statutory medical institution for the treatment of patients	MD – 32	Report of Test or Evaluation of Medical Devices by Medical Device Testing Officer
MD – 19	Licence to import investigational medical device by a government hospital or statutory medical institution for the treatment of patients	MD – 33	Application from a purchaser for test or evaluation of a Medical Device
		MD – 34	Order requiring a person not to dispose of stock in his possession
MD – 20	Application for permission to import small quantity of medical devices for personal use	MD – 35	Receipt for stock of medical devices for record, register, document or material object seized
MD – 21	Permission to import of small quantity of medical devices for personal use	MD – 36	Intimation of person from whom sample is taken
MD – 22	Application for Grant of permission to conduct clinical investigation of an investigational medical device	MD – 37	Receipt for Sample of medical device(s) taken where fair price tendered thereof is refused
MD – 23	Permission to conduct Clinical Investigation	MD – 38	Memorandum to Medical Device Testing Officer
MD – 24	Application for grant of permission to conduct clinical performance evaluation of new *in vitro* diagnostic Medical Device	MD – 39	Application for grant of registration to Medical Device Testing Laboratory for carry out Test or Evaluation of a medical device on behalf of manufacturer
MD – 25	Permission to conduct clinical performance evaluation of new *in vitro* diagnostic Medical Device	MD – 40	Certificate of registration to Medical Device Testing Laboratory for carry out Test or Evaluation of a medical device on behalf of manufacturer
MD – 26	Application for grant of permission to import/manufacture for sale or for distribution of medical device which does not have predicate medical device		
MD – 27	Permission to import or manufacture for sale or for distribution of medical device which does not have predicate Medical Device		
MD – 28	Application for grant of permission to Import or Manufacture for sale or for distribution of new *in vitro* diagnostic Medical Device		

The rule is applicable for substances used for *in vitro* diagnosis and surgical dressings, surgical bandages, surgical staples, surgical sutures, blood and blood components collection bags; mechanical contraceptives (condoms, intrauterine devices, tubal rings), disinfectants and insecticides.

Classifications: The medical devices are classified into four types: Low risk—class A; low moderate risk—class B; Moderate high risk—class C; and High risk—class D.

Class A medical devices have least regulatory requirements and class C or class D medical

Devices have most regulatory requirements. Unlike other countries, our regulation does not permit the manufacturer of imported to classify their products for registration. The CDSCO classifies in our system.

Standards for medical devices: The medical devices must conform to the standards (in the order given below):

- Laid down by the Bureau of Indian Standards (BIS) or as notified by the Ministry of Health and Family Welfare;
- If no standards laid down as described above, the standards laid down by the International Organization for Standardization (ISO) or the International Electro Technical Commission (IEC) or by any other Pharmacopeial Standards;
- Validated manufacturer's standard.

National Accreditation Body and Notified Body: The National Accreditation Board for Certification Bodies under Quality Council of India, Ministry of Commerce and Industry, acts as National Accreditation Body for the purpose of accrediting Notified Bodies. The Central Government may designate any other institution, firm or organization as National Accreditation Body.

The notified bodies, approved by the National Accreditation Body, are empowered to carry out auditing of manufacturing sites of Class A and Class B medical devices to verify the conformity with Quality Management System and other applicable standards.

The notified bodies need to register with the Central Licensing Authority. For carrying out the auditing of manufacturing sites of class C and class D medical devices, the notified bodies with two years of experience in auditing of class A and class B, need to apply for registration. The registration certificate is valid for five years.

Medical Device Testing Officer: The Government designates a Government Analyst as Medical Device Testing Officer.

Medical Device Officer: The Government designates Drugs Inspector as Medical Device Officer.

Central Medical Device Testing Laboratory: It functions as the Appellate Laboratory in addition to the usual function of testing and evaluation of medical devices. The Central Government may designate a Laboratory, accredited by the National Accreditation Body for Testing and Calibration Laboratories, as Central Medical Device Testing Laboratory.

Manufacturing Licence (for Sale) and Licencing Conditions: Two separate types of licences are given: one for manufacturing (including loan licence) for class A and class B Medical Devices (issued by State Licencing Authority), and the other for class C and class D medical devices (issued by Central Licencing Authority)

Power of Central and State Governments	
Central Government	*State Government*
1. DCGI is the Licencing Authority. But the power of Licencing Authority may be delegated to any officer of CDSCO not below the rank of Assistant Drugs Controller.	1. State Drugs Controller is the licensing Authority. The power of State Licencing Authority may be delegated to a subordinated officer not below the rank of Assistant Drugs Controller.
2. Deals with: • Import of all classes of medical devices; • Manufacture of class C and class D medical devices; • Clinical investigation and approval of investigational medical devices; • Clinical performance evaluation and approval of new *in vitro* diagnostic medical devices; • Coordination with state licencing authorities	2. Deals with: • Manufacture for sale or distribution of class A and class B medical devices; • Sale, stock, exhibit or offer for sale or distribution of medical devices for all classes.

State Licencing Authority issues license when an applicant satisfies the quality management requirement. There is no requirement of site visit or inspection. In a similar way, the Central Licencing Authority issues licence for manufacturing of class C and class D medical devices but there is need of inspecting the manufacturing sites by a team of officers of at least two medical device officers and notified body (if required).

Conditions of Licence

- Conditions prior to grant of licence:
  - Manufacturing facility need to to conform with Quality Management System;
  - Employment of competent technical staff: The staff have one of the following qualifications and experiences:
    - Degree in Engineering in relevant branch/Degree in Pharmacy/Degree in Science in appropriate subject with not less than 2 years experience in manufacturing or testing of medical devices; OR
    - Diploma in Engineering in relevant branch/Diploma in Pharmacy with not less than 4 years of experience in manufacturing or testing of medical devices.
  - Employment of analyst: The competent technical staff having one of the above qualification and having experience of 2 years in testing of medical devices may be appointed for attesting and analysis of medical devices.
- Conditions after issue of licence:
  - Licence is to be produced on demand;
  - "The occurrence of any suspected unexpected serious adverse event and action taken thereof" need to be informed within 15 days of such occurrence;
  - To test or get tested each batch of product for compliance with the standard prior to release;
  - Maintain an audit or inspection book;
  - Maintain at least one batch of each product for reference at least for a period of 180 days after the expiry;
  - Maintain the records of manufacturing and sales;
  - Devices for sale must be accompanied by package insert or insert manual;
  - If manufacturing is closed or suspended for 30 days or more, this should be informed to the Licencing Authority.
- Validity of Licence: 5 years unless suspended or cancelled.

Test Licence to manufacture for test/ evaluation/clinical investigation: Small quantities of all types of devices are permitted with Licence from Central Licencing Authority. The following documents are to be submitted along with application:

- Brief description of the medical device;
- List of equipment, instruments;
- List of qualified personnel;
- Copy of manufacturing licence;
- Approval letter for research or development from any government organization;
- Conditions of licence:
  - Maintain the records of manufacturing;
  - Uses for the purpose only;
  - Allow the Medical Device Officer to inspect.
- Validity of licence: 3 years unless suspended or cancelled.

Import for manufacture or sale: The provision is simplified. There is no need of registration certificate for registration of foreign manufacturer, its manufacturing site and the products. The company needs to appoint an agent in India who would apply for import licence.

The agent with a licence for manufacture or sale may apply to CLA seeking import licence. When the CLA has reason to believe that the quality of medical device is comprised and there is necessity of evaluation, the cost of the evaluation would be borne by the applicant.

If the CLA needs to have the inspection of overseas manufacturing site, the applicant has to pay the cost.

- When the medical device has 'free sale certificate' from the regulatory authority of country: Australia, Canada, Japan, European Countries or USA, Licence would be issued;
- If import is intended from other countries: the licence for class C and class D medical devices would be issued only after establishing their safety and performance though clinical investigation in India;
- If import is intended for class A and class B medical devices, the licence would be issued after establishing the safety and performance through review of published literatures; or through clinical investigation in the country of origin;
- Conditions of Licence:
  - Produce Licence on Demand;
  - Action Take report is to be submitted if there are adverse reports appear like adverse reaction, withdrawal or quality issues;
  - Stop the despatch or marketing immediately, if adverse reports appear;
  - Withdraw from the market if directed;
  - Inform the CLA within 30 days if there is any change in the overseas manufacturer; This prevents the possibilities for two different importers to import different products manufactured at the same manufacturing site.
  - Consignment must be accompanied by in voice or statement;
  - If for sale, it must be accompanied by package inserts or user manual;
  - Recall the product if directed, when the CLA has the reason to believe the product is not in conformity with standard.
- Validity of Licence: 5 years unless suspended or cancelled.

Single Window Clearance: All applications for import, manufacture, sale or distribution and clinical investigation, irrespective of central or state's jurisdiction, have to be made through single on-line portal of Central Government.

Test Licence for Import for Test / Evaluation/ Clinical Investigation: The Central Licencing Authority decides the quantity to be permitted and issues licence on receipt of application with required documents.

Conditions of Licence

- The imported devices should be exclusively used for the purpose for which imported: Test, evaluation or investigation;
- Maintain all activities;
- Consignment is to be accompanied by in voice or statement;
- If imported material not used, is to be exported back or destroyed;
- Validity of the licence is for 3 years.

The small quantity of investigational medical devices, which is usually not allowed to import, is permitted to be imported by the Government Hospital or Statutory Medical Institution for the use of patients suffering from life threatening situation or disease requiring unmedical need. The Central Licencing Authority is the concerned authority for issuing licence for the purpose on application of Medical Officer through Medical Superintendent of the hospital. The hospital has keep record and use them only for the purpose for which import permission given.

Import for Personal Use: The small quantity of medical device, which is usually prohibited, can be imported for personal use under the following conditions:

- It is the part of passenger's personal baggage and meant for personal use;
- It is declared as personal baggage to the customs;
- The quantity does not exceed than what is prescribed;
- It should be accompanied by the invoice or statement.

The Central Licencing Authority grants licence after application.

Shelf Life and Import: The following categories are permitted to import:

- Shelf life is of less than 90 days: Allowed for import if more than 40% residual shelf life at the date of import;
- Shelf life is of more than 90 days but less than a year: Allowed for import if more than 40% residual shelf life at the date of import;
- Shelf life is of more than one year: Allowed for import of more than 60% residual shelf life at the date of import.

Labelling of medical devices: The following particulars need to be printed in indelible ink on the label:

- Name of the medical device;
- Details necessary for the user to identify the device and its use;
- Name of manufacturer and address of manufacturing premises where the device has been manufactured;
- Correct statement about the net quantity in terms of weight, measure, volume, number of units, and the number of the devices contained in the package expressed in metric system;
- Month and year of manufacture and expiry (alternately the label needs to have the shelf life of the product): In case of sterile devices, the date of sterilization may be given as date of manufacture of the device;
- If the device is made up of stable materials such as stainless steel or titanium, and supplied non-sterile or in case of medical equipment or instruments or apparatus, the date of expiry may not be necessary;
- Provide an indication that the device contains medicinal or biological substance;
- Distinctive batch number or lot number preceded by the word "Lot No." or "Lot" or "Batch No." or "B. No.";
- Special storage or handling conditions applicable to the device;

- If the device is supplied as a sterile product, its sterile state and the sterilisation method;
- Warnings or precautions to draw the attention of the user of medical device;
- Label the device appropriately, if the device is intended for single use;
- Overprint on the label of the device, the words "Physician's Sample—not to be sold", if a medical device is intended for distribution to the medical professional as a free sample;
- Manufacturing licence number (if not imported) by preceding the words "Manufacturing Licence Number" or "Mfg. Lic. No." or "M. L";
- In case of imported devices, by way of stickering, printed, the import licence number, name and address of the importer, address of the actual manufacturing premises and the date of manufacture: The label may bear symbols recognised by the Bureau of Indian Standards or International Organisation for Standardisation (ISO).

In addition to the labelling requirement as specified in Medical Device Rules, the requirements specified under Legal Metrology Rules for Pre-packaged Commodities should also be complied. This would be effective from 01 January 2018 unless exempted.

Sale Licence: There is no separate provision for sale of medical devices. The provision related to "sale of drugs other than homeopathic medicines' is applicable for medical device.

AYURVEDIC, SIDDHA AND UNANI (ASU) DRUGS

When the Drugs Act (later amended as Drugs and Cosmetics Act) was first enacted in 1940, the Ayurvedic, Siddha, and Unani systems of medicines were kept out of purview of this legislation. This exemption continued till 1964 when the Act was amended to exercise control over the medicines of these systems through Drugs and Cosmetics (Amendment)

Act 1964. However, the rules for controlling the provision of the Act were laid down in 1970.

The Drugs Act was basically enacted to control the allopathic medicines, the system which was introduced by the British for their benefits. Though ASU medicines were in practice but to a lesser extent and it was believed that such systems do not require any control as they are safe. Everything natural means safe was the understanding. With time, the ASU medicines were patronised and there have been rapid strides in production of such medicines in the commercial sector. It has been felt that unless a quality control discipline is introduced through a central legislation, the consumers or the public are likely to be cheated which may lead to distrust on the public on these proving systems of medicines.

Ayurvedic system of medicines is perhaps one of the ancient systems of medicines and has been in practice for around 3000 years or so. While Ayurvedic system is known to have its origin from Veda (Rig Veda) and practiced by Aryans, the Siddha system is traced back to Dravidian origin. The Unani system of medicine owes its origin to Greek but was introduced into India by Arabs. Though ASU medicines have their origin to the ancient cultures, they do have scientific basis like modern allopathic medicines. The Government of India (GOI) has been taking several measures promoting such heritage with high curative values for the benefit of mankind. One of noticeable step is the creation of Department of AYUSH within the Ministry of Health at the central level. Though central authority in drugs regulation is the DCGI, much coordination with respect to legislation and its control is supervised by the Department of AYUSH.

The provision of the Act and the Rules that controls ASU medicines is very similar to control measures available for allopathic medicines.

Standards of ASU Medicines

The first schedule of Drugs and Cosmetics Act specifies the names of books of Ayurvedic, Siddha and Unani Tibb systems of medicines which are recognised as authoritative books. It lists 54 books in Ayurveda, 30 books in Siddha and 14 books in Unani Tibb system.

- The drugs included in Ayurvedic Pharmacopoeia need to be complied with the standards for identity, purity, and strengths as given in the current edition of Ayurvedic Pharmacopoeia.

- The upper limit of self-generated alcohol in Asavas and Aristar should not exceed 12% v/v.

- Only permitted excipients such as additives, preservatives, antioxidants, colouring agents, flavouring agents, alternate sweeteners with specified standards or grade can be used. Preservatives, alternate sweeteners and colouring agents need to be mentioned on the label of the product.

Import of ASU Medicines

The ASU medicines are indigenous to India and there are very little chances of importing these medicines into this country. At present no specific guideline is available. However, the raw materials for manufacturing of these medicines are imported. But the quality of imported substances is ensured by experts before permitting import.

Export of ASU Medicines

As worldwide there are good demands for these medicines, India exports these medicines in good quantities. The importing country insists on WHO GMP certification (WHO GMP is a misnomer). In order to comply with this requirement, GOI initiated the process of issuing Certificate of Pharmaceutical Products (COPP).

As the heavy metal content of these medicines raised an alarming concern, the government made it mandatory for testing of these medicines for heavy metal content before permitting their export.

The labels and packages or containers of ASU medicines for export need to be in compliance with the requirements of the importing country. But the following particulars must appear:

Amendment Procedure for the Drugs and Cosmetics Act

Being Central Act, the Government of India is only empowered to amend the provision of the Act or Rules. The state governments have no power in this regard.

Drafting a bill giving the specific proposed amendment by the Ministry of Health and Family Welfare

↓

Circulation of bill to other concerned ministries for their comments and agreements

↓

Revision of bill (if required based on suggestions of different ministries) and placing before cabinet

↓

Submitted to President after cabinet's approval seeking permission to introduce the bill in the Parliament

↓

Introduction of the bill either in Lok Sabha or Rajya Sabha by the Union Health Minister

↓

Debate or discussion in both the houses of Parliament and passing in each house

↓

The bill becomes an Act

↓

The Amendment Act comes into force after President's Assent

If a bill needs detailed consideration, it may be referred either of the houses to a joint parliamentary committee (JPC) consisting members of both the houses. The JPC after detailed deliberations on the bill submits reports and revises the bill. The revised bill is then considered by the Parliament. Drugs and Cosmetics (Amendment Bill) 2007 proposed the creation of Central Drugs Authority was rejected by the parliamentary committee.

Amendment to Drugs and Cosmetics Rules

Preparation of draft amendment by DCGI for all drugs other than ASU

(Adviser Department of AYUSH for ASU drugs)

↓

Placing before the respective DTAB for consideration and agreement
(DTAB too can also propose its own amendment)

↓

After approval of DTAB, it is forwarded to the Health Ministry for acceptance

↓

Referred to the Ministry of Law for examination and vetting

↓

Ministry of Health publishes the draft amendment in the Gazette of India for public comments

↓

Considering the comments the ministry revises or finalises the draft amendment

↓

Publication of the final amendment in the Gazette of India

↓

The Amendment is enforced

In emergency situation, the Government of India can publish draft amendments and finalises without consulting DTAB. But DTAB is needed to be consulted within 6 months of Amendment.

a. Name of the Ayurvedic/Siddha/Unani drug (single or compound formulation).
b. The name, address of the manufacturer and the manufacturing license number.
c. Batch or lot number.
d. Date of manufacture including date for "Best for Use Before".
e. Main ingredients (if required by importing country).
f. The products not specified in first Schedule (authoritative books) or Schedule E-(I) (list of poisons in these systems): If the importer does not require the name and address of manufacturer, then the label should bear a code number approved by the Licensing Authority appointed by state government (usually drugs controller for ASU medicines).

Manufacture of ASU Drugs (for sale)

A. Manufacturing is permitted with license only. A separate license is necessary for each manufacturing premise.
B. The licensing authority (LA) is appointed by the state government. The drugs controller of the state for ASU drugs is usually the licensing authority. Application for grant of license with prescribed fees is to be made to the LA and the license is issued within a period of three months subject to compliance with the following requirements:
   a. Manufacturing is carried out following Good Manufacturing Practices (Schedule T).
   b. Manufacturing is conducted under the direction and supervision of a full time competent technical staff possessing one of the following qualifications:
      i. A degree in Ayurveda or Ayurvedic Pharmacy, Siddha or Unani system of medicine.
      ii. Diploma in ASU system.
      iii. Graduate in Pharmacy or Pharmaceutical Chemistry or Chemistry or Botany with at least two years experience in manufacture of Ayurvedic or Siddha or Unani medicine.
      iv. Vaid or Hakim registered in a state register of practitioners of indigenous systems of medicine having experience of at least four years in manufacturing of Siddha or Unani drugs.
      v. Pharmacist in Ayurvedic (including Siddha) or Unani systems of medicines having experience of not less than eight years in the manufacture of Ayurvedic, Siddha or Unani drugs. The competent technical staff must have respective qualification such as qualification in Ayurveda, Siddha or Unani Medicines.
   c. The licensee maintains the records of details of manufacturing and of tests of raw materials and finished products.
   d. The licensee allows the inspection by drugs inspector to manufacturing premises and to inspect finished products.
   e. The licensee maintains an inspection book.
C. The license is valid for three years from the date of issue or renewal. The renewal application is to be submitted before expiry or within one month of expiry. However, if the renewal of application is not made within three months of expiry, the license is treated as expired.

License must for Producers of Chawanprash:

The Supreme Court has held that manufacturer of popular Ayurvedic Health Tonic, Chawanprash, cannot use agriculture produce like "gur, amla and ghee" for its production without proper license obtained from the authority. The top court ruled that though "gur, amla and ghee" are agriculture produce free from any control, but when they are used by manufacturers in Ayurvedic medicines their purchase from the market has to be under license as per provision of Drugs and Cosmetics Act.

Procedure for Cancellation or Suspension of License

• The LA may issue show cause notice giving 15 days time from the receipt or if it is believed that the licensee has failed to comply with the condition of license or provision of the Act and may then cancel or suspend the license.

- The licensee may appeal to the state government against the order of LA within three months of receipt of such order. The decision of the state government is final.

Labelling and Packing

The following particulars should be conspicuously mentioned on the label or the package must have:

I. The true list of all the ingredients used with their quantity. Where the number of ingredients is too large to be accommodated on the label, they need to be printed separately and enclosed with the packing.

II. A reference to the method of preparation.

III. Caution: "To be taken under medical supervision" is to be written in both in English and Hindi if the product is for internal use or contains substances listed as poisons.

IV. Other particulars in inedible ink:
   a. The name of the drug as mentioned in specified authoritative books.
   b. Net content in terms of weight, volume in metric system.
   c. The name and address of the manufacturer.
   d. "The manufacturing License Number" or "Mfg. Lic. No." or "ML".
   e. "Batch No." or "Batch" or "Lot Number" or "Lot No." or "Lot".
   f. The date of manufacture.
   g. "Ayurvedic Medicine" or "Siddha Medicine" or "Unani Medicine" as the case.
   h. "For external use only" if the medicine is for external application.
   i. "Physician's Sample. Not to be sold", if the product is intended for free distribution to the medical profession.

Packing Size and Alcohol Content

- Preparation (Asavas) with high content of alcohol as base: For Kapur Asava, Ahiphenasava, Mrgamadasava, the maximum size of the packing is 15 ml.

- Preparations containing self-generated alcohol:
   - Mritsanjivani Sura: Maximum alcohol content: 16% v/v, maximum size of pack: 30 ml.
   - Mahadrakshava: Maximum alcohol content: 16% v/v, maximum size of pack: 120 ml.

Prohibition from Manufacturing

- Manufacturing is not allowed except in accordance with the standard prescribed in relation to that drug.
- The following are prohibited from manufacturing:
   - Misbranded, adulterated, or spurious ASU drugs.
   - Patent or proprietary medicines if the true list of all ingredients is not displayed on the label.
   - Manufacturing is not in accordance with the conditions of license

This is not applicable to Vaidyas and Hakims who make medicines for their own patients. Similar to allopathic medicines, this provision is not applicable for manufacturing small quantities of any ASU drug for the purpose of examination, test or analysis.

- The central government is empowered to prohibit manufacturing of any ASU drug likely to cause any risk to human beings or animals or does not have therapeutic value claimed.

Like allopathic medicines, there are two Advisory statutory bodies: ASU DTAB, and ASU DCC.

Sale of ASU Medicines: There is no regulation and no license is necessary. But the procured drugs for sale should have been manufactured under a license.

Ayurvedic, Siddha and Unani DTAB: The ASU DTAB constituted by the central government to advise the central government and the state governments on technical matters arising out of administration of the ASU provision of Drugs and the Cosmetics

Act. The ASU DTAB is constituted with the following:

I. Ex Officio Members

i. The Director General of Health Services.

ii. The Drugs Controller General (India).

iii. The Principal Officer in the Ministry of Health dealing with Indian System of Medicine.

iv. The Director of Central Drugs Laboratory.

II. Nominated Members

v. Government Analyst nominated by the central government.

vi. One Pharmacognocist nominated by the central government.

vii. One Phyto-Chemist nominated by the central government.

viii. Two from Ayurvedic Pharmacopoeia Committee, one each from Unani Pharmacopoeia Committee and Siddha Pharmacopoeia Committee nominated by the central government.

ix. One teacher in Dravyaguna, and Bhaishajya Kalpana nominated by the central government.

x. One teacher ILM–UL–ADVIA and TAKLIS–WADAWASAZI nominated by the central government.

xi. One teacher in Gunapadam nominated by the central government.

xii. One person representing each industry (A,S,U) nominated by the central government.

xiii. One person each from among the practitioners of A,S,U nominated by the central government.

The central government appoints a member as Chairman and also appoints a secretary and other staff. The nominated members hold office for three years but are eligible for re-nomination. With the approval of the central government, the Board can make bye-laws fixing a quorum and regulating its own procedure.

The Ayurvedic, Siddha and Unani Drugs Consultative Committee (ASU DCC): The ASU DCC is constituted by the central government to advise the central government, the state governments, and ASU DTAB on any matter for the purpose of securing uniformity of administration throughout India. The DCC is constituted with two nominated members of central government and one nominated member of each state government.

Central Drugs Laboratory for ASU Drugs: The Pharmacopoeial Laboratory of Indian Medicines located at Ghaziabad functions as CDL for ASU drugs. It has the following functions:

- To develop Pharmacopoeial standards and draft monographs and amendments along with standardised methods for ASU drugs;

- To act as Central Appellate Drug Laboratory for testing ASU drugs;

- To analyse or test samples sent by custom authorities or court;

- To maintain reference museum and herbarium for the drugs used in ASU system;

- To run a training centre for quality control methods in ASU systems of medicines;

- To carry out other duties as assigned by the central government.

Procedure for Sending Sample

- Samples for testing should be sent to the Director of Pharmacopoeial Laboratory of Indian Medicines by registered post in sealed packet. The packet should contain the memorandum in Form 1A.

- The packet and the outer cover should be market with a distinguishable number.

- The copy of the memorandum in prescribed form (Form 1A) and the specimen impression used to seal the packet should be separately sent by registered post to the Director.

Procedure for CDL

- On receipt of the packet, authorised officer should open and record the condition of the seal on the packet.

- After test or analysis send the report along with full protocols of the test applied forthwith in Form 2A.
- The certificate or report should be signed by the Director or any Central Government authorised officer.

Government Analyst: The Central Government and the State Governments appoint Government Analysts for the respective areas.

Qualifications

- Qualifications prescribed for Government Analyst for Allopathic Medicines.
- A recognised degree in Ayurveda, Siddha or Unani as required and has not less than three years postgraduate experience in the analysis of drugs under the control of a Government Analyst or Chemical Engineer or Head of the approved institution.

Duties

- To analyse or test samples of ASU drugs sent by Drugs Inspectors, any person or other authorities of the Central or State Government and submit reports.
- To forward the reports of analytical and research work with a view to their publication at the discretion of the Government.

Procedure to send Sample

- The sample for test or analysis should be sent by registered post or by hand in a sealed package along with a memorandum in Form 18 A. The outer cover should address to the Government Analyst.
- The package and the outer cover should be marked with a distinguish number.
- The copy of the memorandum and the specimen impression of the seal used to seal the packet should also be sent by the registered post or by hand.

Procedure for Government Analyst

- On receipt of the package, the Government Analyst or an officer authorised by him will open the package and record the conditions of the seal on the package.

- On completion of test or analysis, three copies of the report is to be sent: One to the sender in Form 13 A, One to the Controlling Authority and One to the DCGI.

State Drug Licensing Authority for ASU Drugs: The State Governments appoint Licensing Authorities for their jurisdiction. The following are the qualifications prescribed for appointment as Licensing Authority:

- Recognised Degree in Ayurvedic/Siddha/Unani Medicines.
- BPharma (Ayurveda) of a recognised university.
- At least five years experience:
    - in the Ayurveda/Siddha/Unani drug manufacturing, or
    - testing of ASU drugs, or
    - enforcement of provisions related to ASU drugs of Drugs and Cosmetics Act, or
    - teaching or research or clinical practice of ASU system.

Drugs Inspector: The Central Government or the State Governments appoint inspectors having prescribed qualification. No person with financial interest in the manufacture or sale of any drug can be appointed. Every inspector is treated as a public servant. The following qualifications are prescribed:

- Qualifications as prescribed for allopathic medicines and has undergone practical training in the manufacture of ASU drugs; or
- Approved Degree in Ayurvedic or Siddha or Unani System of Medicines; or
- Approved Degree in Ayurvedic Pharmacy; or
- Approved Diploma in Ayurveda, Siddha or Unani systems.

Duties of Inspectors: To inspect the manufacture of ASU drugs:

- To inspect at least twice a year all premises licensed to manufacture and to satisfy

Offences and penalties relating to ASU medicines

Offences	Penalties (First offence)	Penalties (Subsequent offences)
Manufacture of adulterated, misbranded drugs or without a valid license	Imprisonment extendable to 1 year with fine not less than 20 thousand rupees or three times the confiscated value, whichever is more.	Imprisonment is extendable up to 2 years and with fine not less than 50 thousand rupees or three times the confiscated value, whichever is more.
Manufacture of spurious drugs	Imprisonment of not less than 1 year but extendable up to 3 years and with fine not less than 50 thousand rupees or three times the confiscated value, whichever is more.	Imprisonment of not less than 2 years extendable up to 6 years and with fine not less than 100 thousand rupees or three times the confiscated value, whichever is more.
Manufacture of prohibited drugs	Imprisonment which is extendable to 3 years and with fine of 50 thousand rupees or three times the confiscated value, whichever is more.	
Contravention to any other provision	Imprisonment extendable to 6 months and with fine not less than 10 thousand rupees.	Imprisonment extendable to 1 year and with fine not less than 20 thousand rupees or three times the confiscated value, whichever is more.
Penalty for vexatious search or seizure	Fine extendable to 1 thousand rupees.	

The trial of offences can be done at a court inferior to that of Metropolitan Magistrate or First Class Judicial Magistrate. The Central Government or State Governments may designate special Session Court(s) as Special Courts to try offences relating to adulterated and spurious drugs. The Court may, on the application of drugs inspector, direct the details of the offender like name, place of residence, offences, and penalties imposed to be published on conviction. This can be done at the expense of such convicted person and published in newspapers.

Validity Periods of Various Licences (unless suspended or cancelled)

Licence/Approval	Validity period
Import Licence	3 Years
Registration Certificate for Import	3 Years
Manufacturing/Loan Licence	No limit of validity if continuing retail fees for every five years.
Sale Licence	No limit of validity if continuing retail fees for every five years.
Registration of Ethics Committee	3 Years
Operation of Blood Bank	5 Years
For carrying out testing of cosmetics on behalf of licensee for manufacturing	5 Years
For carrying out testing of ASU medicines on behalf of licensee for manufacturing	3 Years
Certificate of GMP for ASU medicine	5 Years

himself/herself that the conditions of the license are observed.
- To send the report of inspection forthwith to the controlling authority indicating whether or not the conditions of license are observed.

- To take samples and send them for test or analysis.

- To institute prosecutions in respect of violations of the provisions of Act and the Rules.

ISM Wing of Kerala to order Stop Production of Musli Power Xtra for Violation of D and C Rules, (Pharmabiz, Dated 29 October 2009)

Chennai, 29 Oct: The ISM Wing of Directorate of Drug Control of Kerala will be issuing an order to stop manufacturing and marketing of Musli Power Xtra by Kunnath Pharmaceuticals in Ernakulam for violation of provisions under the Drugs and Cosmetics Rules for the last few years. The proposed action follows an inspection of the company's factory at Moovattupuzha last week. The ISM Wing is also processing action against the company as per the norms of Drugs and Magic Remedies (objectionable advertisement) Act, 1955, it is learnt. The ISM action is subsequent to complaints received from public including leading Ayurvedic doctors against the company alleging manufacture and sale of spurious drugs. Following the inspection of the factory, the Company has been given an oral stop production order The drug inspector said that Kunnath Pharmaceuticals was manufacturing and marketing the product, Musli Power Xtra, claimed to treat infertility in both men and women throughout India and outside by giving wide publicity. The product was said to be formulated from Safed Musli (Chlorophytum Borivilianum) known as Indian herbal aphrodisiac. The company was charging ₹ 750 for a bottle containing 30 capsules and ₹ 1500 for a bottle of 60 capsules. He said the company had claimed that a capsule a day could boost the fertility among people. According to the drug inspector, the approval for the production of Musli Power Xtra was given for a formulation in which the main ingredient indicated was the seed of 'Nilappana' (Curculigo orchioides). But the company was producing the drug with Safed Musli for which no license was given to the company as it was not contained in the Indian pharmacopoeia at the time of issuing the license. He said that as per Section 33 EE A (d) of D & C Act, any drug which has been substituted wholly or in part by any other drug or substance could come under the provisions of Spurious Drugs Act. The Drugs and Magic Remedies (objectionable advertisement) Act clearly specifies the prohibition of advertisement for certain drugs, especially in the category of drugs described as aphrodisiac. The inspector said that the state drug authorities had warned the company not to advertise or put on label the term 'aphrodisiac' directly or indirectly with any other word or phrase to attract people. But the company has been giving extensive publicity for the product substantiating its power in increasing the potency of men and women. The official said that on inspection of the Batch Manufacturing Record (BMR) at the factory it was found that the company's use of Safed Musli for the production of the drug was a digression of what is given in the formula approved by the department. They were buying the extracts of the Safed Musli from Elixir Extracts Pvt Ltd, Moovattupuzha. He said the punishment for this violation involves three years imprisonment and a fine of ₹ 50,000. When contacted, Dr K C Abraham, managing director of Kunnath Pharmaceuticals, said that there is no need of separate license for manufacturing ayur-vedic drugs and he got the license from the authorities years before. Dr John also said that the managing director of the company is neither a qualified person nor has any degree in any discipline. (Later two cases were filed by the drugs control department).

GMP Certificate Issue

The GMP (Schedule M) compliance is mandatory for manufacturing license. But there is no provision or procedure to issue the GMP certificate to the companies following or complying with GMP under Drugs and Cosmetics Rules. This has been clarified by the Central Public Information Officer of CDSCO in response to a Right to Information (RTI) application. It is also clarified that Drug Manufacturing Unit with a valid license is considered as GMP compliant Unit.

(*Source:* Pharmabiz dated 20 August 2010)

On the other hand, there is specific provision under the Rules to issue GMP for Ayurvedic, Siddha and Unani Drugs. This certificate can be issued to licensees who comply with the requirements of GMP as laid down in Schedule T.

(*Source:* Under Section 155 B of Drugs and Cosmetics Rules 1945)

DCGI slaps show cause notice on GSK for Running HPV ad in Media (Pharmabiz Date (24/12/09)

Mumbai, 24 Dec: The Drug Controller General of India (DCGI) has eventually issued a show cause notice to the Glaxo SmithKline (GSK) for launching an advertisement campaign in the national media on cervical cancer vaccine without taking prior approval from his office. In the show cause notice, the DCGI has asked GSK to explain within 10 days the reasons for such an ad in the media, failing which the DCGI will proceed to take action against company. DCGI sources said that the action includes withdrawal of licenses issued to the GSK's cervical cancer vaccine Cervarix, which the company had launched in the Indian market recently. The DCGI notice to the GSK said that the company has violated Rule 106, Schedule J of the Drugs and Cosmetics Act, 1940 under which the drug company cannot advertise any drugs. For launching the advertisements, the companies need to take prior permission from the DCGI and in the GSK's case, no such permission was given by the DCGI.

(*Source:* Pharmabiz)

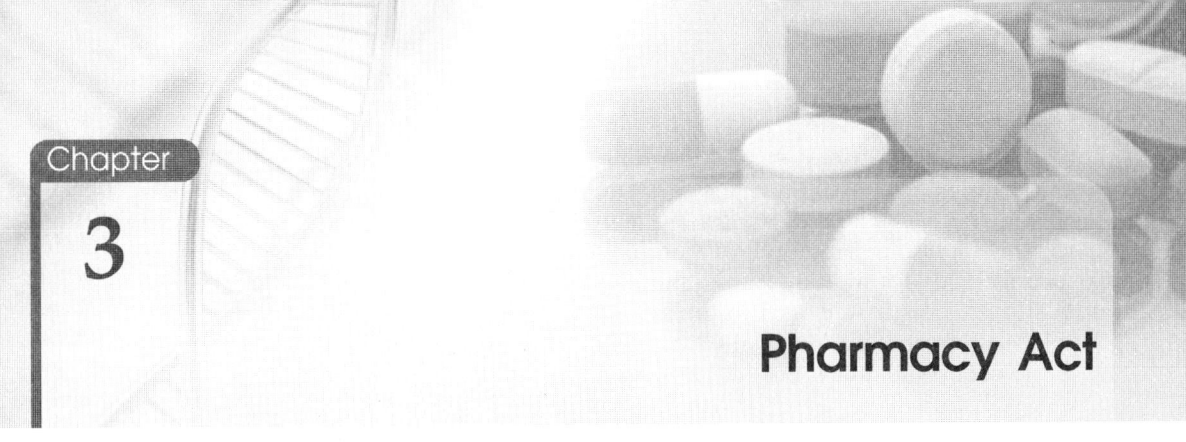

Pharmacy Act

"No man ever reached to excellence in any one art or profession without having passed through the slow and painful process of study and preparation."

— *Horace*

After reading this chapter, you should be able to understand and appreciate:
- Need and mechanism available for regulating the pharmacy profession
- Constitution and functions of Pharmacy Council of India and State Pharmacy Council
- Education regulation
- Minimum qualification for teachers in pharmacy institutions regulation
- Pharmacy practice regulation
- Registration of pharmacists
- Administrative procedure for implementing the Act.

There was no restriction on the practice of profession of pharmacy in pre-independent British India, anybody could enter into the profession even without having any education or knowledge on the subject of pharmacy or related discipline. The dispensing and compounding was practiced by such persons having no adequate training and such practice was causing great harm to the health systems and the public. On the other hand, in other countries there was legislation which was controlling the practice of profession of pharmacy through prescribing minimum standard of education for practicing the profession.

With these backgrounds, the Government of India thought of bringing a change to control the profession of pharmacy and the Pharmacy Bill 1947 was introduced in the legislature and the bill was passed with modification suggested by Select Committee and received assent on 4th March 1948. This is the Pharmacy Act 1948 and it has undergone several amendments with time.

The main objective of Pharmacy Act is to make better provision for the education and practice of pharmacy through constitution of pharmacy councils. The Act extends to the whole of India except the state of Jammu and Kashmir. Though the Act came into force immediately, certain provisions relating to state pharmacy council, registration of pharmacists, and miscellaneous provision were made operative at different times as the state governments notified. These provisions were even operative partially in some areas of states as there was territorial changes occurred due to reorganization of states on 1st November 1956.

The National Council for Human Resource in Health (NCHRH): NCHRH is proposed to be established by the health ministry as an overarching regulatory authority in the country to reform the current regulatory framework in medical education and enhance the supply of skilled personnel to the healthcare sector in the country. Once in place, the NCHRH will be the overarching regulatory body for all the premier medical educational institutions and autonomous regulatory bodies like Medical Council of India (MCI), Pharmacy Council of India (PCI), Nursing Council of India (NCI), Dental Council of India (DCI) and the proposed Central Councils for Paramedical and Allied Medical Sciences Education.

It will prescribe standards with a view to have proper planning and coordinated development of medical and allied health education throughout the country and maintain national live electronic register of medical and allied health professionals.

As per the draft bill, the administration of the Council will consist of a Secretariat headed by a Secretary-General who will be appointed by the Council for a fixed term of three years. Under this secretariat, seven departments, each for separate categories like Medicine, Pharmacy, Nursing, Dentistry, Rehabilitation and Physiotherapy, Public Health and Hospital Management and Allied Health Sciences, will be established and headed by a director for regulatory purposes.

In every state, there will be separate bodies constituted by the Council for each administrative department which will be known as Registration and Ethics Board with name of the state in front and the department's name in the end. These bodies will replace the existing State Councils. These boards have to maintain a live electronic register of professionals in the state of the respective Department to be known as 'State Register of (name of the Department) and which will be linked to the National Register of Human Resources in Health maintained by the Council. Each Board will comprise a president, a vice-president and not less than 10 members out of which three will be women candidates. There will be a nominee of the state government also.

The Pharmacy Council of India has brought all levels of Pharmaceutical Education under its umbrella. All levels Pharmacy Education (Diploma, Degree, Pharm.D. and Master programmes) are also with AICTE control. It is almost certain that the dual control (PCI and AICTE) is likely to continue at least for sometimes even though it appears to have some common understanding between the two bodies. Even the proposal of merging two bodies: AICTE and University Grants Commission is under active consideration of Government of India. The pharmacy practice regulation is also notified. The council has also specified the minimum qualification of teachers for pharmacy institutions. Earlier, teachers' qualification was specified for Diploma in Pharmacy and Doctor of Pharmacy in their respective regulation. The University Grants Commission too specified the qualification for pharmacy teachers along with VI pay revision. The AICTE has too specified the qualification requirement for pharmacy teachers.

Composition and Constitution of Central Council (Pharmacy Council of India)

The central government constitutes the Central Council called Pharmacy Council of India with the following members:

1. Six members elected by University Grants Commission (UGC) of Indian University or affiliated colleges granting degree or diploma in pharmacy. Out of these members, there shall be at least one teacher of each of the subjects: pharmaceutical chemistry, pharmacy, pharmacology and pharmacognosy.

2. Six members nominated by the central government of whom at least four should possess degree or diploma in pharmacy and practicing pharmacy or pharmaceutical chemistry.

3. One member elected from among themselves by the members of Medical Council of India.

4. Director General Health Services: Ex-officio. If he is unable to attend, a person authorized by him in writing may attend the meeting.

5. Drugs Controller, India: Ex-officio. If he is unable to attend, a person authorized by him in writing may attend the meeting.

6. Director of Central Drugs Laboratory: Ex-Officio.
7. A Representative of University Grants Commission.
8. A representative of All India Council for Technical Education (AICTE).
9. A registered pharmacist representative of state pharmacy council who is elected among the members of state pharmacy council.
10. A registered pharmacist representative of each state nominated by the state government.

Earlier there was provision for having a nominated member (not elected) from each union territory government from among the persons eligible for registration.

The first Pharmacy Council of India was constituted under the Act on 9th March 1949 with Dr KC KE Raja as First President nominated by Government of India. The Golden Jubilee year was celebrated in 1999 throughout the country. The Council has also celebrated 60th Anniversary Celebration in which Her Excellency the then President of India Srimati Pratibha Devisingh Patil graced on 9th July 2010. Dr. B. Suresh, Vice Chancellor of JSS University, Mysore, is the President currently (2017). He has been the president for three successive terms. He is perhaps the most dynamic President so far the Council had and is successful in bringing many innovative reforms in Pharmaceutical Education and Profession.

The Pharmacy Council of India (PCI) is a corporate body having perpetual succession and a common seal with a power to acquire and hold movable and immovable property.

The composition of PCI as on 24th April 2017 (http://www.pci.nic.in/CouncilMembers/CentralCouncil.aspx accessed on 24 April 2017)

Nomination by University Grants Commission

1. **Prof Lakshmi Kanta Ghosh**
   Department of Pharmaceutical Technology
   Jadavpur University, Kolkata

2. **Prof Shivajirao Kadam**
   Vice-Chancellor, Bharati Vidyapeeth
   University Lal Bahadur Shastri Marg
   Pune - 411 030 (Maharashtra)

3. **Prof Karan Vashisht**
   Department of Pharmacognosy CAS,
   University Institute of Pharmaceutical Sciences
   Punjab University Chandigarh

4. **Prof B Suresh**
   Vice-Chancellor, JSS University, JSS Medical Institutions Campus, Sri Shivarathresshwara Nagara
   Mysore - 570 015 (Karnataka)

5. **Prof MD Karvekar**
   1449, Sector 7, 4th Main 21st Cross
   HSR Lay Out
   Bangalore - 560 1026.

6. **Dr BP Srinivasan**
   (Ex-Director) Delhi Institute of Pharmaceutical Science & Research
   C-1533 Green Field Colony
   Faridabad - 121 003 (Haryana)

Nominated by the Central Government

1. **Shri Ashwani Khajuria, S/o Shri Shyam Lal Khajuria** Vinayaka Mission Research Foundation, H. No. 146, Ward No.1, Near Sports Stadium Udhampur (Jammu and and kashmir)

2. **Shri Raj Kumar Chauhan, S/o Shri Zile Singh Chauhan** Pharmacist CGHS Wellness Centre Kali Bari
   New Delhi - 110013.

   Prof V Ravichandran
   Director
   National Institute of Pharmaceutical Education and Research, NIPER-Kolkata at Indian Institute of Chemical Biology, No 4, Raja SC Mullick Road, Jadavpur
   Kolkata - 700032 (West Bengal)

Elected by Medical Council of India

Dr Bharat Agrawal
Shop No. 125, Third Floor, Dawabazar, RNT Marg, Indore, Madhya Pradesh

Ex-Officio Members

1. Director General of Health Services, Nirman Bhawan
   New Delhi - 110 011

2. Drugs Controller General (India), FDA Bhawan, Kotla Road
   New Delhi - 110 002

(Contd...)

(Contd...)

3. Director, Central Drugs Laboratory, 3 Kyd. Street Kolkata - 700 016 (West Bengal)

Representative of UGC

Prof OP Kalra
Principal
University College of Medical Sciences
(University of Delhi) and Guru Teg Bahadur
Hospital Dilshad Garden
Delhi - 110 095

Representative of AICTE

Dr NR Sheth
Professor, Department of Pharmaceutical
Sciences, Saurashtra University,
Saurashtra University Campus,
Saurashtra University, Saurashtra
Rajkot - 360 005 (Gujarat)

Elected by State Pharmacy Council

1. **Andhra Pradesh**
Shri M Venkata Reddy
503, Venkateswara Arcade, Plot 178,
Near Indian Overseas Bank Moti Nagar
Hyderabad - 500 018 (Andhra Pradesh)

2. **Arunachal Pradesh**
Shri Gebomb Tayeng Assistant Drugs
Controller Directorate of Health Services
Naharlagun
Arunachal Pradesh

3. **Assam**
Sri Nabin Ch. Baruah
Lecturer
Institute of Pharmacy Assam Medical College
Dibrugarh - 786 002 (Assam)

4. **Bihar**
Vacant

5. **Chhattisgarh**
Sri Ajay Singh Rajput
C/o Ajay Medical Durg Road Kohka Chowk,
Kohka, Bhilai District: Durg (Chhattisgarh)

6. **Goa**
Sri Santosh P. Fondekar
B-S-2, Sabnis Monarch
Caranzalem - 403 002, (Goa)

7. **Gujarat**
Shri Chhaganbhai Nanjibhai Patel
Professor and Principal
Department of Pharmaceutical Chemistry
Shri Sarvajanik Pharmacy College
Mehsana - 384 001 (Gujarat)

8. **Haryana**
Mr Ved Prakash # 770, Sector-1, Narnaul
Dist: Mahendergarh (Haryana)

9. **Himachal Pradesh**
Sri Sanjeev Pandit President, HP Chemist
and Druggist Association
Prop. of M/S Pacific Chemists
63, The Mall Shimla - 171 001

10. **Karnataka**
Shri MS Nagaraj No. 387
10th Cross, 2nd Phase, 1st Stage,
Manjunathanagar,
Bangalore - 560 010 (Karnataka)

11. **Kerala**
Sri B Rajan TC 18/2043(9)ABRA 343 A,
Annoor Thirumala
PO Thiruvananthapuram - 695006

12. **Maharashtra**
Shri JS Shinde
Shinde Bldg. Maratha Kolsewadi
Narveeer Tanaji Chowk
Kalyan (E) - 421304

13. **Manipur**
Shri Sougrakpam Lokendrajit Singh
Office of The Chief Medical Officer Senapati
District, Senapati
Manipur - 795106

14. **Meghalaya**
Shri Antony Laloo
Directorate of Health Services (MI)
Health Complex,
Red Hill Laitumkhrah Shillong, Meghalaya

15. **Mizoram**
Dr H Lalhlenmawia
Deptt. of Pharmacy
Regional Institute of Paramedical and
Nursing Sciences
Zemabawk - 796 001

16. **Nagaland**
Sri Khele Thorie Quality Manager
Nagaland State AIDS Control Society
Directorate of Health and Family Welfare,
Ruziezou
Kohima - 797 001
(Nagaland)

17. **Odisha**
Shri Deba Prasad Pati
At: Tanarapa Sason PO: Barabati
Dist: Cuttack - 754100, Odisha

(Contd...)

(Contd...)

18. **Punjab**
Sh. Harbans Singh
H. No. 190, Anand
Nagar - A, Gurudwara Street,
Patiala Punjab

19. **Rajasthan**
Sri Ajay Phatak
I/160, SFS Agarwal Farm Mansarovar
Jaipur - 302 020 (Rajasthan)

20. **Tamil Nadu**
Prof B Jayakar
Head
Vinayaka Missions's College of Pharmacy
Kondappanaickanpatty
Salem - 636 008
(Tamil Nadu)

21. **Tripura**
Shri Bimal Kanti Chakraborty
Ramnagar Road No. 5
P. O.: Ramnagar
Agartala
Tripura - 799002

22. **Uttar Pradesh**
Sri SN Srivastava Gauri Dutta
Dharamshala Road,
Near Chitragupta Mandir, Gandhinagar,
Basti - 272 001 (UP)

23. **Uttarakhand**
Mr Virendra Singh Panwar
Pharmacist District Hospital, Pauri
Distt. Pauri Garhwal
(Uttarakhand)

24. **West Bengal**
Dr R Debnath
6F Shubham Plaza 83/1 Beliaghata Main Road
Kolkata - 700 010
(West Bengal)

25. **Delhi**
Sri Inder Singh Chauhan
D-1, West Jyoti Nagar,
Gali No. 9, Loni Road, Shahdara
Delhi - 110 094

26. **Pondicherry**
Sri VM Mounnissamy
Reader in Pharmacy
College of Pharmacy
Mother Theresa Post-Graduate and Research
Institute of Health Sciences (MTPG & RIHS)
Gorimedu, Indira Nagar
Puducherry - 605006

Nominated by State Governments

1. **Andhra Pradesh**
Shri PV Appaji
Director General Pharmaceutical Export
Promotion Council of India
101, Aditya Trade Centre, Ameerpet,
Hyderabad - 500 038
(Andhra Pradesh)

2. **Arunachal Pradesh**
Mrs. Banu Otem Dai Senior Lecturer
Deptt. of Herbal Remedies and Cosmetology
Rajiv Gandhi Polytechnic
Itanagar Arunachal Pradesh

3. **Assam**
Mrs S Das
Head
Institute of Pharmacy Gauhati Medical College
Guwahati (Assam)

4. **Bihar**
Sri Kumar Ajay
Lecturer
Govt. Pharmacy Institute
Agamkuan
Patna - 800 007 (Bihar)

5. **Chhattisgarh**
Dr Shailendra Saraf
Professor and Director,
Dean, Faculty of Technology
Institute of Pharmacy
Pt. Ravishankar Shukla University
Raipur - 492 010 (Chhattisgarh)

6. **Goa**
Shri Salim A. Veljee
Deputy Director
Directorate of Food and Drugs Admns
Old IPHB Building, Altinho,
Panaji - 403001 (Goa)

7. **Gujarat**
Sri HG Koshia
Commissioner
Office of the Commissioner
Food and Drugs Control Administration,
Gujarat State, Block No. 8,
1st Floor
Dr. Jivraj Mehta
Bhawan, Gandhinagar - 382010

8. **Haryana**
Shri Gurcharan Singh S/o Shri Joginder
Singh H. No. 4, Sector-8, Part-II
Karnal (Haryana)

(Contd...)

(Contd...)

9. **Himachal Pradesh**
   Sri Navneet Marwaha
   Licensing Authority
   HP Office of the Assistant Drug Controller
   Sai Road Baddi, Tehsil Nalagarh
   Dist - Solan

10. **Jharkhand**
    Sri Awdhesh Oraon
    Lecturer
    Govt. Pharmacy Institute
    Bariatu, Ranchi - 9 (Jharkhand)

11. **Karnataka**
    Dr FV Manvi
    No. 34, "Santrupti",
    Jadhav Nagar
    TV Centre Road
    Belgaum - 590001 (Karnataka)

12. **Kerala**
    Dr MK Unnikrishna Panicker
    Anaswara
    TC16/502 (10, EVRA - 71)
    Jagathy
    Thiruvananthapuram
    Kerala - 695 014

13. **Madhya Pradesh**
    Shri Neeraj Upmanyu
    Professor and Principal School of Pharmacy
    and Research
    People's University
    Bhanpur Bypass Road
    Bhopal - 462037 (Madhya Pradesh)

14. **Manipur**
    Sri N. Rimot Kumar Meetai Wangkhei
    Khunou
    Soibam Leikai
    Imphal East
    Manipur - 795005

15. **Maharashtra**
    Shri Vijay Pandurang Patil
    President
    Maharashtra State Pharmacy Council ES IS
    Hospital Compound
    Lal Bahadur Shastri Marg
    Mulund (W)
    Mumbai - 400080

16. **Meghalaya**
    Shri Devistone Swer
    Assistant Drugs Controller
    Licensing and Controlling Authority Health
    Complex

Directorate of Health Services (MI)
Red Hill Road,
Laitumkhrah,
Shillong - 793003

17. **Mizoram**
    Sri Pu Lalsawma
    Asstt. Drugs Controller Directorate of Health
    Services
    Mizoram

18. **Nagaland**
    Sri S. Lithungo Lotha, Addl. Asstt. Drugs
    Controller, Directorate of Health & Family
    Welfare
    Kohima Nagaland

19. **Odisha**
    Shri Annada Sankar Das
    661, Tankapani Road
    Bhubaneshwar - 751014
    (Odisha)

20. **Punjab**
    Shri Jagjot Singh
    S/o S. Harcharan Singh
    M/s Bahia Medical Store
    VPO-Nathana
    Dist: Bathinda (Punjab)

21. **Rajasthan**
    Mr Naveen Sanghi
    D-115, Siwad Area
    Mangal Marg, Bapu Nagar
    Jaipur - 302015 (Rajasthan)

22. **Tamil Nadu**
    Dr. N. Narayanan
    Plot 22, 3rd Street, (Near Vodafone Tower)
    Kuberan Nagar Extn., Madipakkam
    Chennai - 600091

23. **Tripura**
    Sri Soumen Paul Majumder
    Deputy Drugs Controller I/C, Government of
    Tripura
    Agartala (Tripura)

24. **Uttar Pradesh**
    Sri Uttam Chandra Mishra
    S/o Sh. Rameshwar Prasad
    Malhotra Nivas, City Montessari Inter
    College
    Opp. Lucknow Chowk, Hardoi Road,
    Lucknow
    (Uttar Pradesh)

(Contd...)

25. **Uttarakhand**
Dr Preeti Kothiyal, (Formerly Professor,
Faculty of Pharmacy. DIT, Dehradun)
Presently Principal, Division of
Pharmaceutical Sciences
Sri Guru Ram Rai Institute of Technologyand
Sciences Patel Nagar,
Dehradun (Uttarakhand)

26. **West Bengal**
Dr Amalendu Basu
Additional Director of Technical Education
Bikash Bhawan
Salt Lake
Kolkata - 700149 (West Bengal)

27. **Andaman and Nicobar**
Ms. M. Chandrika
Chief Pharmacist, and G.B. Pant Hospital
Portblair - 744104 (A and N)

28. **Chandigarh**
Sri Sunil Kumar Chaudhary
Drugs Control Officer
Chandigarh Administration
Govt. Multi Specialty Hospital
Sector - 16
Chandigarh - 160016

29. **Dadra and Nagar Haveli**
Shri Ramanga Lingeshware Rao
Pharmacist Administration of Dadra and
Nagar Haveli
UT Office of the Medical Superintendent
Shri Vinoba Bhave Civil Hospital
Dadra and Nagar Haveli
Silvassa

30. **Delhi**
Shri Atul Kumar Nasa
Assistant Drugs Controller
Drugs Control Department
Govt. of NCT of Delhi, F-17, Karkardooma
New Delhi - 110 032

31. **Lakshadweep**
Sri CM Mohammed
Store Superintendent, Medical Dte.,
Lakshadweep,
Kavaratti - 673555

32. **Puducherry**
Dr V Gopal
Professor and HOD, College of Pharmacy,
Mother Theresa Post Graduateand Research
Institute of Health Sciences (MTPG & RIHS
Gorimedu, Indira Nagar
Puducherry - 605006

33. **Daman and Diu**
Shri Dharmesh N. Agrawal
Drugs Inspector, Fort Area
Primary Health Centre
Moti Daman - 396220 (UT)

President and Vice President of PCI

The President and Vice President are elected
by the members of the council from among
themselves. They can hold office for a period
not exceeding five years and not extending
beyond the expiry of membership of the
council. However, being members of the
council, they are eligible for re-election. In
case, the term of office (as member) expires
before the expiry of the full term for which he
is elected as president or vice president, he
can continue to hold office if he regains the
membership either by election or nomination.

The nominated and elected members hold
office for a term of five years from the date of
nomination or election or until his successor
has been duly nominated or elected, whichever is longer. The nominated or elected
member has the liberty to resign the membership by writing to the president. The seat of
such member is treated as vacant.

If the elected or nominated member absents
without excuse from three consecutive meeting
of the council, then it is treated as if he has vacated
his seat. Similarly if the member is elected under
UGC from among the teachers, Medical Council
of India from among its members, State
Pharmacy Council from among the registered
pharmacists, and if he ceases to become the
member of these organizations, then his seat
is also treated as vacant. The casual vacancy
in the central council can be filled by fresh
nomination or election and such members can
hold office only for the remaining period of
the term against whom he is nominated or
elected. The members of the central council
are eligible for re-nomination or re-election.

Staff

The central council has a registrar (appointed)
who acts as secretary too to the council. The
council has power to appoint other officers
and servants as necessary to carry out its

function. With previous sanction of the central government the council can fix the rate of remuneration and allowances to be paid to the President, Vice President, and other members of the council; the pay and allowances and other conditions of services of officers and servants of the council.

Executive and Other Committees

The central council has provision of an Executive Committee consisting of the President and Vice President and five other members elected by the central council from among its members. The president of the council is the chairman of the executive committee. A member of the executive committee holds office until the expiry of the term as member of the council. He is eligible for re-election. The central council has provision to constitute other committees too for general or other purposes for a period not exceeding five years. It may co-opt persons as members of such committee who are not the members of central council.

Composition of Executive Committee of Pharmacy Council of India as on 24 April 2017 (http://www.pci.nic.in/CouncilMembers/Executive Committee.aspx accessed on 24 April 2017)

President	**Prof B Suresh** Vice-Chancellor, JSS University Sri Shivarathresshwara Nagar Mysore - 570 015 (Karnataka)
Vice President	**Dr Shailendra Saraf** Professor and Director Dean, Faculty of Technology Institute of Pharmacy Pt. Ravishankar Shukla University Raipur - 492010 (Chhattisgarh)
Members	**1. Prof MD Karvekar** # 1449, Sector 7, 4th Main 21st Cross, H.S.R. Lay Out Bangalore - 560102 (Karnataka) **2. Prof B Jayakar** Head Vinayaka Missions's College of Pharmacy Kondappanaickanpatty Salem - 636 008 (Tamil Nadu)

(Contd...)

(Contd...)

3. Sri HG Koshia
Commissioner
Office of the Commissioner,
Food & Drugs Control
Administration, Â
Gujarat State
Block No. 8, 1st Floor
Dr. Jivraj Mehta Bhawan
Gandhinagar - 382010 (Gujarat)

4. Sri Ajay Phatak
I/160, SFS Agarwal Farm
Mansarovar
Jaipur - 302020 (Rajasthan)

5. Sri Inder Singh Chauhan
D-1, West Jyoti Nagar
Gali No. 9
Loni Road
Shahdara Delhi - 110094

Education Regulation (ER)

Subject to the approval of the central government, the central council frames regulations prescribing the minimum standard of education required for qualification as a pharmacist. The education regulation may prescribe:

a. The nature and period of study and practical training to be undertaken before admission to an examination;

b. The equipment and facilities to be provided for students undergoing approved courses of study;

c. The subjects of examination and the standards therein to be attained;

d Any other conditions for admissions.

The central council is required to submit copies of the draft of the proposed education regulation to all state Governments inviting comments. The comments of the state governments received within three months of submission of draft should be taken into consideration before submitting the education regulation or amendments to the central government. The Education Regulation is required to be published in the official gazette. The executive committee reports to the central council on the efficacy of ER and recommend amendments as necessary.

The ER becomes operative once the state government notifies in the official gazette at any time after constitution and consultation with the state council. However, if no declaration is made, the ER becomes effective in the state on the expiry of three years from the date of constitution of the state council.

Currently the following regulations are framed under Education Regulation:

1. *Education regulation 1991*: This Governs the Diploma in Pharmacy Programme. Diploma in Pharmacy is a two-year Programme.

2. *Pharm D Regulation 2008*: This governs the Doctor of Pharmacy Programme. The PharmD Programme is of six years duration and PharmD (Post Baccalaureate) is of 3 years duration.

3. *Bachelor of Pharmacy (Practice) Regulation 2014*: This governs the two years programme for Diploma in Pharmacy qualified working pharmacists.

4. *The Bachelor of Pharmacy Course Regulation, 2014*: This governs the four years [Eight Semesters] B. Pharm. Programme.

5. *The Master of Pharmacy Course Regulation, 2014*: This governs the two years [Four Semesters] M. Pharm. Programme.

6. *Minimum Qualification for Teachers in Pharmacy Institutions Regulation 2014*: This provides the details of qualification and experience required for teachers at different levels of pharmacy programmes.

Qualification of Teachers

The regulation specifies the qualification of teachers of various programmes at different levels. The present text does not intend to give full details but intends to give the entry level qualification. For full details, the readers can refer the regulation.

In addition to the qualification specified in the Table, the teacher is required to be the registered pharmacist. Only pharmacy teachers' qualification is mentioned. Non-pharmacy qualified teachers are not included in the Table.

Pharmacy Practice Regulation

The Pharmacy Practice Regulations, 2015, is gazetted on 15th January 2015 giving a legal status to the various activities of professional pharmacists. Though the Indian pharmacists have been providing a lot of services, their services are not recognized as professional services. The pharmacists are just termed either as seller or supplier of medicines. The present regulation would open up new avenues for the pharmacists to provide services like patient counselling, identifying drug use related issues and activities related to promoting safe and effective use of medicines with a professional fee. Notification of Pharmacy Practice Regulation is a milestone in the profession similar to implementation of Education Regulation. At the time of writing the text, there are only

Course/level of institution	Qualification at entry level as teacher	Qualification and Experience of Principal or Head of the Institution
Diploma course	1. PCI recognised PG course OR PharmD degree OR 2. PCI recognised BPharm with 3 years professional experience [Lecturer]	• PCI recognised PG course in any discipline of pharmaceutical sciences OR Doctor of Pharmacy Degree • 5 years of teaching experience
BPharm./ MPharm./ PharmD.	1. First Class BPharm with MPharm in appropriate branch. OR 2. PharmD [Lecturer/Assistant Professor] Lecturer after 2 years of experience will be designated as Assistant Professor	• First Class BPharm with MPharm. in appropriate branch. OR • PharmD • PCI recognised PhD degree • 15 years experience in teaching or research out of which 5 years must be in a position of Professor or Head of the Department

two states: Kerala and Haryana have reported to have started implementing the provision of the regulation.

The salient points of the Pharmacy Practice Regulation are:

- The professional pharmacists (or practitioners) are divided into four basic types: Community pharmacists, hospital pharmacists, drug information pharmacists and clinical pharmacists based on their professional roles.

- In addition to defining the roles and duties of various pharmacists, it has elaborated the job positions and qualification requirements for pharmacists in healthcare system like hospitals. The regulation outlines positions of pharmacists in hospital pharmacy practice as Pharmacist (new recruitment), Senior Pharmacist (Promotion avenue for Diploma Pharmacists with four years of experience or direct recruitment with B Pharm. or Pharm D. qualification), Chief Pharmacist (Promotion avenue for Diploma Pharmacists with ten years of experience or B. Pharm. with five years of experience or direct recruitment with M Pharm. or Pharm D. qualification). While the regulation defines the role and qualification needed for community pharmacists, hospital pharmacists and drug information pharmacists, it is silent for clinical pharmacists.

- The regulation has provision of professional fees for professional services but need to be declared before providing such services. It makes it obligatory for the pharmacists to maintain patients' medical records in the format suggested. This documentation of complete record would help pharmacists to avoid hypersensitive drug reactions improving patient safety. This even may give rise to the concept of family pharmacist.

- For renewal of registration, the pharmacist has to attend at least two refresher courses of at least one day duration in a span of five years.

- The role of pharmacy inspectors is specified.

The people were under the impression that under the Pharmacy Practice Regulation, the pharmacists can start their clinics for diagnosis and treatment. The message on this were widely circulated in social media, i.e. mail, etc. The PCI has to intervene on this and clarified that there is no such provision. Under the said Regulations, the registered pharmacist is required to dispense medicines on the prescription of a Registered Medical Practitioner and can counsel the patient or care giver on medicine to enhance or optimize drug therapy.

While the pharmacy practice regulations bring new hope for the professional pharmacists, the regulation implementing authorities must initiate the process to implement in letter and spirit. There should be effective surveillance to monitor the implementation. It would have been perhaps more appropriate to increase the penalty for the offences relating to non-adherence to regulations and malpractices.

Approval and withdrawal of Approval of the Courses

Any authority in state which conducts a course of study for pharmacists or hold examination in pharmacy is required to apply to the central council for approval of the course as approved course for the admission to an approved examination or approval of the said examination for the purpose of qualifying for registration as a pharmacist. The authority concerned needs to furnish details of course or training or examination as the case to the council periodically.

Withdrawal of Approval

When the EC reports to the central council that the approved course or examination is not in conformity with ER, the central council issues notice to the authority concerned informing its intention to withdraw the approval. The authority concerned can make representation to the council through the state government within three months from the receipt of the notice. After consideration of representation and comments of the state government, the council may declare its decision to withdraw the approval or continue approval.

Other Qualifications for Registration

If the central council is satisfied that a qualification in pharmacy granted outside the territories to which Pharmacy Act extends has requisite skill and knowledge, then it declares such qualification to be approved one for registration. Indian citizens possessing such qualifications are treated as qualified for registration. However, citizens of other countries possessing such qualification may be permitted if the country allows the persons of Indian origin holding such qualification to enter and practice the profession of pharmacy in that country.

Central Register

The central council maintains a register of pharmacists known as central register containing the names of all persons registered as pharmacists in the state council. The state council is required to supply five copies of the register as soon as after first April of every year. The registrar of the state council should inform the addition or amendments to the register to central council without delay. It is the duty of the registrar of the central council to revise the central register and publish in the gazette of India. The central register is deemed as public document.

The registrar of the central council enters the name of person following the receipt of registration in the register of the state.

Inspection

The executive committee of the council appoints inspectors to:

1. Inspect any institution which provides an approved course of study;
2. Attend at any approved examination;
3. Inspect any institution whose authorities have applied for approval of course of study or examination and attend at any examination of such institutions.

An inspector attending at any examination should not interfere with the conduct of examination, but should report the executive committee on the sufficiency of every examination he attends and on other matters as required. The executive committee forwards the copy of every such report to the authority or institution concerned. On receipt of the comments from the said authority or institution, the executive committee forwards the copy with the comments to the central government and to the state government concerned.

The central council is required to furnish copies of its minutes of the executive committee and the annual report of its activity to the central government. The central government may publish such reports.

The central council is required to maintain proper accounts and other relevant records and prepare an annual statement of accounts as specified by the central government in consultation with the Comptroller and Auditor General of India (CAG). The accounts of the council is audited annually by CAG or by any person authorized by him. The expenditure incurred in connection with the audit is payable by the council to the CAG. The CAG or person authorized by him has same rights, privileges, and authority as available for auditing of government accounts. He has the right to demand the production of books of accounts, connected vouchers and other documents and papers. The accounts so certified together with audit report are required to be forwarded to the central council and who in turn forward the same with its comments to the central government.

Power to Make Regulations

The central council has the power to make regulations with the approval of central government. Such regulations may be related to the management of the property of the council; the manner in which elections to be conducted; the summoning and holding the meeting of central council, the time and places of such meeting, the conduct of business there at and the number of members necessary to constitute a quorum; the functions of the executive committee, the summoning and holding meeting, the time and places of such meeting, the number of members necessary to constitute a quorum; the powers and duties of President and Vice President; the qualification, the term of office and the powers and duties of the Registrar, Secretary, Inspectors and other officers and servants of the central council including the amount and nature of security to be furnished by the registrar or any other officer or servant; the manner in which the central register to be maintained.

Every regulation made under this Act is required to be laid before each house of Parliament as soon as after it is made. If both houses agree in making modification in the regulation or both houses agree that regulation should not be made, the regulation thereafter will have modified form or be of no effect.

State Pharmacy Council

Constitution and Composition: The state government constitutes a state council consisting of the following members:

a. Six members elected from among themselves by the registered pharmacists of the state;

b. Five members nominated by the state government out of which at least three should possess prescribed degree or diploma in pharmacy or pharmaceutical chemistry or are registered pharmacists;

c. One member elected from among themselves by the members each medical council or the council of medical registration of the state;

d. The Chief Administrative Medical Officer of the state–Ex-Officio. If he is unable to attend any meeting, a person authorized by him in writing can attend;

e. The officer in charge of Drugs Control Organization of the state–Ex-Officio. If he is unable to attend any meeting, a person authorized by him in writing can attend;

f. The Government Analyst–Ex-Officio. If more than one government analyst, the government appoints one.

Interstate Agreements

Two or more state governments may enter into an agreement:

a. For the constitution of a joint council for all participating states; or

b. The state council of one state shall serve the needs of the other participating state. In such a situation the membership of the state council is augmented by not more than two members of whom one should be a person possessing a prescribed degree or diploma in pharmacy or pharmaceutical chemistry or a registered pharmacist nominated by each of the other participating state governments;

c. For the apportionment between the participating states of the expenditure in this regard;

d. Determine which of the participating state government shall exercise the several function of the state government under the Act;

e. Provide for consultation between the participating state governments;

f. Make such incidental and ancillary provisions as necessary.

An agreement made is required to be published in the official gazettes of the participating states.

Composition of Joint State Councils

A joint state council consists of the following members:

a. Not less than three and not more than five members as decided in the agreement elected from amongst themselves by the registered pharmacists of each participating state;

b. Not less than two and not more than four as decided in the agreement nominated by each participating state government. More than half of the members should possess prescribed degree or diploma in pharmacy or pharmaceutical chemistry or are registered pharmacists;

c. One member elected from amongst themselves by the members of each medical council or the council of medical registration of each participating state;

d. The chief administrative medical officer of each participating state—Ex-Officio. If he is unable to attend any meeting, a person authorized by him in writing can attend;

e. The officer in charge of drugs control organization of each participating state— Ex-Officio. If he is unable to attend any meeting, a person authorized by him in writing can attend;

f. The government analyst of each participating state—Ex-Officio. If more than one government analyst, the government appoints one.

Every state council (or joint state council) is a corporate body having perpetual succession and a common seal, with power to acquire or hold movable and immovable property.

President and Vice President of State Council

The President and Vice President of State Council are elected by the members from amongst themselves. However, the state government nominates a person to become the president for the five years from the first constitution of the state council. If such person is not a member of the council, he is treated as an additional member. He shall hold office at the pleasure of the state government.

They can hold office for a period not exceeding five years and not extending beyond the expiry of membership of the state council. However, being members of the state council, they are eligible for re-election. In case, the term of office (as member) expires before the expiry of the full term for which he is elected as president or vice president, he can continue to hold office if he regains the membership either by election or nomination. Any dispute regarding election is to be referred to the state government and its decision is final.

A nominated or elected member can hold office for a period of five years from the date of nomination or election or until his successor has been duly nominated or elected, whichever is longer. A nominated or elected member may any time resign membership by writing to the president. The seat of such members becomes vacant there-

upon. If the elected or nominated member absents without excuse from three consecutive meeting of the state council, then it is treated as if he has vacated his seat. Similarly if the member is elected and ceases to be registered pharmacist or ceases to be the member of Medical Council or Council of Medical Registration as the case is, then his seat is also treated as vacant. The casual vacancy in the state council can be filled by fresh nomination or election and such members can hold office only for the remaining period of the term against whom he is nominated or elected. The members of the state council are eligible for re-nomination or re-election. The council cannot be questioned on the ground merely of existence of vacancy or defect in the constitution of state council.

The state council with previous sanction of the state government appoints a Registrar who acts as secretary. If decided by state council, he can function as Treasurer too. For the first four years from the first constitution of the state council, registrar is appointed by the state government who shall hold office at the pleasure of state government. With the prior sanction of the government, the state council can appoint other officers and servants and fix the salaries and allowances and other conditions of service of secretary and other staff. It can fix the rates of allowances payable to the members of the state council.

Pharmacy Inspectors

A state council with the previous sanction of the state government may appoint inspectors with the prescribed qualification (qualification as prescribed by Kerala State Pharmacy Council: Degree or Diploma in Pharmacy with degree in any discipline; has 10 years of experience in government or public sector; registered as pharmacist in Kerala State Pharmacy Council) to:

- Inspect any premises where drugs are compounded or dispensed and submit a written report to the registrar;
- Enquire whether a person engaged in compounding or dispensing of drugs is a registered pharmacist;

- Investigate any complaint made in writing in respect of any contravention of the Act and report to the registrar;
- Institute prosecution under the order of executive committee of the state council;
- Exercise any other power necessary for carrying out the provision of the Act related to state council, registration and other provisions like penalty.

Willfully obstructing an inspector in the exercise of the powers conferred on him is punishable with imprisonment for extending up to six months or with fine not exceeding one thousand rupees, or with both. Every inspector is deemed to be a public servant.

At present (2017) perhaps only two states: Kerala and Maharashtra have utilized the provision of appointing pharmacy inspectors. Karnataka has discontinued the appointment of inspectors reported to be due to administrative reasons. Some other states' council have made attempt and initiated discussion with the respective state governments.

There are confusions and conflicts between the power and functioning of Pharmacy Inspectors and Drugs Inspectors. The job responsibilities of pharmacy inspectors are mentioned above. Most of the retail units are licensed for selling medicines (not dispensing as required for pharmacy license). Please refer to the Chapter on Drugs and Cosmetics Act to see various types of retail sale licenses. The conflict is on 'Selling' and 'Dispensing'. The Chemists Associations argue that they have the license for sale.

Maharashtra's Pharmacy Inspectors have identified cases of violation of Pharmacy Act. In one case, the offending doctor has been convicted of being an abettor which implies hiring unqualified person as a pharmacist in his clinic. The offending Osmanabad based medical practitioner was let scot-free by the Judicial Magistrate First Class (JMFC), Osmanabad in the first place. The doctor was later on convicted by the Aurangabad bench of High Court based on a fresh appeal filed by MSPC against the JMFC verdict as per the provisions of the

Pharmacy Act, 1948 (*Source*: Pharmabiz. August 27, 2013]

The State Council constitutes an Executive Committee consisting of the President and Vice President and any other members elected by the State Council from amongst members. The President of the state council is the chairman of the executive committee. A member of the executive committee holds office until the expiry of his term as a member of the state council. Subject to his membership of the council, he is eligible for election. The executive committee exercises powers and duties provided in the Act and as prescribed.

The state council is required to furnish reports, copies of minutes, minutes of the executive committee, and abstracts of its account to the state government as the state government requires. The copies of all these documents should be sent to the central council. The state government may publish such documents as it may think.

Registration of Pharmacists

The state government is required to prepare a register of pharmacists soon after the provision of registration of pharmacist takes effect. Once the state council is constituted, it assumes the duty of maintaining the register. The register should include the following particulars:

- The full name and residential address of the registered person;
- The date of his first admission to the register;
- His qualification for registration;
- His professional address and name of the employer if employed;
- Such other particulars as prescribed.

Preparation of First Register

The state government is required to constitute a Registration Tribunal, by notifying in the official gazette, for preparing the first register and fixes a date on or before which the application for registration with prescribed fees should be made to the Registration Tribunal. On examination of the application, if the Tribunal is satisfied of applicant's qualification for registration (described later), direct the entry of the name of the applicant on the register. Such register once published by the state government, aggrieved person may appeal against the decision of the tribunal to an authority appointed by the state government, within sixty days of publication. The register will be amended based on the decision of the authority and a registration certificate can be issued to persons whose name is entered in the register. Upon constitution of the state council, register is given into its custody. The state government may direct the all or part of fees collected for payment to the council.

Qualification for Entry on First Register

A person of eighteen years old residing or carrying out the business or profession of pharmacy in the state can apply for entry in the first register if:

a. Holds a degree or diploma in pharmacy or pharmaceutical chemistry or a chemist and druggist diploma of an Indian university or a state government or a prescribed qualification granted by an authority outside India, or

b. Holds a degree of an Indian university other than degree in pharmacy or pharmaceutical chemistry, and has been engaged in the compounding of drugs in a hospital or dispensary or other place in which drugs are regularly dispensed on prescription of medical practitioners for a total period of not less than three years, or

c. Has passed an examination recognized as adequate by the state government for compounders or dispensers, or

d. Has been engaged in the compounding of drugs in a hospital or dispensary or other places in which drugs are regularly dispensed on prescription of medical practitioners for a total period of not less than five years prior to the date notified for inviting application for entry in the first register.

The provision of preparing first register is no longer valid. In a significant judgment, SC in its order of July 6, 2017 stated that First Register prepared by erstwhile Bihar will be treated as the First Register for Jharkhand and Bihar. There is no need for preparing the first register again.

The issue of preparing first register by the Jharkhand Government began with creation of new state curving out of erstwhile Bihar (2000). The Jharkhand High Court too struck down the attempt of preparing first register. Then, the final order came from SC.

The first register allows the registration of even those who do not have formal pharmacy qualification as notified by Government of India under Education regulation 1991.

Qualification for Subsequent Registration

After the date fixed inviting application for entry into the first register or before the implementation of education regulation in the state, a person of eighteen years old residing or carrying out the business or profession of pharmacy in the state may get his name registered if he:

a. Satisfied the conditions prescribed with prior approval of the central council; or when no condition prescribed, the condition for registration in the first register is satisfied. He must have passed the matriculation examination or an examination prescribed as being equivalent.

b. Is a registered pharmacist in another state;

c. Possess qualification approved under qualification granted, outside the territory to which the act extends, for registration. He must have passed the matriculation examination or an examination prescribed as being equivalent.

After the implementation of Education Regulation in the state, a person of eighteen years old residing or carrying out the business or profession of pharmacy in the state may get his name registered if he:

a. Has passed the approved examination; This may be Diploma in Pharmacy, Bachelor of Pharmacy or PharmD.

b. Is a registered pharmacist in another state;

c. Possess qualification approved under qualification granted, outside the territory to which the Act extends, for registration. He must have passed the matriculation examination or an examination prescribed as being equivalent.

Special Provision for Registration

I. of Certain Persons

The state council may permit the registration of:

a. The names of displaced persons who have been carrying on the business or profession of pharmacy as their principle means of livelihood from a date prior to 4th day of March 1948 and who satisfy the condition for registration for entry in first register (Displace person means any person who on account of the setting up of the dominions of India and Pakistan or on account of civil disturbances or the fear of such disturbances in any area forming part of Pakistan has left or been displaced from his place on or after 1st day of March 1947 and since then been residing in India.);

b. The names of citizens of India who have been carrying on the business or profession of pharmacy in any country outside India and who satisfy the condition for registration for entry in the first register;

c. The names of persons who resided in an area which has subsequently become a territory of India and who satisfy the condition for registration for entry in the first register;

d. The names of persons who carry on business or profession of pharmacy in the state and satisfied the conditions for registration for entry in the first register; or have been engaged in the compounding of drugs in a hospital or dispensary or other place in which drugs are regularly dispensed on prescription of medical practitioners for a total period of not less than five years prior to the date fixed for inviting application by registration tribunal for the first registration;

e. The names of persons who were qualified for registration immediately before the 1st day of November 1956 but not qualified for registration in a state to which the place where he resided or carried out the business or profession of pharmacy now belonged.

f. The names of persons who were registered in a state as it existed immediately before the 1st day of November 1956; who by reason of the area in which they resided or carried on their business or profession of pharmacy having become part of a state as formed on that date, reside or carry on such business or profession in the latter state;

g. The names of persons who reside or carry on their business or profession of pharmacy in area in which the provision of registration takes effect after the commencement of ''e Pharmacy (Amendment) Act, 1959 and who satisfy the condition for registration in the first register. This special provision was in operation for a period of two years from the commencement of Pharmacy (Amendment) Act 1959. The state government had the powers to extend this provision for a period(s) not exceeding two years in aggregate.

II. for displaced persons, repatriates and other persons:

A state council may permit the registration of:

a. The names of persons who possess the qualification (degree or diploma in pharmacy or pharmaceutical chemistry or a chemist and druggist diploma of an Indian university or a state government or a prescribed qualification granted by an authority outside India; or has passed an examination recognized as adequate by the state government for compounders or dispensers) and were eligible for registration between the closing of the first register and the date when the education regulations came into effect;

b. The names of persons approved as qualified persons before 31st December 1969 for compounding or dispensing of medicines under Drugs and Cosmetics Act 1940 and the rules.

c. The names of displaced persons or repatriates who were carrying on business or profession of pharmacy as their principal means of livelihood in any country outside India for a total period of not less than five years from a date prior to the date of application for registration.

The first two provisions are in operation for a period of two years from the commencement of the Pharmacy (Amendment) Act 1976.

(Displaced person means any person who on account of civil disturbances or fear of such disturbances in any area now forming part of Bangladesh has left or been displaced after 14th day of April 1957 but before 25th day of March 1971.

Repatriate means any person of Indian origin who on account of civil disturbances or the fear of such disturbances in any area now forming part of Burma, Sri Lanka, or Uganda or any other country has left or been displaced after 14th day of April 1957 and has since then been residing in India.)

Registration Process and Removal from Register

Upon publication of the first register and constitution of the state council, interested person with required qualification for registration needs to apply to the registrar of the council with prescribed form of registration. If the registrar is of the opinion that the applicant has satisfied the conditions for registration, he enters the name of the applicant and issues a certificate of registration in the prescribed form. If a person name is removed from the register of any state, his name can be considered for entry in register only with the approval of the state council recorded at a meeting. Any person whose application is rejected by the registrar, may appeal to the state council within three months from the date of rejection and the decision of the state council is final.

The registered pharmacist has to pay the renewal fees annually to the state council for continuing registration but should be paid before the 1st day of April of the year to which it is related. The provisions for paying lifetime fees is abolished. The Pharmacy Practice Regulation mandates the minimum of two refresher courses in five years for renewal of registration.

On payment of renewal fees, the registrar issues a receipt and the receipt is the proof of registration. When the renewal fee is not paid by due date, the names can be removed from the register. Once removed, it can be restored on such conditions as may be prescribed.

A registered pharmacist is entitled to have his further degree such as degree or diploma in pharmacy or pharmaceutical chemistry entered in the register by paying the prescribed fee.

- The name of the registered pharmacist can be removed from the register by the order of the Executive Committee if it is satisfied, after giving him a reasonable opportunity of being heard or after an enquiry, in case:
- His name has been entered by error or on account of misrepresentation of suppression of a material fact; or
- He has been convicted of any offence or has been guilty of any infamous conduct in any professional respect which in the opinion of Executive Committee renders him unfit to be kept in the register; or
- A person employed by him for the purpose of his business of pharmacy or employed to work under him in connection with any business of pharmacy has been convicted of any offence or has been guilty of any such infamous conduct. This is applicable only if EC is satisfied that:
  - The registered pharmacist has committed the similar offence or infamous conduct within previous twelve months;
  - Any person employed by registered pharmacist has committed similar offence or had infamous conduct during previous twelve months and the registered pharmacist had knowledge of such previous offence or infamous conduct;

– The offence or infamous conduct continued over a period and the registered pharmacist had knowledge of the continuing offence or infamous conduct;

– The offence is under the Drugs and Cosmetics Act and the registered pharmacist or the persons employed by him or under his control has not used due to diligence in enforcing compliance.

The removal from the register may be permanent or for specific period. The order of removal is subject to confirmation by the state council—does not take effect until the expiry of three months from the date of confirmation. A person aggrieved by the order and confirmation by the state council may appeal to the state government within thirty days of receiving confirmation communication. The order of the state government is final. The registered pharmacist whose name has been removed is required to surrender his certificate of registration to the Registrar and the name of such person will be published in the official gazette.

The state council may order the restoration of the names in the register whose name has been removed upon payment of prescribed fees. But if the appeal against the removal order is rejected by the state government, such persons' name cannot be re-entered unless confirmed by the state government. The order of refusing to enter a name on the register or removing a name from the register cannot be questioned in any court.

When a certificate is lost or destroyed, there is a provision of issuing duplicate certificate of registration upon payment of prescribed fee.

The register containing names of registered pharmacists was printed after the 1st day of April subsequent to the commencement of Pharmacy (Amendment) Act, 1959. The register is required to be printed every year after the 1st day of April showing all additions and other amendments. It is to be made up to date at least three months before ordinary elections to the state council. The copies of the register are made available on payment of prescribed fees.

Registration Procedure

(http://www.tnpc.ac.in/home.html, accesed on 31 December, 2017)

For Fresh Registration— Documents Required:
- D Pharm qualification
  - Transfer certificate
  - 10th and 12th mark sheets
  - Course-cum-conduct certificate
  - Provisional/Diploma Certificate
  - D Pharm—all mark sheets
  - 500 hours hospital training certificate
  - Any address proof–Aadhar Card, Voter ID, Ration Card, PAN Card or any certificate issued by Govt. Authorities.
  - Recently taken color passport size photograph
- B Pharm qualification
  - Transfer certificate
  - 10th and 12th mark sheets
  - Course—cum-conduct certificate
  - Provisional/Degree certificate
  - B Pharm—all mark sheets
  - Any address proof—Aadhar Card, Voter ID, Ration Card, PAN Card or any certificate issued by Govt. Authorities.
  - Recently taken color passport size photograph
- Pharm D qualification
  - Transfer certificate
  - 10th and 12th Mark Sheets
  - Course–cum-conduct certificate
  - Provisional/degree certificate
  - Pharm D all mark sheets
  - Internship certificate issued by the Head of the Hospital
  - Any address proof—Aadhar Card, Voter ID, Ration Card, PAN Card or any certificate issued by Govt. Authorities.
  - Recently taken color passport size photograph

Fees Required

- D Pharm—Rs. 1800/–
- B Pharm—Rs. 2300/–
- Pharm D—Rs. 3300/–

Process:

- Fill the online application form
- Scan and upload all the above certificates to the application form
- Scan and upload the image of your photograph:
  - (a) Photo size W 30 mm × H 35 mm: File size up to 100 kB
  - (b) Signature size W 55 mm × H 10 mm: File size up to 30 kB
- Submit the application form—you will receive an Application Approval e-mail after verification of your documents
- Log in and book your appointment date and time

Renewal of Registration

Procedure for Renewal of Registration Certificate:

- Pay the Fees as detailed below and keep ready the payment particulars: For 5 years– Rs. 500/–
- Fill the online application form
- Scan and upload the image of your photograph:
  - (a) Photo size W 30 mm × H 35 mm File size up to 100 kB
  - (b) Signature size W 55 mm × H 10 mm File size up to 30 kB
- Submit the application form
- You will receive E-Mail with a Renewal Receipt
- Print the Renewal

Penalty for Falsely Claiming Registered Pharmacist

Person whose name is not entered in the state register, but pretends to be so, he or she shall be punishable on the first conviction with fine which may extend to five hundred rupees and on the subsequent conviction with imprisonment extending to six months or with fine not exceeding one thousand rupees or with both. The use of descriptions: Pharmacist, chemist, pharmaceutist, dispenser, dispensing chemist, or any combination of such words is reasonably calculated to suggest of falsely claiming as registered pharmacist.

Dispensing by Unregistered Persons

The state government notifies a date after which no person other than a registered pharmacist is permitted to compound, prepare, mix, or dispense any medicine on the prescription of a medical practitioner. Where on such date is notified by the state government, this provision will take place on the expiry of a period of eight years from the commencement of the Pharmacy (Amendment) Act, 1976. Dispensing by medical practitioner for his own patients or with special sanction of the state government for the patient of another medical practitioner is not covered under this provision. This indicates that we can have dispensing doctors. Contravention of this provision of the act is punishable with imprisonment for a term which may extend to six months, or with a fine not exceeding one thousand rupees or with both.

The Section 42 of the Pharmacy Act provides exclusive rights to dispense medicines (except situation mentioned above under dispensing by unregistered person). The Kerala High Court has held that the government order enabling junior public health nurses to dispense drugs cannot be sustained under the law. The court also directed the state government to take necessary steps to dispense drugs through qualified pharmacists in accordance with law.

Earlier, The Director of Health Services, Government of Kerala, issued order for dispensing by the junior public health nurses.

[Source: The New Indian Express, Kochi Edition, Date 15 October 2017]

Failure to Surrender Certificate of Registration

Any person, whose name has been removed from the register, fails to surrender without sufficient cause shall be punishable with fine which may extend to fifty rupees.

Payment of Part of Fees to Central Council

The state council has to pay a sum of equivalent to one-fourth of the total fees realized by the state council during the previous financial year to the central council before the end of June each year.

Appointment of Commission of Enquiry

Whenever it appears to the central government that the central council is not complying with any provision of the act, it may appoint a Commission of Enquiry consisting of three persons: Two of them are appointed by central government and one being the judge of a High Court and one is appointed by the council. The commission enquires the matters and submits report to the central government with its recommendation. The central government may accept the report or remit the same for modification or reconsideration. On acceptance of recommendation, the central government may order the central council to take remedial measures as recommended. If the council fails to comply with the order within the specified time, the central government may issue necessary order to give effect of the recommendations.

Similarly the state government has power to appoint Commission of Enquiry on functioning of State Pharmacy Council.

Power to Make Rules

The state government may make rules to carry out with respect to provision of registration, constitution of the council, and other aspects by notification in the Official Gazette. Every rule made by the state government is required to be laid before the state legislature as soon after it is made. These rules are usually related to:

- The management of the property of the state council, maintenance and audit of its accounts;
- The manner in which the elections are conducted for constitution of the state council or joint state council;
- The summoning and holding of meeting of the state council, the time and places at which such meetings shall be held, the conduct of business and the number of members necessary to form a quorum;
- The power and duties of the president and vice president of state council;
- The constitution and functions of the executive committee, the summoning and holding of meeting, the places and times at which such meetings will be held, number of members necessary for quorum;
- The qualifications, the term of office, powers and duties of the Registrar, other officers and servants of the state council including the amount and nature of security to be given by the treasurer;
- The qualifications, powers and duties of an inspector;
- The particulars to be stated and the proof of qualifications to be given in application for registration;
- The conditions for registration, fees payable and the charges for supplying the copies of register;
- The format of certificate of registration;
- The maintenance of a register;
- The conduct of pharmacists and their duties in relation to medical practitioners, public and the profession of pharmacy.

Education Regulation, 1991 and Amendment Regulation, 1996: Salient Points

- Minimum qualification required for registration as pharmacist is pass in Diploma in Pharmacy and successful completion of practical training or any other course as approved by Pharmacy Council of India.
- Minimum qualification for admission into Diploma in Pharmacy Course: A pass in any of the following examination with Physics, Chemistry, Biology or Mathematics:
  - Intermediate examination in science,
  - First year of three year degree course in science,
  - 10 + 2 examination in science,
  - Pre-degree examination,
  - Or any other examination as approved by PCI.
- Duration of Diploma in Pharmacy Course: Two academic years with working day not less than 180 days per year and practical training of 500 hours spread over a period of not less than 3 months.

- Course conducting authority and examining authority must approved by the PCI.
- Examination: 20 marks sessional for both theories and practical papers and remaining 80 in final examination. Pass marks: 40% separately in theory and practical but inclusive of sessional marks. Securing 60% marks in aggregate in one attempt yield a first class while securing 75% marks in any subject yield a distinction in that subject. There are provisions of improvement of sessional marks.
- Practical Training: After appearing part– II (final) examination, the student needs to undergo training in:
  - Hospitals/Dispensaries run by Central/State Governments/Municipal Corporation/Central Government Health Scheme and Employees State Insurance Scheme.
  - A Pharmacy, Chemist and Druggist licensed under the Drugs and Cosmetics Rules, 1945.
  - Drugs manufacturing Unit licensed under the Drugs and Cosmetics Act, 1940 and rules made thereunder.
  - Any other hospital or dispensary approved by PCI.

In 2008, a new registrable qualification has been introduced: Pharm D regulations are framed under the Act.

At present person possessing either approved Diploma in Pharmacy, Bachelor of Pharmacy and Pharm D are eligible for registration.

Pharmacists cannot give Injections

A pharmacist qualified with Diploma in Pharmacy is running a medical shop in Tirunelveli District of Tamil Nadu. He had been giving injections to patients as prescribed doctors. When police objected to this practice, the pharmacist approached Madurai Bench of Madras High Court for permission to administer injections to patients.

While dismissing the petition the court observed that those who had completed pharmacy course should only dispense medicines, as per the rules. Therefore, they cannot be permitted to administer injections, the judge said, dismissing the petition.

(The New Indian Express, Puducherry Edition dated 30 August 2009).

Pharmacy Council regulates the education, training and registration of pharmacists. But once registered, his/her profession will not be controlled by the Pharmacy Council but by the Authorities administering Drugs and Cosmetics Act and the Rules thereunder.

4

Narcotic Drugs and Psychotropic Substances Act

"Don't do drugs because if you do drugs you'll go to prison, and drugs are really expensive in prison."

— *John Hardwick* `

"It is easier to find man who will volunteer to die, than to find those who are willing to endure pain with patience."

— *Julius Caesar*

After reading this chapter, you should be able to understand and appreciate:

- Abuse of drugs and other substances
- International Treaties on Drug Abuse and its Prevention
- Control mechanisms for narcotic drugs and psychotropic substances including essential narcotic drugs.
- Procedure for handling Essential Narcotic Drugs for Medical Purpose.
- Procedure for cultivation, manufacture, sale and export of opium.
- Procedure for import, export and transhipment of narcotic drugs and psychotropic substances.
- Administrative procedures for implementing the Act.

Drug use and abuse are as old as perhaps mankind itself. Human beings have always had a desire to eat or drink substances that make them feel relaxed, stimulated or euphoric. Humans have used drugs of one sort or another for thousand of years. Wine was used at least from the time of early Egyptians; narcotics from 4000 BC; and medicinal use of marijuana has been dated to 2737 BC in China.

The use of cannabis plant for a variety of purposes has long existed in India. The cannabis has a strong religious association as a gift from Lord Shiva to his followers. It is linked to the religious festivals like Shivaratri, Krishna Ashtami, and participation in bhajan sessions. Occasions like Holi, the festival of colours, are not complete without the sharing of bhang—a drink made with cannabis. Opium has also been used for sociocultural reasons in different parts of the country. It has been offered at harvest festival in a ceremony called Akha Teej, intended to strengthen family marital clan bonds and put aside old feuds. Cannabis was known to increase concentration during meditation, hence was used by Hindu saints. Its use was widespread in religious places like Hardwar, Varanasi, Puri, etc. The use of cannabis is also mentioned in Atharva Veda. Opium use becomes popular during Mughal period.

Cannabis has long been used along with other ingredients to treat rheumatism, migraine, malaria and cholera; to relieve fluxes, facilitate surgical operations; to relax nerves; restore appetite; for general well being; and is also considered beneficial for the functioning of heart and liver. The ancient Greek and Egyptian societies used extracts from the opium poppy to quiet children, among other things. The Greek physician Galen prescribed opium for headache, deafness, epilepsy, asthma, coughs, fevers, "women's problems," and for melancholy moods. It has been recognized as excellent pain reliever. Similarly, coca has been used to produce euphoria, hyperactivity and hallucinations and later its medicinal properties were discovered and used as cough syrup and tonics.

While the majority of the human societies throughout history have practiced recreational drug use in various forms, the problem of addiction was recognized gradually. The addiction becomes a social problem which led to a lot of complications and antisocial activities. It was the government's responsibility to curb drug abuse and at the same time allow the use of these drugs for research and treatment. With time to time various laws were enacted: Opium Act 1857 and Opium Act 1878. The problem of drug abuse was not just restricted to any one country but was a global problem. In order to address this global issue, the second International Opium Conference at Geneva, called Geneva Convention, was held in 1925 to take appropriate measures to suppress the contraband traffic and abuse of dangerous drugs especially obtained from opium, cannabis and coca. India participated in the convention and being one of the signatories, the Government of India passed the Dangerous Drugs Act 1930 with an aim to control certain operations relating to these drugs and vesting the authority in the central government.

India again participated in UN 1961 Single Convention on Narcotic Drugs at New York where it was decided to eradicate culturally ingrained patterns of drug use, including those involving cannabis and opium. Indian delegations at the UN had long objected to the proposed policy of international cannabis prohibition but made little headway.

The drug abuse pattern has changed with time. Tourism has contributed to a diversi-fication of drug use patterns. In the mid and late 1970s, it was noticed to have new forms of drug taking behaviour. The Indian cities have been introduced to new foreign drugs like Heroin. The relative easy availability of foreign drugs in comparison to opium contributed to a shift in drug use of choice. The wide spectrum of drugs was made available like mescaline, psilocybin, tetrahydro-cannabinol, LSD, etc. The Single Convention treaty was not able to have adequate control over these new substances. A separate Convention on Psychotropic Substances was held in 1971. But it is reported that 1971 convention though closely resembles the single convention, it has less rigorous provision for the so-called psychotropic substances. A new dimension of problem associated with the drug abuse is transmission of HIV/AIDS and other blood borne diseases through injection of drugs. In order to keep pace with time and situations and as part of international obligation, Government of India passed a new legislation, Narcotic Drugs and Psychotropic Substances Act 1985.

The principal acts: Opium Act 1957, Opium Act 1878 and Dangerous Drugs Act 1930 have certain deficiencies in controlling illicit drug traffic and drug abuse at national and international level:

- The scheme of penalties is not sufficiently deterrent to meet challenges of well-organized gangs of smugglers.
- It does not provide investigating officers of number of important agencies like narcotics, customs, central excise, etc. with power of investigation of offences under various laws.
- The regulation does not comply with international treaties signed by government at later period.
- Psychotropic substances are not covered under these laws. It does not comply with international treaty, convention on Psychotropic substances 1971.

In view of the above, a comprehensive legislation, the Narcotic Drugs and Psychotropic Substances (NDPS) Act 1985 was enacted to consolidate and amend the existing laws relating to narcotic drugs, strengthen the existing controls over drugs of abuse, considerably enhance the penalties for trafficking offences, make provisions for exercising effective control over psychotropic substances and it came into force on 16th September 1985. It extends to the whole of India. **The Act is administered by the Department of Revenue, Ministry of Finance, Government of India. In addition, there are two other Ministries of Government of India too involved. Narcotic Control Bureau falls under the Home Ministry and Drug Demand Reduction is handled by Ministry of Social Justice and Empowerment.** A number of agencies both at the Centre and in the States have been empowered to enforce the provisions of the Act. These agencies include the Department of Customs and Central Excise, the Directorate of Revenue Intelligence, the Central Bureau of Narcotics and the Central Bureau of Investigation at the Central level and State Police and Excise Departments at the State level. The Union Ministries of Social Justice and Empowerment and Health are responsible for the demand reduction aspects of drug law enforcement which broadly covers healthcare and the deaddiction, rehabilitation and social reintegration of addicts.

The central or the state governments are empowered to make rules under the Act but should have regard to International Conventions.

Some Significant Measures taken Under NDPS Act 1985

- Punishment: Up to one year of imprisonment or a fine which may extend to 20 thousand rupees for the consumption of substances described under the act.
- Punishment: Imprisonment may be for a term of six months or a fine extendable to ten thousand rupees, or both for consumption of cannabis products other than the bhang.
- Quantity of possession: 250 milligram of heroin, 5 gram of opium, 5 grams of charas or hashish, 500 grams of ganja and 25 milligrams of cocaine can lead to arrest for trading in drugs.

The criminalization of drug use and the increasing rates of arrest for possessing small quantities of drugs led to widespread criticism of this harsh legislation. A study of 2001 based on Tihar jail inmates reported that 325 persons were arrested under NDPS 1985 out of total arrest of 1910 because of possession of small quantities of drugs meant for personal consumption. As a consequence of reassessment of the act in 2001 resulted in amendments relating to length of imprisonments and the quantity and the type of drug seized. In case of traditional drugs, only individuals in possession with large quantities of cannabis can be arrested for drug trafficking and face imprisonment. There were further changes in the law in 2002 creating two categories of drug possession: small quantities and commercial quantities. For trafficking in commercial quantities, the punishment specified is imprisonment for more than 20 years and a fine varying between one lakh rupees and two lakh rupees. The categorization of quantity varies according to substance seized; for hashish, a small quantity means less than 100 grams and commercial quantity as 1 kilogram and above. Similarly for heroin, a small quantity is below 5 grams and commercial quantity above 250 grams.

The issue of illegal drug use is souring in India with passage of time. The problem has been the major setback in evolution of India as a developed economy. The use of illicit drugs has increased with more than three million drug addicts across the country. Cannabis, Heroin, Opium, Methamphetamine and Hashish are most common examples. In 2016, the national capital recorded the highest number of drug seizures in the country. Early this year (2017), a survey revealed that 70,000 children in Delhi alone are drug addicts.

It is reported that in spite of amendment to the Act, some problems still persist such as any form of use remains a criminal offence which can result in imprisonment for a period of six months. Such an offence seems to be unrealistic in our country where use of cannabis and opium has cultural and religious association across many states. The process of searching is the most pivotal step in the procedure as it provides the base for setting the case. The task needs to be done in most patient way by the most trusted officer as in many cases innocent people are penalized without any reasonable cause. As per the statistics, around 64,734 drug trafficking cases have been reported in last four years out of which many are false and frivolous [The Narcotic Drugs and Psychotropic Substances (Amendment) Bill 2016—Bill number 225 of 2016].

Milestones in Control of Drug Abuse Legislations

- Opium Act 1857.
- The single convention on Narcotic drugs, 1961 (amended by the protocol of 25 March 1972).
- Opium Act 1878.
- Dangerous Act 1930.
- Convention on Psychotropic Substances, 1971.
- Narcotic Drugs and Psychotropic Substances Act 1985 and Rules 1985.
- Convention against the illicit in Narcotic Drugs and Psychotropic Substances, 1988.
- Prevention of Illicit Traffic in Narcotic Drugs and Psychotropic Substances Act, 1988.
- Narcotic Drugs and Psychotropic Substances (Amendment) Rules 2014—Provision of export outside the state.
- Narcotic Drugs and Psychotropic Substances (Amendment) Act 2014—concept of essential narcotics introduced.
- Narcotic Drugs and Psychotropic Substances (Amendment) Rules 2015— Provision relating to import into or export to outside India.
- Narcotic Drugs and Psychotropic Substances (Amendment) Rules 2015— Provision related to possession to use of essential narcotic drugs.
- Notification of essential narcotic drugs on 5th May 2015.

Authorities and Officers

The central government takes the following measures for preventing and combating abuse of and illicit traffic of narcotic drugs and psychotropic substances:

- To coordinate the actions by various officers, state governments, and other authorities.
- To meet obligations under International Conventions.
- To assist the concerned authorities in foreign countries and concerned International organizations.
- To take steps for identification, treatment, education, after care, rehabilitation and social re-integration of addicts.
- Other measures as the Government deems necessary including constituting authority for implementing the Act and the Rules.

Officers of the Central Government

- Narcotics Commissioner and other subordinate officers like Deputy Narcotics Commissioner, Assistant Narcotics Commissioner, Superintendent, District Opium Officer, Inspector and Sub-Inspector: The Narcotic Commissioner may authorize any subordinate officer to exercise his power subject to direction by the central government.

Power and Duties of the Various Officers of the Central Government

1. **Narcotics Commissioner (NC):** The Narcotics Commissioner is the Head of the Department [Central Bureau of Narcotics (CBN)] and undertakes overall supervision and control overall activities of the Department. NC or the subordinate officers exercise all powers and perform all functions relating to the superintendence of the cultivation of opium poppy and production of opium. He has been empowered to:
   - Specify terms and conditions and functions of Lambardar (of a village) designated by the District Opium Officer.
   - Withhold or cancel a license already issued to a poppy cultivator and specify the manner of destruction of opium poppy.
   - Specify the records to be maintained by the Lambardar and also specify further checks by such officers over the measurement conducted by the proper officer.
   - Specify records to be maintained by the Lambardar for weighment of daily produce of opium of the cultivator.
   - To issue instructions for delivery of opium, produced by the poppy cultivators.
   - Specify the manner under which the opium produce is to be weighed,

examined and classified according to its quality and consistence.

- To hear the appeal of any cultivator aggrieved by any decision or order made or passed relating refusal, withholding or cancellation of a license for opium cultivation by the Deputy Narcotics Commissioner.
- Allocate Medicinal (Excise) Opium to various State Excise Authorities for the purpose of distribution to the registered opium addicts.
- License the manufacture of 'manufactured drug' (all coca derivatives, medicinal cannabis, opium derivatives and poppy straw concentrate) and specify the conditions of license.
- Issue Import certificate. (No Narcotic Drugs and Psychotropic Substances specified in schedule can be imported into India without import certificate).
- Issue Export Authorization. (No Narcotic Drugs and Psychotropic Substances specified in schedule can be exported out of India without Export Authorization).
- Grant 'No Objection Certificate' for export of eight Precursor Chemicals and import of three Precursor Chemicals under Export and Import Policy of Directorate General of Foreign Trade (DGFT).
- Register the Import Contract for import of poppy seeds under the Export–Import policy issued by the Department of Commerce, Ministry of Commerce and Industry.

Responsibilities of Central Bureau of Narcotics

- Supervision over licit cultivation of opium poppy in India spread across 22 districts in states of Madhya Pradesh, Rajasthan and Uttar Pradesh.
- Preventive and enforcement function especially in three poppy growing states.
- Investigation of cases under NDPS Act 1985 and filing of complaint in the Court.
- Action for tracing and freezing of illegally acquired property which is liable for seizure or freezing or forfeiture.
- Issue of licenses for manufacture of synthetic narcotic drugs.

- Issuance of Export Authorisations/Import Certificate for export/import of Narcotic drugs and Psychotropic Substances.
- Issuance of No Objection Certificate (NOC) for import/export of a selected number of Precursor Chemicals.
- Registration of import contracts with the Narcotic Commissioner, Gwalior, prior to import. Import of Poppy Seeds are permitted only from Australia, Austria, France, China, Hungary, the Netherlands, Poland, Slovenia, Spain, Turkey and Czech Republic on production of an appropriate certificate from the Competent Authority of the exporting country that the opium have been grown licitly or legally in that country.

The Narcotic Control Bureau (Ministry of Home Affairs): Though the Narcotic Drugs and Psychotropic Substances Act itself does not create the Narcotic Control Bureau (NCB), it has been constituted by the central government under the provision of the Act on 17th, March, 1986. It is the apex coordinating agency. It takes measures with respect to:

- Co-ordination of actions by various offices, state governments and other authorities under NDPS Act, Customs Act, Drugs and Cosmetics Act and any other law in force.
- Implementation of the obligation in respect of countermeasures against illicit traffic under various international conventions and protocols that are in force at present or which may be ratified or acceded to by India in future.
- Assistance to concerned authorities in foreign countries and concerned international organizations to facilitate coordination and universal action for prevention and suppression of illicit traffic in these drugs and substances.
- Coordination of actions taken by other concerned Ministries, Departments and Organizations in relation to matters relating to drug abuse.

It also functions as Enforcement Agency through its field units located at Ahmedabad, Mumbai, Kolkata, Chandigarh, Delhi, Imphal, Jammu, Jodhpur, Lucknow, Chennai and Thiruvananthapuram. The zonal units collect and analyse data related to seizure of Narcotic Drugs and Psychotropic Substances, study trends, modus operandi, collect and disseminate intelligence and work in close cooperation with the Customs, State Police, and other law enforcement agency.

2. **Deputy Narcotics Commissioner (DNC):** There are two DNCs at Headquarters, Gwalior, designated as (i) DNC (Administration) and (ii) DNC (Enforcement). The DNC (Enforcement) controls and supervises the technical section, opium section and also the enforcement function. The DNC (Enforcement) also exercise supervision over the Preventive and Intelligence Cells located at New Delhi and Guwahati. The field DNCs located at Neemuch, Kota and Lucknow supervise the work and function of the opium divisions and the Preventive and Intelligence cells in the state of Madhya Pradesh, Rajasthan and Uttar Pradesh respectively.

The field DNCs also functions as an Appellate Authority in the matters relating to refusal, withholding or cancellation of a license for opium poppy cultivation by the District Opium Officer. They can withhold or cancel such license already issued.

3. **Assistant Narcotics Commissioner (ANC):** The ANCs work directly under the respective DNCs. The field ANCs, for sufficient reasons to be recorded in written, can withhold or cancel a license already issued for cultivation of opium poppy.

4. **Superintendent (Preventive):** The Superintendent (Preventive) is the overall incharge of Preventive and Intelligence Cells.

5. **District Opium Officer (DOO):** The DOO is the Licensing Authority for licit opium poppy cultivation. He also supervises all functions and duties relating to licensing/cultivation, measurement and test-measurement of poppy fields, preliminary weighment and weighment/procurement of opium produce in respect of all cultivators in his jurisdiction. He also performs enforcement functions.

6. **Inspector:** The inspector looks after all the work relating to cultivation as well as enforcement work. He has also been entrusted to perform the functions relating to search, seizures and investigation.

7. **Sub-inspector:** A sub-inspector in the opium division is the incharge of a Range. His primary duty is to undertake measurement of area of all the licensed fields, to ensure that there is no cultivation of opium poppy without a license. At the time of weighment, the sub-inspector assists the DOO and attends other works relating to procurement of opium, dispatch of opium consignment to Government Opium Factories. The sub-inspector also attends the enforcement work and other works as assigned. He has also been entrusted to perform the functions relating to search, seizures and investigation.

The Narcotic Drugs and Psychotropic Substances Consultative Committee

The central government constituted "The Narcotic Drugs and Psychotropic Substances Consultative Committee" to advise the Central Government on matters relating to the administration of the Act. The Committee consists of a Chairman and other members not exceeding 20. The Committee has the power to regulate its own procedure and meets periodically as required by the government. The Committee may appoint sub-committee if required taking persons even if they are not the member of Committee.

Officers of the State Government: The State Government may appoint officers with designations as it thinks fit for the purpose of this Act. The District Police, the Railway Police, the Prohibition Enforcement Wing, Narcotics Intelligence Bureau (NIB), and CID under the control of state government enforce the law. At present the NIB is headed by the Superintendent of Police (Government of Tamil Nadu 2011).

National Fund for Control of Drug Abuse: The fund has been created under the Act. Amounts obtained through selling forfeited properties are credited to this Fund. This Fund are also added any amounts appropriated by the Parliament and any contributions from other agencies and organizations. This Fund can be applied by the central government to meet the expenditure incurred in connection with the measures taken for:

a. Combating illicit traffic in narcotic drugs, psychotropic substances or controlled substances;
b. Controlling the abuse of narcotic drugs and psychotropic substances;
c. Identifying, treating, rehabilitating addicts;
d. Preventing drug abuse;
e. Educating public against drug abuse;
f. Supplying drugs to addicts where such supply is a medical necessity.

Applications for sanction of money out of the Fund should be submitted in the prescribed form to the Joint Secretary (Rev), Department of Revenue, Ministry of Finance, North Block, New Delhi. The governing body of the fund chaired by Additional Secretary (Rev) can sanction amounts up to ₹ 10 lakhs and larger amounts can be sanctioned by the Finance Minister.

Prohibition, Control and Regulations

Prohibition: The following operations are prohibited:

- Cultivation of any coca plant or gather any portion of coca plant.
- Cultivation of the opium poppy or any cannabis plant.
- Production, manufacturing, possessing, selling, purchasing, transporting, warehousing, using, consuming, importing (interstate), exporting (interstate), importing into India, exporting from India or transshipping any narcotic drug or psychotropic substance except for medical or scientific purposes.

However, some of the operations are permitted with license or authorization. They are discussed later. The provision is not applicable for export of poppy straw for decorating purpose.

The following activities relating to property derived from offences are also prohibited:

- Converting or transferring any property knowing that such property is derived from an offence committed under the Act for the purpose of concealing or disguising the illicit origin of the property or assisting any person in the commission of an offence or to evade the legal consequences.
- Concealing or disguising the true nature, source, location, disposition of any property knowing that such property is derived from an offence committed under the Act.

Power of Central Government and State Governments	
Central Government	*State Government*

1. Permit and regulate:
  • The cultivation, or gathering any portion of coca plant, or production, possession, sale, purchase, transport, import interstate, export interstate, use of consumption of coca leaves.
  • The cultivation of the opium poppy.
  • The production and manufacture of opium and production of poppy straw.
 	
  • The sale of opium and opium derivatives from the central government factories for export from India or sale to state government or to Manufacturing Chemists.
 	
  • The manufacture of manufactured drugs (other than prepared opium) but not including manufacture of medicinal opium or any preparation containing any manufactured
	1. Declares any place to be the warehouse where owner will take deposit of poppy straw that is legally imported interstate and intended for export.
	  • Also to regulate the safe custody of such poppy straw warehoused and the removal of such poppy straw for sale or export.
	  • To levy fees for such warehousing and to prescribe the manner and the period for disposing of the warehoused poppy straw in default of payment of fees.
	2. Provides the limit for issuing Licenses for cultivation of any cannabis plant.

(Contd...)

(Contd...)

Central Government	State Government
drug from materials which the maker is lawfully entitled to possess.	3. Ensures that the cultivation of cannabis plant by licensee only.
• The manufacture, possession, transport, import interstate, export interstate, sale, purchase, consumption or use of psychotropic substances.	4. Ensures that all cannabis produce be delivered to the authorized officers.
• The import into India and export from India and trans-shipment of narcotic drugs and psychotropic substances.	5. Fixes the price to be paid to the cultivators for delivered cannabis.
2. To fix from time to time the limits within which license may be given for the cultivation of opium poppy.	6. Prescribes the forms, conditions of license, fees to be charged and officers to issue license.
3. Ensure that all opium, the produce of the land are delivered by the cultivators to the authorized officers of central government.	
4. To prescribe forms and conditions of various licenses; fees to be charged; authorities for issuing license, withholding, refusing or cancelling and authorities for hearing appeal.	
5. To prescribe procedure for weighing, examining, and classifying according to its quality and consistence by authorized officers.	
6. To fix the price to be paid to the cultivators for the opium delivered.	
7. To prescribe procedure for the weighment, examination and classification of the opium received at the factory and adjusting the price of the produce based on quality and consistency examination; authorities for taking decision with regard to weighment, examination, classification, adjusting the price; authorities for hearing appeal.	
8. Ensure that adulterated opium delivered by the cultivator but detected at the factory are confiscated by the authorized officers.	
9. Prescribe forms and conditions of license for the manufacture of manufactured drugs and the authorities for issuing such license and fixing charges for it.	
10. Prescribe the forms and conditions of licenses or permits for the manufacture, possession, transport, import interstate, export interstate, sale, purchase, consumption or use of psychotropic substances; the authorities for issuing such licenses or permits; the fees to be charged.	
11. Prescribe the ports and other places at which any kind of narcotic drugs or psychotropic substances be imported or exported or transshipped; the forms and conditions of such certificates, authorizations or permits; the authorities for issuing such orders and the fees to be charged.	
12. Regulate any controlled substance used in the production of any narcotic drug or psychotropic substance in public interest through licenses, permits including production, manufacture, possession, transport, import interstate, export interstate, sale, purchase, consumption, use, storage, distribution, disposal or acquisition.	

• Acquiring, possessing or using knowingly any property which was derived from an offence committed under the Act.	If the person possessing the drugs or substances does not carry himself but

Offences and Penalties (Narcotic Drugs and Psychotropic Substances Act)

Offence	Penalty
Cultivation of opium, poppy straw, cannabis or coca plants without license	Rigorous imprisonment up to 10 years and fine up to ₹ 1 lakh
Embezzlement of opium by licensed cultivator	Rigorous imprisonment of 10 to 20 years and fine of ₹ 1 to 2 lakh (regardless of the quantity)
Production, manufacture, possession, sale, purchase, transport, import interstate, export interstate or use of drugs	Small quantity—rigorous imprisonment up to 6 months or fine up to ₹ 10,0000 or both. More than small quantity but less than commercial quantity—rigorous imprisonment up to 10 years and fine up to ₹ 1 lakh Commercial quantity—rigorous imprisonment of 10 to 20 years and fine of ₹ 1 to 2 lakh **Small and commercial quantities are defined for each drug separately through a notification.**
Import, export or transshipment of narcotic drugs and psychotropic substances	Same as above
External dealings in NDPS, i.e. engaging in or controlling trade whereby drugs are obtained from outside India and supplied to a person outside India	Rigorous imprisonment of 10 to 20 years and fine of ₹ 1 to 2 lakh (regardless of the quantity)
Knowingly allowing one's premises to be used for committing an offence	Same as for the offence
Violations pertaining to controlled substances (precursors)	Rigorous imprisonment of 10 to 20 years and fine of ₹ 1 to 2 lakh (regardless of the quantity)
Financing traffic and harbouring offenders	Rigorous imprisonment of 10 to 20 years and fine of ₹ 1 to 2 lakh (regardless of the quantity)
Attempts, abetment and criminal conspiracy	Same as for the offence
Preparation to commit an offence	Half the punishment for the offence extendable to one and half of the maximum term
Repeat offence	One and half times the punishment for the offence. Death penalty in some cases
Consumption of drugs	Cocaine, morphine, heroin—rigorous imprisonment up to 1 year or fine up to ₹ 20,000 or both Other drugs—imprisonment up to 6 months or fine up to ₹ 10,000 or both Addicts volunteering for treatment enjoy immunity from prosecution
Punishment for violations not elsewhere specified	Imprisonment up to 6 months or fine or both

entrusts the same to some other person for carriage in a car, then that person (driver of the car) would be the person who transports the said drugs and the person who directs him to do so would be the abettor of the offence of transporting.

The central government may permit the cultivation of any coca plant or gathering of any portion or the production, possession, sale, purchase, transport, import interstate, export interstate or import into India of coca leaves for use in the preparation of any flavouring agent containing no alkaloid.

Similarly there are provisions in which the central government allows cultivation of cannabis plant for industrial purpose for obtaining fibre or seed or for horticulture purpose.

The narcotic drug, psychotropic substance, coca plant, the opium poppy or cannabis plant cannot be liable to be distrained or attached by any person for the recovery of any money under any order or decree of any court or authority.

The central and the state governments are empowered to establish centres for identification, treatment, etc. of addicts and for supply of narcotic drugs and psychotropic substances where such supply is a medical necessity.

There are several ministries, departments are involved in the administration of this NDPS Act. The power of central government and state government is already described. It is necessary to know the corresponding departments of various activities under the Act and the Rules. The important activities and the corresponding department of central and state governments are given for easy learning.

Sl. Number	Activities	Government/Department/Organization
1	Drug law enforcement	**Central Government** 1. Narcotics Control Bureau 2. Central Bureau of Narcotics 3. Directorate General of Revenue Intelligence 4. Commissionerates of Customs 5. Commissionerates of Central Excise 6. Coast Guard **State Governments** Vary from State to State, usually: 1. State Police 2. State Excise Officers
2	Identification and destruction of illicit opium and cannabis crops	**Satellite survey of suspected areas** Central Economic Intelligence Bureau (CEIB) coordinates the survey and shares the information with NCB and CBN **Central Government** 1. Narcotics Control Bureau, MHA, GOI 2. Central Bureau of Narcotics, Gwalior, DoR, GOI **State Governments** Vary from State to State, usually: 1. State Police 2. State Excise Officers
3	Framing rules to regulate various activities relating permit, control and regulate (Rule 9)	Department of Revenue, Ministry of Finance, Government of India
4	Framing rules to regulate various activities relating to permit, control and regulate (Rule 10)	State Government
5	Licensing and supervision of cultivation of opium poppy	Central Bureau of Narcotics, Gwalior
6	Licensing of manufacture of narcotic drugs	Central Bureau of Narcotics, Gwalior
7	Drying and export of opium	Chief Controller of Factories, New Delhi
8	Extraction of alkaloids from opium	Chief Controller of Factories, New Delhi
9	Import of alkaloids of opium	Chief Controller of Factories, New Delhi
10	**Allocation** of INCB approved estimates of narcotic drugs as quotas and subsequent monitoring	Central Bureau of Narcotics, Gwalior
11	Supply of samples of narcotic drugs to testing labs, training institutions, etc.	Chief Controller of Factories, New Delhi

(Contd...)

(Contd...)

Sl. Number	Activities	Government/Department/Organization
12	Control on sale, use, consumption, movement, etc. of narcotic drugs	State governments usually through their State Excise Departments
13	Control on import and export of narcotic drugs and psychotropic substances and precursors	Central Bureau of Narcotics, Gwalior
14	Registration of import contracts for poppy seeds	Central Bureau of Narcotics, Gwalior
15	Regulation of manufacture, trade, etc. of psychotropic substances	State Drugs Controllers under the NDPS Rules read with Drugs and Cosmetics Act and Rules. Narcotics Commissioner for import and export
16	Receipt and monitoring of returns regarding controlled substances under the NDPS (Regulation of Controlled Substances) Order, 1993	Narcotics Control Bureau, MHA, GOI
17	Controlled delivery operations	Director General, Narcotics Control Bureau
18	Seizure, freezing and forfeiture of properties of drug traffickers, their relatives and associates	Competent Authority appointed under the NDPS Act (Delhi, Chennai, Mumbai and Kolkata, presently)
19	Management of properties seized or forfeited	Administrator appointed under the NDPS Act (Delhi, Chennai, Mumbai and Kolkata, presently)
20	Supply of opium to addicts	State Governments, usually through the State Excise Departments
21	Regulation of poppy straw	State Governments subject to guidelines dated 30th November 2009 of the Department of Revenue, Government of India.
22	Drug demand reduction through NGOs engaged in drug de-addiction and rehabilitation of addicts	Ministry of Social Justice and Empowerment, Govt. of India
23	Training personnel of NGOs in drug demand reduction	National Institute of Social Defence under the MSJ & E
24	Preventive education	Ministry of Social Justice and Empowerment
25	Treatment of drug addicts through Government hospitals	Ministry of Health and Family Welfare, GOI
26	Training doctors in drug demand reduction	National Drug Dependence Treatment Training Centre, AIIMS, New Delhi
27	Drug demand reduction activities at the State level	Social Welfare Departments of the States
28	Treatment of addicts through State Government hospitals	Health Departments of the States
29	Testing of samples of seized drugs	1. Central Revenue Control Laboratory 2. Laboratories of Government Opium and Alkaloids Works (GOAW) 3. Central Forensic Science Laboratories 4. State Forensic Science Laboratories of different States

(Contd...)

(Contd...)

Sl. Number	Activities	Government/Department/Organization
30	Training of personnel in drug law enforcement	1. National Academy of Customs, Excise and Narcotics (NACEN) 2. National Police Academy 3. State Police Training Schools 4. National Institute of Criminology and Forensic Sciences 5. CRCL 6. Narcotics Control Bureau (NCB)
31	Filing of returns to the International Narcotics Control Board and the Commission on Narcotic Drugs	Narcotics Control Bureau, MHA, GOI
32	Compilation of seizure statistics from different agencies	Narcotics Control Bureau, MHA, GOI
33	Exchange of live information on import and export of drugs and precursors with the competent authorities of other countries and with the INCB	Central Bureau of Narcotics, Gwalior
34	Access to morphine/opioids for cancer/pain relief and palliative care	Ministry of Health & F. W., Government of India, Health Department of States, State Drug Controllers, and Chief Controller of Factories

Restrictions over External Dealings: No person is permitted to engage in or control any trade involving procurement from outside India or supply to outside India without authorization from the central government and conditions imposed by that state government.

Offences and Penalties	
Offence	*Penalty*
Cultivation of opium, cannabis or coca plants without license	Rigorous imprisonment—up to 10 years + fine up to Rs.1 lakh
Embezzlement of opium by licensed farmer	Rigorous imprisonment—10 to 20 years + fine Rs. 1 to 2 lakhs (regardless of the quantity)
Production, manufacture, possession, sale, purchase, transport, import inter-state, export inter-state or use of narcotic drugs and psychotropic substances	• Small quantity—rigorous imprisonment up to 1 year or fine up to Rs. 10,000 or both • More than small quantity but less than commercial quantity—rigorous imprisonment. up to 10 years + fine up to Rs. 1 Lakh • Commercial quantity—Rigorous imprisonment 10 to 20 years + fine Rs. 1 to 2 Lakhs
Import, export or transhipment of narcotic drugs and psychotropic substances	Same as above
External dealings in NDPS, i.e. engaging in or controlling trade whereby drugs are obtained from outside India and supplied to a person outside India	Rigorous imprisonment 10 to 20 years + fine of Rs. 1 to 2 lakhs (Regardless of the quantity)

(Contd...)

(Contd...)

Offence	Penalty
Knowingly allowing one's premises to be used for committing an offence	Same as for the offence
Violations pertaining to controlled substances (precursors)	Rigorous imprisonment up to 10 years + fine Rs. 1 to 2 lakhs
Financing traffic and harboring offenders	Rigorous imprisonment 10 to 20 years + fine Rs. 1 to 2 lakhs
Attempts, abetment and criminal conspiracy	Same as for the offence
Preparation to commit an offence	Half the punishment for the offence
Inappropriately dealing with property derived from offences	Rigorous imprisonment of not less than three years extendable to 10 years with /without fine
Repeat offence	One and half times the punishment for the offence. Death penalty in some cases.
Consumption of drugs	Cocaine, morphine, heroin—rigorous imprisonment up to 1 year or fine up to Rs. 20,000 or both. Other drugs—imprisonment up to 6 months or fine up to Rs. 10,000 or both. Addicts volunteering for treatment enjoy immunity from prosecution
Punishment for violations not elsewhere specified	Imprisonment up to six months or fine or both

Small and Commercial Quantities of Common Drugs		
Drug	Small quantity	Commercial quantity
Amphetamine	2 grams	50 grams
Buprenorphine	1 gram	20 grams
Charas/Hashish	100 grams	1 kg
Cocaine	2 grams	100 grams
Codeine	10 grams	1 kg
Diazepam	20 grams	500 grams
Ganja	1 kg	20 kg
Heroin	5 grams	250 grams
MDMA	0.5 gram	10 grams
Methamphetamine	2 grams	50 grams
Methaqualone	20 grams	500 grams
Morphine	5 grams	250 grams
Poppy straw	1 kg	50 kg

There is a thin line between the preparation for and an attempt to commit an offence. A culprit first intends to commit an offence, then makes preparation for committing it and thereafter attempts to commit the offence. If the attempt succeeds, he has committed the offence; if he fails, he is said to have attempted to commit the offence. Attempt to commit an offence, therefore, can be said to begin when the preparations are complete and the culprit commences to do something with the intention of committing the offence and which is a step towards the commission of the offence.

While deciding for offence under preparation to commit an offence, it is not enough to make out a case of mere preparation. It is necessary to establish that if not prevented by circumstances independent of his will, the person was determined to carry out his intention to commit offence.

No sentences awarded under this Act can be suspended or remitted or commuted. While imposing a punishment higher than the minimum term of imprisonment or amount of fine, the following factors are required to be taken into consideration:

- The use or threat of use of violence or arms by the offender;
- The fact that the offender holds a public office and that he has taken advantage of that office in committing the offence;
- The fact that the minors are affected by the offence or the minors are used for the commission of the offence; (The question of the age of the person is relevant not for the purpose of determining his guilt but only for the purpose of punishment which he should suffer for the offence);
- The fact that office is committed in an educational institution or social service facility or in the immediate vicinity or in other place to which school children and students resort for educational, sports and social activities;
- The fact that the offender belongs to organized international or any other criminal group which is involved in the commission of the offence; and
- The fact that the offender is involved in other illegal activities facilitated by commission of the offence.

The Code of Criminal Procedure is not applicable to a person convicted of an offence under this Act unless the person is less than 18 years of age or that the offence is committed by the licensee or his servants.

Security for Abstaining from Commission of Offence: Whenever any person is convicted of an offence punishable under the Act and convicting court is of opinion that it is necessary to require such person to execute a bond for abstaining from the commission of any offence under this Act, the court may order him to execute a bond in prescribed form for a sum proportionate to his means, with or without his sureties, for a period not exceeding three years.

The bond becomes void if the conviction is set aside.

Constitution of Special Courts: The Government is empowered to constitute, by notification in the Official Gazette, necessary numbers of Special Courts for the purpose of speedy trial of offences under the Act. The Special Court consists of a single judge appointed by the Government with the concurrence of the Chief Justice of the High Court. A Session Judge or An Additional Session Judge is qualified for appointment as Judge for Special Court.

Offences triable by Special Courts: The following offences can be tried by Special Courts:

- All offences under the Act which are punishable with imprisonment for a term of more than three years;
- When the accused is forwarded to the Magistrate and the person is detained in custody for a period not exceeding fifteen days by Judicial Magistrate and seven days by Executive Magistrate and such Magistrates forward the case to Special Court;
- Upon perusal of a police report or complaint made by an officer of central or state government, the Special Court takes cognizance of the offence without the accused being committed to it for trial;
- Offences for which the accused is additionally charged (in addition to the offence under the Act).

The investigation relating to offences and relating to embezzlement of opium by cultivator, external dealing in narcotic drugs and psychotropic substances, and financing illicit traffic and harbouring offenders should be completed within one hundred and eighty days. In case, the investigation is not completed, the Special Court may extend the period of investigation up to one year on the report of the Public Prosecutor indicating the progress of the investigation and the specific reasons for the detention of the accused beyond the period of one hundred and eighty days.

The offences punishable under the Act for a term of not more than three years may also be tried summarily.

The Code of Criminal Procedure is applicable to the Special Court and the Special Court has the status of Session Court. The person conducting prosecution in the Special Court is deemed to be a Public Prosecutor.

Cognizable and Non-Bailable Offences:

- Every offence punishable under the Act is cognizable;
- The accused punishable for at least two offences relating to embezzlement of opium by cultivator, external dealing in narcotic drugs and psychotropic substances, and financing illicit traffic and harbouring offenders or involving commercial quantity be given no bail unless:
  - The Public Prosecutor has given an opportunity to oppose the application for such release.
  - The Court is satisfied that the accused is not guilty of such offence and he is not likely to commit any offence while on bail.

Both the tests: There are reasonable grounds for believing that the accused is not guilty of offence and he is not likely to commit offence during bail, must be satisfied before bail can be granted. The cases should be tried as early as possible because normally the accused are not released on bail.

Offences by Companies: When an offence has been committed by a company, every person in charge of and was responsible to the company at the time of the offence is deemed to be guilty of the offence. He is liable to be proceeded against and punished accordingly. However, such person is not liable to any punishment if he proves that the offence was committed without his knowledge or that he had exercised all due diligence to prevent the commission of such offence.

When it is proved that the offence has been committed with the consent or connivance of, or is attributable to any neglect on the part of any director, manager, secretary, or other officer of the company, then they are deemed to be guilty of that offence.

Power of Court to Release Certain Offenders on Probation

- When an addict is found guilty of an offence relating to consumption of narcotic drug or psychotropic substance or offences relating to small quantity of any narcotic drug or psychotropic substance, the Court after considering his age, character, antecedents or physical or mental condition, with his consent may direct his release for undergoing medical treatment for de-toxification or de-addiction from a hospital or an institution maintained or recognized by government. He has to enter into a bond in the prescribed form with or without sureties to appear and furnish the report of his medical treatment and to get abstained from committing further offence within one year.
- Based on medical report, the Court may direct to release the offender for a period not exceeding three years. On his failure to abstain from committing further offence, he will be called upon to receive sentence during such period.

Power of Court to publish names, place of business, etc. of certain offenders: Where any person is convicted of offences relating to poppy straw, coca plant and leaves, prepared opium, opium poppy and opium, embezzlement of opium, cannabis plant and cannabis, manufactured drugs and preparations, psychotropic substances, import–export, external dealing, allowing premises for offences, attempt to commit offence, abetment and criminal conspiracy and preparation to commit offence, the Court may publish the name and place of business or residence, nature of contravention of the convicted person in newspaper.

However, such publication shall not be made until the period for preferring an appeal against the order has expired without any appeal or such appeal is disposed of. The expenses of publication are recoverable from the convicted person as if it were a fine imposed by the Court.

Procedure

Power to Issue Warrant and Authorization

- Metropolitan Magistrate or Magistrate of the First Class or Magistrate of the Second Class especially empowered by the State Government to issue warrant for arrest or search.

- Gazetted rank officer of the department of central excise, narcotics, customs, revenue intelligence or any other department of the central government including paramilitary forces or the armed forces as empowered or officer of the revenue, drugs control, excise, police or any other department of state government is empowered to authorize any officer subordinate to him but superior in rank to a peon, sepoy or a constable to arrest or search as required. He himself also is empowered to arrest or search.

Power of Entry, Search, Seizure and Arrest without Warrant or Authorization

The following officers are empowered to:

a. Enter into and search any building, conveyance or place;

b. In case of resistance, break open any door or remove any obstacle to entry;

c. Seize drug or substance and materials used in manufacture, animal or conveyance;

d. Detain search and arrest.

1. Any officer superior in rank to peon, sepoy or constable of the departments of central excise, narcotics, customs, revenue intelligence or any other department of central government including paramilitary forces or armed forces as empowered;

2. Any other officer of the revenue, drugs control, excise, police or any other department of state government as empowered.

The officer should have reason to believe that the offence has been committed may act between sunrise and sunset. If the officer believes that the search warrant or authorization cannot be obtained without affording opportunity for the concealment of evidence or facility for the escape of an offender, he may enter and search such building, conveyance or enclosed place anytime between sunset and sunrise after recording the grounds of his belief.

When an officer takes down any information in writing or records grounds for his belief need to send a copy of this record to his immediate official superior within 72 hours. In order to bring transparency as well as to protect innocent persons getting into trouble, the government proposed audio-visual recording of post-entry search, seizure and entry.

Power of Seizure and Arrest in Public Place

The public place means any public conveyance, hotel, shop or any other intended for use or accessible to public.

Any officer mentioned above either of central government or state government is empowered:

a. Seize narcotic drug or psychotropic substances or controlled substance in any public place if he has reason to believe an offence has been committed. He may seize the other materials including animal or conveyance, document, liable to confiscation.

b. Detain and search any person believed to have committed offence and arrest if such person if found in possession of unlawful of substances.

Power of entry, search, seizure and arrest in offences relating to coca plant, opium poppy and cannabis plant: The procedures followed for narcotic drugs and psychotropic substances are applicable.

Procedure where seizure of goods liable to confiscation is not practicable: The authorized officer may serve the order to the owner or person in possession of goods not to remove or deal with such goods without the previous permission of the officer concerned.

Duty of land owner to give information of illegal cultivation: The landholder needs to inform any illegal cultivation of opium poppy, cannabis plant or coca plant in his land to the officers mentioned (under power of entry, search, seizure and arrest without warrant or authorization) or any police officer. The landholder is liable to punishment if he knowingly ignores to give information.

Duty of certain officers to give information of illegal cultivation: The government officers, panch, sarpanch, any village officer should provide immediate information about the illegal cultivation of opium poppy, cannabis plant or coca plant to the police officer or officers mentioned (under power of entry, search, seizure and arrest without warrant or authorization). On delibe-rately ignoring to provide information invites punishment.

Power of attachment of crop illegally cultivated: The Metropolitan Magistrate, First Class Judicial Magistrate, Magistrate especially empowered by state government or the gazette officers mentioned (under power of entry, search, seizure and arrest without warrant or authorization) are empowered to order attachment or destroy of any opium poppy, cannabis plant or coca plant which are believed to have illegally cultivated.

Power to stop and search conveyance: The officers authorised for entry, serach, seizure and arrest without warrant or authorisation are empowered to stop and search conveyance if there are reasons to suspect that any animal or conveyance is used for the transport of narcotic drug or psychotropic substance in contravention to the Act or Rule. In case of aircraft, it may be compelled to land.

Power to undertake controlled delivery: The Director General of Narcotic Control Bureau or any officer authorised by him may undertake controlled delivery of any consignment to any destination in India or to a foreign country, in consultation with competent authority of the country concerned.

Conditions for searching of persons: The officers empowered for entry, search, seizure and arrest without warrant or authorisation, while searching person(s), should take such person without unnecessary delay to the nearest authorised Gazetted Officer or Magistrate, if such person requires. The officer may detain the person until he is brought to the Gazetted Officer or the Magistrate. The Gazetted Officer or the Magistrate orders their discharge, if no ground is found or else, will allow search. The female must be searched by female only.

The Code of Criminal Procedure 1973 is applicable to warrants, arrests, searches and seizures.

Disposal of persons arrested and articles seized: The arresting officer is required to inform the arrested person about the reason of the arrest. Every arrested person, article seized should be forwarded without unnecessary delay to the Magistrate by whom the warrant was issued. The arrested person and seized article should be forwarded to the officer-in-charge of the nearest police station or to the officer empowered (Department of Central Excise, Narcotics, Customs, Revenue Intelligence or Border Security Force) without unnecessary delay.

The state governments are also empowered to invest any officer of the department of drugs control, revenue or excise or any other officer with the power of an officer-in-charge of a police station for investigation of offences under the Act.

Police to take charge of articles seized and delivered: The officer-in-charge of police station should receive and keeps goods and articles seized and delivered to him. He should allow the accompanying officer to affix his seal to such articles or to take samples. The samples so taken should also be sealed with a seal of officer-in-charge of the police station.

Presumption of possession of illicit articles: In trials, it may be presumed, unless and until the contrary is proved, that the accused has committed an offence in respect of possession of the followings:

a. Any narcotic drug or psychotropic substance;

b. Any opium poppy, cannabis plant or coca plant growing on any land which he has cultivated;

c. Any apparatus specially designed or any groups of utensils specially adopted for the manufacture of any narcotic drug or psychotropic substance; or

d. Any material which has undergone any process towards the manufacture of a narcotic drug or psychotropic substance, or any residue left of the material from which any narcotic drug or psychotropic substance has been manufactured.

Obligation of officers to assist each other: The law enforcing officers described under **power of entry, search, seizure and arrest without warrant or authorization** should assist each other in carrying out the provision of the act.

Report of arrest and seizure: The law enforcing officer who makes arrest or seizure is required to make a report within 48 hours of every arrest or seizure to his immediate superior.

Punishment or vexatious entry, search, seizure or arrest: The authorized person (officer) is punishable with imprisonment for period extendable to six months or with fine up to one thousand rupees, or with both if:

- Without reasonable ground of suspicion enters or searches, or causes to be entered or searched, any building, conveyance or place;
- Vexatiously and unnecessarily seizes the property of any person on the pretence of seizing or searching for any narcotic drug or psychotropic substance or other articles;
- Vexatiously and unnecessarily detains, searches or arrests any person.

The person wilfully and maliciously giving false information causing arrest or search is punishable with imprisonment extendable to two years or with fine or with both.

Failure of officer on duty or his connivance at the contravention of the provision of the Act: Any officer ceases or refuses to perform or withdraws from duties without written permission or lawful excuse is punishable with imprisonment up to one year or with fine or both. The officer, if wilfully aids or connives at the contravention of the provision of the Act and Rules is punishable with imprisonment up to five years and also with fine.

Liability of illicit drugs, substances, plants, articles and conveyances to confiscation: The narcotic drug, psychotropic substance, plant, material or conveyance in respect of which an offence has been committed is liable to confiscation.

The goods used for concealing illicit drugs or substances are liable to confiscation too. The sale proceeds of illicit drugs or substances are also liable to confiscation.

Procedure in making confiscation: Irrespective of accused being convicted or acquitted or discharged, the trial court decides whether the seized articles or things are liable to confiscation and if required, orders confiscation.

When article or thing is liable to confiscation, but the person committed the offence is not known or cannot be found, the trial court decides confiscation according to the following procedure:

- No order of confiscation should be passed until the expiry of one month from the date of seizure, or without hearing any person who claims the right;
- For article or thing other than narcotic drug, psychotropic substance, the opium poppy, coca plant or cannabis plant, is liable to speedy and natural decay: the Court may direct the sale at any time if the sale proceeds benefit the owner.

The person not convicted but claims the right to property of confiscated materials may appeal to the Session Court against the order of confiscation.

The central or the state governments are empowered to make rules for disposal of confiscated articles and provide for rewards to officers and informers.

Power to Tender Immunity from Prosecution

- The central or the state government may tender immunity to such person from prosecution for any offence under this Act or Rules or Indian Penal Code on condition of his making a full and true disclosure of the whole circumstances relating to contravention. The reason for having such opinion of giving immunity should be recorded in writing.
- Such person to whom tendered immunity make him immune from prosecution for any offence.

- If it appears to the central government or the state government that the person has not complied with conditions of immunity or wilfully conceals or gives false evidence, the immunity tendered can be withdrawn.

Presumption as to documents in certain cases: When any document is produced or furnished by any person or has been seized from the custody or control of any person; or has been received from any place outside India (duly authenticated) is tendered as evidence, the Court presumes the same as evidence unless the contrary is proved.

Power to call for information: The authorized officer of the central or the state government is empowered to call for information and requires any person to produce or deliver any document or thing or to examine any person in connection with the contravention of provision of legislation.

The officers concerned are granted the privilege of the non-disclosure of the source of information relating to the commission of offence.

Protection of action taken in good faith: The officers of the central government or the state government are granted immunity from civil and criminal proceedings for exercising their powers or discharging their functions or for anything done or intended to be done in good faith.

ESSENTIAL NARCOTIC DRUGS

The Government has notified certain narcotics as essential narcotic drugs in an attempt to improve their access for medical and scientific purposes. They are: Methyl morphine, Ethyl morphine and their salts (including Donine) (Except the preparations containing not more than 100 mg per dosage unit); Fentanyl and its preparations; Dihydrocodeinone, its salts and preparations; 4:4—diphenyl-6-dimethylamino–heptanone-3, its salts and preparations; Morphine, its salts and preparations, containing more than 2% morphine; and Dihydroxy Codeinone, its salts and preparations.

The provisions of these drugs are different from other narcotic drugs. The provisions related to possession, transport and other aspects are described below. The manufacture, possession, transport, import—interstate, export—interstate, sale, purchase, and consumption are regulated under licence or permit of the state government. **The state Drugs Licensing Authority (usually called State Drugs Controller) is the concerned authority.**

Manufacturing: The manufacturing license conditions are similar to license of manufacturing synthetic manufactured drugs. The state Drugs Controller is the Licensing Authority.

Possession: The maximum limit of possession by:

- Individual—one time sold or dispensed amount;

- Registered medical practitioner for his practice but not for sale—[unless more quantity authorized]. The medical practitioner needs to keep accounts;

Drug	Quantity	Drug	Quantity
Morphine, its salts and preparations containing more than 0.2%	500 mg	Dihydrocodeinone, its salts and preparations	320 mg
Methyl morphine (codeine), salts and preparations excluding not more than 100 mg of the drug per dosage unit	2000 mg	Fentinyl and its preparations	Two transdermal patches one each of 12.5 µg per hour and 25 µg per hour
Dihydroxy codeinone, salts and preparations	250 mg		

- Registered Medical Institutions—as authorized. The Government run health facilities including those of local bodies with one registered medical practitioner having at least a degree in medicine or dentistry and have training in pain relief, palliative care or substitution in opioid therapy are deemed to be recognized institutions—they do not require to apply for recognition. The private institutions do require to apply to state drugs controller. The institute needs to designate the medical officer, called designated medical officer who would be responsible.

Kerala: Any institution wising to dispense oral morphine must have at least one registered medical practitioner with a minimum period of 10 days training in palliative care.

The name of the designated medical officer will be endorsed on the certificate of recognition. The recognized medical institution needs to submit its annual requirement to the state drugs controller by 30th November of the preceding year. If requirements are more, the institution can submit the revised estimate and keep accounts of increased use with justification.

The expired drugs are to be disposed of in presence of nominated officer of the state drugs controller.

Home care facility can be provided if the patient is registered with the health institution. The designated medical officer has keep all accounts.

- *Any other person*: The Drugs Controller of the state may authorize in charge of education institute or persons engaged in research; pilot of an aircraft or captain of a ship; person in charge ambulance or first aid station or first aid.
- *Licensed chemists*: As authorized. They need to have licence from State Drugs Controller.
- *Manufacturer*: Quantity as specified in Drug Licence.
- *Government opium factory*: No Limit

Inter-state movement: The persons permitted to possess essential narcotic drugs are allowed to have inter-state export and import of the permissible quantity.

Transport: The transport is permitted with consignment note. The consignment note is not necessary if accompanied by sale documents like cash memo.

Transmission by post, courier, rail or road is permitted. The manufacturer, licensed dealer or licensed chemist are permitted to transmit on the following conditions: Sending only by registered post; accompanying by declaration containing names of consignor and consignee, contents in detail, license or authorization number of the consignee, consignee should maintain the accounts of use.

Sale: Manufacturer or licensed dealer can sell (other than prescription) can sell licensed dealer, licensed chemist, registered medical practitioner, persons authorized by state government and recognized medical institutions.

The licensed chemist can sell only on prescription. The prescription should be in writing, dated and signed by the registered medical practitioner with full name, address and registration number. The prescription should also mention the name and address of the patient, quantity of essential drugs to be supplied with daily dose and period of use.

Self-prescription is not acceptable. The condition of retail license is similar to the license issued for sale of other drugs.

Appeal: The appeal against the decision of the Drugs Controller can be made to the concerned Secretary of the government within 60 days of receiving order.

Morphine Use and Access in India

In spite of being the one of the largest producers of opium, there has been very limited access to morphine for medical use for pain management. More than one million new cases of cancer are diagnosed annually in India. Millions of cancer patients are dying of pain just because of poor access to these pain management specially morphine.

The major barriers to this poor access are identified as:

- *Stringent NDPS legislations*: NDPS rules vary from state to state requiring complicated and lengthy licencing procedure for procurement of morphine. There was a need of five separate licences.
- *Harsh punishment*: There has been fear of punishment in the event of small discretion of stock. Very few pharmacies have retail licence for sale of morphine and other medicines. Schedule X drugs require strict compliance
- Inadequate number of trained healthcare professionals [Medical Professionals and Nurses]. There has been no proper weightage of palliative care in medical and nursing curriculum.

The NDPS Amendment and changes incorporating the provision of Essential Narcotic Drugs, it is expected that there will be improvement of access to morphine for palliative care. The amendment enables medical institutes to procure morphine by obtaining a single licence from the State Drugs Controller rather than five. Kerala has better (though not full access) access to morphine compared to other states due to development of palliative care system in the state.

There is a move to legalise the Medical Use of Marijuana (Draft National Policy for Drug Demand Reduction).

OPIUM POPPY CULTIVATION AND PRODUCTION OF OPIUM AND POPPY STRAW

The opium poppy cultivation is prohibited but are cultivated on behalf of Central Government under a License issued by the Central Bureau of Narcotics (CBN). At present, the licit opium cultivation is permitted in selected tracts in three traditionally opium growing states: Madhya Pradesh, Uttar Pradesh and Rajasthan. Licenses to cultivators to cultivate opium poppy are issued in terms

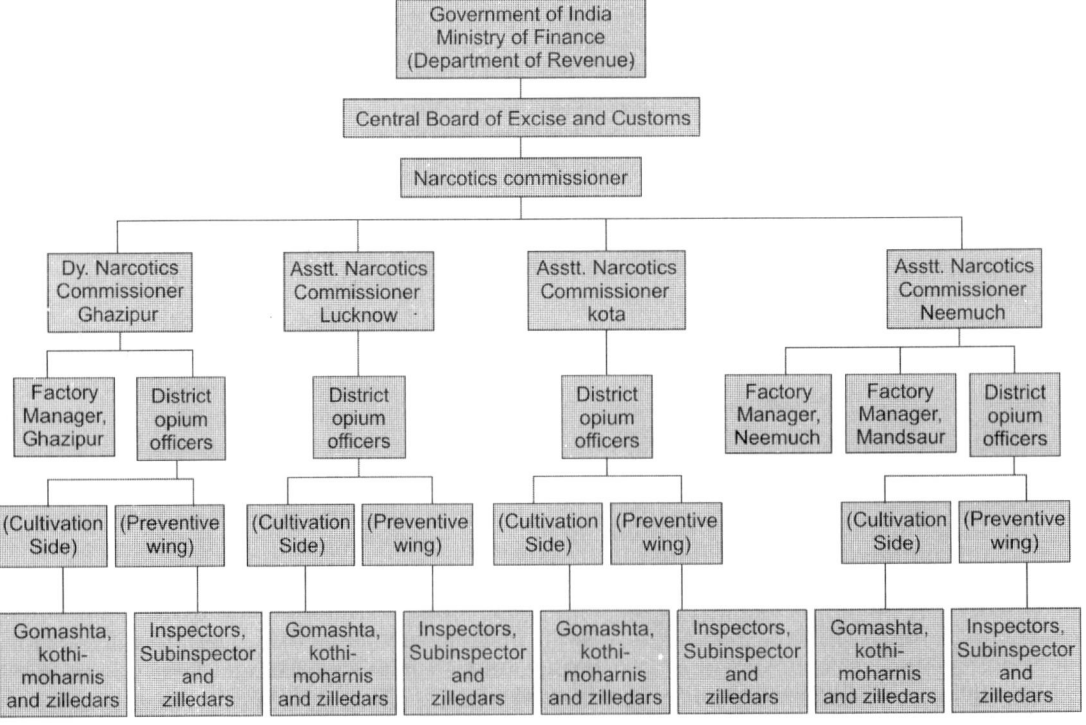

Administrative set up concerned with production and manufacture of opium.

of General Conditions relating to grant of license. The license for cultivation of opium poppy is granted by the District Opium Officer on receipt of a payment of fee of ₹ 25/- only. Normally the settlement operation is held in the month of October–November every year.

General Conditions for grant of license for cultivation of opium (1st day of October 2015 to 30th day of September 2016) (The Gazette of India: Extraordinary, October 5, 2015):

1. Place of cultivation: Notified tract.
2. Eligibility for cultivation: The following are eligible for a license:
   a. Cultivators who had cultivated opium poppy during the crop year 2014–2015 and tendered an average yield of opium of not less than 56 kg/hectre in the state of Madhya Pradesh and Rajasthan and an average yield of opium of not less than 52 kg/hectre in the state of Uttar Pradesh.
   b. Cultivators who ploughed back their entire opium poppy crop cultivated during the crop year 2013–2014 and 2014–2015 but not similarly ploughed in 2012–2013 under the supervision of CBN.
   c. Cultivators whose appeal against refusal of license has been allowed after the last date of settlement in the crop year 2014–2015.
   d. Cultivators who cultivated opium poppy in the crop year 2012–2013 or during any subsequent crop year and were eligible for a license in the following crop year, but did not voluntarily obtain a license for the following crop year, did not actually cultivate opium poppy due to any reason.
   e. Cultivators who are the legal heirs of deceased eligible cultivators. (The District Opium Officer decides one legal heir in case of more than one legal heir).
3. **Conditions of License:** No cultivator is granted license unless he/she satisfies that:
   a. Cultivator did not exceed the area licensed during the crop year 2014–2015 beyond the '5% Condonable Limit' allowed by the licensing policy.

   b. Cultivator did not resort any time to illicit cultivation of opium poppy and was not charged for any offence under the NDPS Act and Rules.
   c. Cultivator did not violate any departmental instructions issued by CBN/NC during the crop year 2014–2015.
   d. Cultivator did not tender adulterated opium or inferior quality [Inferior Quality means: Opium with morphine strength of less than 0.9% as dry basis; ash content of over 4.5%; any amount of starch, sugar, gum tannin, etc.].
4. **Maximum Area:** (100 Ares = 1 hectare)
   a. All eligible cultivators—10 Ares.
      – The cultivators who tendered average yield of 58 kg/hectre and above— 15 Ares.
      – The cultivators who tendered average yield of 60 kg/hectre and above— 20 Ares.
      – The cultivators who tendered average yield of 65 kg/hectre and above— 25 Ares.
      – The cultivators can cultivate in an area less than the licensed area.
   b. Cultivators can sow opium in not more than 2 plots.
5. **Forewarning:**
   a. A minimum qualifying yield (MQY) of 58 kg/hectre in Madhya Pradesh and Rajasthan and 52 kg/hectre in Uttar Pradesh must be tendered during the crop year 2015–2016 to become eligible for a license to cultivate opium poppy in the following year (2016–2017).
   b. Morphine content of the opium tendered during 2015–2016 may become the basis for payment for the crop year 2015–2016 and eligible for license in crop year 2016–2017.
   c. Cultivators who had fully ploughed back their entire poppy during crop year 2013–2014 and 2014–2015 would not be entitled for license in the crop year 2016–2017, if they also uprooted their crop fully in the crop year 2015–2016.

d. Cultivators, whose opium for the crop year 2015–2016 is found to be 'water mixed' and of consistency lower than 55 degrees will not be eligible for a license in the next crop year 2016–2017.

e. Cultivators whose opium for the crop year 2015–2016 is found to be adulterated and classified as 'inferior' by the Government Opium and Alkaloid Works, Neemuch or Ghazipur will not be eligible for license in the next crop year 2016–2017.

6. **Condonable Limit:** up to 5% in excess of licensed area.

7. **Miscellaneous:**

a. Any cultivator who cultivates opium poppy during 2015–2016 not on his own land but in the land leased from others needs to provide the details of owner of the plot, survey number any other details as directed by the NC.

b. The General Licensing Conditions are without prejudice to the right of the NC/DNC to issue or withhold a license when appropriate.

c. Any field may be taken over for any research that may be conducted by the government directly or in collaboration with any specialized institution or agency. The area taken over for research will not be taken into account while calculating the yield. The cultivator whose filed is selected for research will be considered for license next year if the stipulated MQY is tendered.

d. Any filed may be selected for obtaining poppy straw without extraction of opium. Cultivators whose fields are selected will be eligible for a license for next crop year.

e. The quantity of opium tendered by a farmer will be calculated at 70° consistency, on the basis of analysis by the Government Opium and Alkaloid Works, Neemuch or Ghazipur.

Procedure

1. **Measurement:** From the end of each year, the CBN officers start exercising statutory control. They measure each and every field to check excess cultivation than the licensed area. This exercise is known as measurement. The measurement is conducted by sub-inspector with the help of one sepoy. The condonable limit in respect of excess in cultivated area shall not exceed 5% of the licensed area. The measuring officer is required to record details of the cultivators, area found excess in his field book, joint license and miniature license. The in-charge of the measurement party can get excess cultivation uprooted under his supervision. No panchnama would be drawn but the in-charge of the party would enter the details of the uprooted area in the joint license against the name of the concerned cultivator. In case, the cultivator refuses to uproot excess cultivation, beyond the condonable limit, then a regular panchnama is drawn and the details thereof mentioned in the joint license as well as individual license. In such cases, measures are taken for immediate cancellation of the license of the cultivator and the whole crop uprooted under departmental supervision.

Towards the end of measurement operation, a percentage of these fields is taken up for test measurement to detect any discrepancies.

2. **Crop Damage:** Opium crop may suffer some damage due to natural calamity, rains, hailstorm, plant diseases, etc. Such damage occurs prior to lancing the capsules and post-lancing. To give relief to these cultivators whose opium crop had been damaged due to natural calamities, they are allowed to get their unlanced damaged crop uprooted under departmental supervision. A cultivator can get his damaged crop uprooted before lancing commenced, provided the area to be uprooted is not less than 10% of the plot, subject to the minimum of one Are (100 Ares = 1 hectare). No uprooting is permitted after lancing has commenced in a particular plot. Partial uprooting is permitted but not in patches. For each

partial and full uprooting, panchnama are to be drawn and entry made in the joint as well as individual license.

3. **Collection:** In the month of February–March, the opium capsule is ready for lancing or extraction of opium by incision of opium capsule. That latex that oozes out of the capsule is collected by the cultivator on daily basis and the weight of such opium is recorded in a register called Preliminary Weighment Register (PWR) maintained by the village Lambardar. CBN staff periodically checks the entries in PWR against the physical stock with the cultivator and in case of any discrepancy, action against the cultivator is taken. [The capsule is the most important organ of the plant as it provides raw opium—a milky exudates. It contains about 70% of the total morphine synthesized by the plant. The terminal capsule is, in general, richer in morphine content than the lateral ones. The lancing is the longitudinal or circumferencial cut/incison by an instrument, of the capsule at appropriate stage. The lancing operation is performed by skilled workers in the afternoon so that a crust is formed on the surface of freshly exudated latex due to hot sun.]

4. **Dealing with Excess:** Where excess quantity is recovered of more than 3 kg, appropriate action like seizure, arrest, etc. is initiated.

5. **Procurement (Weighment)**
   Preliminary Weighment: The cultivator is required to produce each day's collection of the opium before the Lambardar. The Lambardar makes arrangement to weigh such opium and makes necessary entries in the records maintained by him. The cultivator and the Lambardar should sign the entries with signature or thumb impression. The proper officer checks the collection and the entry in the register and enquires into the variation.

   By the end of March, the collection of opium from the plant is almost complete. The cultivator is required to produce whole opium of the land cultivated with opium poppy to the District Opium Officer. CBN sets up procurement centres (also known as **Weighment Centres**) for the collection of this opium. The Weighment Centres are normally set up within the vicinity of the growing villages.

6. **Classification of produce:** When the opium is tendered, two very small samples are taken: (i) for hot air oven testing; (ii) for testing the presence of sugar, starch and gum, etc. The oven test method basically comprises drawal of a very small sample from the opium produce of each cultivator and heating of the sample in an oven to evaporate the moisture.

   Then the opium is classified by the District Opium Officer in different grades based on consistence of the opium. The class is announced publicly.

7. **Payment to the cultivator:** Based on the classification, 90% payment to the cultivator is made. [The good opium is then sent to the Government Opium Factory where it is again tested for its consistence, quality, presence of impurities and adulterants by the Chemical Staff. Based on classification, balance payment is made or excess amount recovered.]

8. **Role of Lambardar:** The District Opium Officer designates one of the cultivators of the village as Lambardar. The function of Lambardar is specified by the Narcotics Commissioner.

   a. The measurement of cultivated land is done by the proper officer in the presence of the cultivator and the Lambardar. Lambardar needs to authenticate the entry along with the cultivator in token of having satisfied themselves regarding correctness of the measurement.

   b. The Lambardar makes arrangement to weigh daily produce of the cultivator and make necessary entry in records. He maintains this record with attestation by the cultivator and himself. However, the produce indicated by the Lambardar is subjected to check by the appropriate officer.

c. The weighment, examination and classification of the opium is done by the District Opium Officer in the presence of Lambardar and the cultivator.

d. Where the cultivator is dissatisfied with the classification of District Opium Officer, the aggrieved cultivator may send the sample separately after sealing the produce in the presence of the officer and the Lambardar.

e. When the opium delivered to the District Opium Officer is suspected to be adulterated, it should be separately forwarded to the Government Opium Factory after proper sealing in the presence of the cultivator and Lambardar.

9. **Grievance Redress Mechanisms**:
   a. Where the cultivator is dissatisfied with the classification of opium done by the District Opium Officer, he may have it forwarded to the Government Opium Factory separately, after having it properly sealed in his presence and the presence of the concerned Lambardar.

   b. Person aggrieved by the decision or order of Government Opium Factory may appeal to the Chief Controller of Factories within 30 days of such decision or order.

   c. Relating to Licensing: The aggrieved person has provision to appeal to the Deputy Narcotics Commissioner or Narcotics Commissioner within 30 days from the date of communication of the order.

MANUFACTURE, SALE AND EXPORT OF OPIUM

Manufacture

Opium is manufactured by the Central Government Opium Factories only. These factories are located at Ghazipur (Uttar Pradesh) and Neemuch (Madhya Pradesh) and are independent control of the Chief Controller of Factories, whose headquarters at Gwalior and New Delhi. A part of opium is converted to alkaloids for supply to manufactures of the medicines.

The state governments may permit the manufacture of opium mixtures from lawfully possessed opium.

Sale to State Governments or Manufacturing Chemists

- The sale is only from Government Opium Factory, Ghazipur.
- The sale to the manufacturing chemist is only under a permit of the concerned state government. The permit is issued in quadruplicate: Quadruplicate copy for the issuing authority and the remaining three copies are forwarded to the opium factory. The factory retains the duplicate copy for record, sends the original copy with the consignment of the opium and returns the triplicate copy to the permit issuing authority after endorsement of actual quantity supplied and the date of dispatch.

The price of opium for sale is fixed by the central government.

MANUFACTURED DRUGS

- The manufacture of crude cocaine, ecgonine and its salts and diacetyl morphine and its salts is generally prohibited. However, the drugs can be manufactured by Government Opium Factory or by chemical staff employed under Central Board of Excise and Customs or any person authorized by the Narcotics Commissioner by special license for medical and scientific purposes. The Narcotic Commissioner needs to consult the DCGI before issuing license.

- **Manufacture of natural manufactured drugs:**
  - The manufacture of cocaine hydrochloride is only permissible by the chemical staff employed under the Central Board of Excise and Customs from confiscated cocaine.
  - The manufacture of morphine, codeine, dionine, thebaine, dihydrocodeinone, dihydromorphine, dihydromorphinone, dihydro-hydroxycodeinone, pholocodine

and their respective salts are permissible by the Government Opium Factory.

– The manufacture of medicinal hemp is permissible under a license by the state government.

- **Manufacture of synthetic manufactured drugs:** The manufacture of manufactured drug is prohibited except under and in accordance of license granted by NC. A fee of ₹ 50 is payable in advance for each license.

- **Requirements for issuing license:**
  - The applicant should have license to manufacture, possess, sale and distribution of drugs;
  - Deposited ₹ 5000 as security for the due observance of the condition of the license;
  - Furnished proof of having land, building and other paraphernalia to properly carry out the business including of good financial standing.

    The quantity of drugs permitted to be manufactured is based on quantity allotted by the State Government for processing; quantity required for supply to other firms within or outside the country and the quantity required for reasonable inventory. The total quantity of the drug manufactured during any one year does not exceed the estimated requirements of this country as furnished to the International Narcotics Control Board.

- **Conditions of license**
  - The licensee will not manufacture the drug except from materials which he lawfully possesses.
  - The licensee will ensure security arrangement in the manufacturing premises.
  - The licensee will give at least 15 days notice in writing to the issuing authority on commencing the manufacture; 15 days notice for stopping manufacturing. He should also inform the propose date to recommence manufacture. If the period of cessation of manufacture exceeds 30 days, the licensing authority may prohibit further manufacture.

- The licensee will not possess or sale or distribute the drug other than the rules framed by the state government.
- The licensee will maintain true accounts of all transactions including the accounts of materials used for the manufacture of the drug, the quantities manufactured, sold or disposed off and furnish returns.
- The licensee should allow inspection, by the authorized officer of stocks, materials used, accounts and records of transactions. A serially numbered Inspection Book is to be maintained.
- The licensee can surrender license by giving not less than 15 days time.

- **Suspension or revocation of license:** The issuing authority may suspend or cancel a license in the following conditions:
  - License is transferred or sublet without the prior approval; or
  - In the event of any breach of any condition of license; or
  - Licensee is convicted for offence related to narcotic drugs.

    However, the licensee is given an opportunity to be heard before suspension or revocation of license.

    The licensee may file an appeal against the order of suspension or revocation to the Narcotic Commissioner or the Board within 30 days from the date of communication. Every appeal must be submitted along with the copy of the order. The Appellate Authority after hearing the appeal may pass order confirming, modifying or annulling the decision as it thinks appropriate.

- **Disposal of stocks:** The stocks which may remain in possession of the licensee on the expiry or cancellation or surrendering of license can be disposed of as specified by the Narcotics Commissioner.

IMPORT, EXPORT AND TRANSHIPMENT OF NARCOTIC DRUGS AND PSYCHOTROPIC SUBSTANCES

In general, the import and export of Narcotic Drugs and Psychotropic Substances specified in Schedule I of The Narcotic Drugs and Psychotropic Substances Rules is prohibited. However, the import with import certificate and export with export authorization is permissible for medical and scientific purposes.

The import or export through post office or through bank is prohibited.

Import

- The import of opium, concentrate of opium straw; and morphine, codeine, thebaine and their salts are prohibited except by the Government Opium Factory.
- The importation of narcotic drugs and psychotropic substances can be done with an import certificate. The import can be divided into two types: Import of narcotic drugs and import of psychotropic substances. While applying for import certificate for narcotic drugs, the applicant has to submit the original or certified copy of the excise permit issued by the state government.
- Issue of Import Certificate: The seven copies of the import certificate are issued by the issuing authority.
  - Original and one duplicate copy are supplied to importer. The original copy is meant for sending to the exporting country and the duplicate copy for producing at Customs House, Land Customs Station or Airport where the consignment arrives. The duplicate copy is to be shown at the post office of the delivery if import is by parcel post.
  - The Collector of Customs or the Postmaster makes the necessary entry in the duplicate copy confirming the import and returns the copy to importer. The importer indicates that he has received the goods.
  - The endorsed duplicate copy is to be returned to the issuing authority: through State Excise Department in case of narcotic drugs and through State Drugs Controller in case of psychotropic substances.
  - The triplicate copy is to be sent to the Collector of Customs who in turn

returns the same with endorsement of actual quantity cleared and a copy of export authorization received at the time of receiving consignment.
  - The fourth (quadruplicate) copy is sent to the Excise Authority of the state government in case of narcotic drugs and the copy is to be sent to the State Drugs Controller in case of psychotropic substances.
  - The fifth (quintuplicate) copy is to be sent to the exporting country.
  - The sixth (sextulplicate) copy is to be sent to the DCGI.
  - The seventh (septuplicate) copy is to be retained in the issuing authority's office. The importation of the quantity is allowed in more than one consignment.

Transit: No consignment of any narcotic drugs or psychotropic substance is allowed to be transited through India unless accompanied by the valid export authorization issued by the Government of Exporting Country. However, the small quantities of such narcotic drugs and psychotropic substances essential for medical purposes to individuals can be carried by the ship or aircraft.

Export: Export of specified quantities of narcotic drugs or psychotropic substances or preparations containing such drugs or substances are permitted by Narcotics Commissioner on the basis of special import license issued by the importing country. The shipment of such consignment should be accompanied by special import license duly endorsed by the NC.

Export Authorization:
  - Narcotic Drug: The exporter applicant has to submit the original or authenticated copy of the excise permit issued by the state government.
  - The applicant has also to submit the original import certificate issued by the government of importing country.

The export authorization certificate is issued in five copies:
- The original is for the consignor and has to accompany the consignment;

- The duplicate copy is to be forwarded to the Collector of Customs of the port who will return the copy with endorsement indicating the date of export and the quantity exported;
- The triplicate should be forwarded to the government of importing country;
- The quadruplicate copy should be forwarded to the state's excise authority;
- The quintuplicate copy is for office record.

When the consignment is to be transshipped or transited through other countries, additional copies of the export authorization is to be made and sent to the concerned countries.

Transhipment and Diversion of Consignment: Transhipment at any port is permissible only with permission of the Collector of Customs. The Collector permits only when the consignment is accompanied by the valid export authorization issued by the exporting country.

- The Collector takes due measure to prevent the diversion of such consignment to a destination other than that named in export authorization.
- The Collector of Customs, however, permits diversion to another country on the production of export authorization, as if the diversions are exported from India to the country, or territory of new destination.
- The Collector of Customs informs the issuing authority regarding the actual quantity and the diversion of the consignment. The issuing authority then informs the country from which the export of the consignment originated.

PSYCHOTROPIC SUBSTANCES

- **General Prohibition:** The manufacture, possession, transport, import interstate, export interstate, sale, purchase, consumption and use of psychotropic substances specified in Schedule I are prohibited.
- **Manufacture:**
  - The manufacture of psychotropic substances (not specified in Schedule I) is

permissible under a license from State Drugs Control Authority.
  - The State Drugs Control Authority, usually State Drugs Controller (Licensing Authority) limits the quantity of substances to be manufactured in consultation with DCGI and other factors such as requirements of the whole country, requirements of the state, quantities required to be supplied to outside the state and requirements for reasonable inventory.
  - The quantity to be manufactured in a year is specified in the Licensing Authority.
  - The manufacture of psychotropic substances specified in Schedule I are permitted by the Licensing Authority in consultation with NC.
- **Possession:**
  - The possession of psychotropic substances by individuals is permitted only under license Drugs and Cosmetics Rules 1945.
  - The possession of reasonable quantity by the research institution; or hospital or dispensary maintained or supported by government or local body or by charity or voluntary subscription; or by individuals is permissible as necessary for their genuine scientific or medical requirements or both. However, for individual possession for medical use of more than one hundred dosage units at a time is not permissible.
  - The research institution, hospital and dispensary needs to maintain the record of purchase and consumption of psychotropic substances.
- **Transport:**
  - Transport, import interstate or export interstate is permitted only if the consignment is accompanied by a consignment note.
  - The consignment note should be prepared in triplicate. The original and duplicate copies are to be sent along with the consignment of psychotropic

substances to the consignee. The consignee returns the duplicate copy after endorsing the receipt of quantity in both original and duplicate copy. The consignor makes the necessary entry, based on the duplicate copy received back, on the triplicate copy.

– The consignee and the consignor should keep the consignment note for a period of two years. The consignment notes may be inspected by Central Government Authorized Officer.

- **Special Provision for Medical and Scientific Purposes:**
  - A narcotic drug and psychotropic substance may be used for:
    - Scientific requirement including analytical requirement of any government laboratory or any research institution in India or abroad.
    - Very limited requirements of a foreigner by a duly authorized person of a hospital or any other government approved establishment.
    - The purpose of de-addiction of drug addicts by government or local body or by an approved charity or voluntary organization or by any central government approved institution.
  - The person performing medical or scientific functions should keep records concerning the acquisition and use of these substances. These records are to be preserved for two years.
  - A narcotic drug and psychotropic substance may be supplied or dispensed for use to a foreigner on medical prescription only by the authorized licensed pharmacists or other authorized distributor.

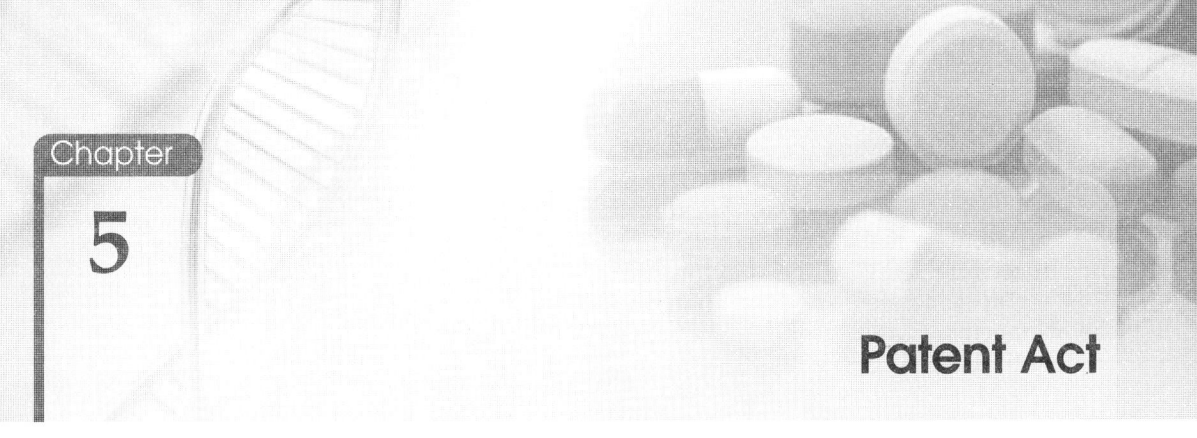

Patent Act

"The Patent System adds the fuel of interest to the fire of genius."

— *Abraham Lincoln*

After reading this chapter, you should be able to understand and appreciate:

- Genesis and revision of Patent Act
- Inventions that are patentable
- Inventions that are not patentable
- Procedure of patenting
- Patent system in other countries
- Provision of compulsory licensing safeguarding the country's interest

Throughout the history of mankind, the inventors or scientists have been rewarded for their hard work, time and resource spent on research in one form or other. This reward motivates or encourages further research leading to more inventions. Granting patent is one such reward. Drug discovery and development is a complex and risky business requiring huge investments. It takes about 10–15 years for developing a new drug costing on an average USD 2.6 billion (2014). Over successive generations, innovations resulting from research have dramatically improved life expectancy and quality of life. However, the benefits of these innovations are not reaching the population with greatest speed. The patent protection is a hindrance to the accessibility of innovations. What is technically possible, however, has not always been accessible. The patent protection often alleged to have threatened the HIV treatment in many countries. Treatment is available but not affordable. A monopoly! The inventions can become property and can therefore be owned and sold, has encouraged scientists and researchers to invent. This allows entrepreneurs and companies to invest in inventions by allowing them to profit from the resulting technologies. On the other hand, it threatens the public health. Thus probably there should be search for balance between making all knowledge freely available within the public domain and granting ownership of valuable discoveries to the inventors. Historically, it has been seen that this balance encourages investment and reinvestment in innovations, although this innovation too infrequently is directed towards the needs of the poor.

The history of patents and patent laws is believed to have started in Italy with a Venetian Statute of 1474 which provided legal protection for 10 years period against potential infringers. The patent law in India can be traced back to British Period and the first legislation was the Act VI of 1856. The objective of this legislation was to encourage inventions of new and useful manufactures and to induce inventors to disclose secret of their inventions. This was repealed and consolidated on many occasions. Later, the Indian Patents and Designs Act, 1911 was introduced replacing all the previous Acts. This Act brought patent administration under the management of Controller of Patents for the first time. This Act was also amended.

Types of Patents

1. Product patents: Claim the Active Pharmaceutical Ingredient (API). They are the strongest patents.
2. Product-by-process patents: Define the product by its process of preparation.
3. Process patents: Claim a new production process for an API.
4. Formulation Patents: Relate to the specific dosage form.
5. Combination Patents: Claim the combination of new or existing medicine.
6. Patent on Product Derivative: Claim a specific form or derivative.
7. Patents containing Markush Claims: Refer to a chemical structure with multiple alternatives.

[*Source*: Patent Situation of Key Products for Treatment of Hepatitis C, Sofosbuvir, World Health Organization, March 2015].

After independence, when it was realised that the Indian Patents and Designs Act, 1911 was not fulfilling its objective and there was a necessity to enact comprehensive patent law owing to substantial changes in political and economic conditions in the country, the Government of India constituted a committee under the Chairmanship of Justice (Dr) Bakshi Tek Chand, a retired Judge of Lahore High Court, in 1949 to review the patent law in India in order to ensure that the patent system is conducive to the national interest. The terms of reference included:

- To survey and report on the working of the patent system in India;
- To examine the existing patent legislation in India and to make recommendations for improving it, particularly with reference to the provisions concerned with the prevention of abuse of patent rights;
- To consider whether any special restrictions should be imposed on patent regarding food and medicine;
- To suggest steps for ensuring effective publicity to the patent system and to patent literature, particularly as regards patents obtained by Indian inventors;
- To consider the necessity and feasibility of setting up a National Patents Trust;
- To consider the desirability or otherwise of regulating the profession of patent agents;
- To examine the working of the Patent Office and the services rendered by it to the public and make suitable recommendations for improvement; and
- To report generally on any improvement that the Committee thinks fit to recommend for enabling the Indian Patent System to be more conducive to national interest by encouraging invention and the commercial development and use of inventions.

The committee submitted its interim report on 4th August, 1949 with recommendations for prevention of misuse or abuse of patent right in India and suggested amendments of the Patents and Designs Act, 1911 on the lines of the United Kingdom Acts. The committee also observed that the Patents Act should contain clear indication to ensure that food and medicine and surgical and curative devices are made available to the public at the cheapest price commensurate with giving reasonable compensation to the patentee.

Based on the recommendation of the committee, the 1911 Act was amended in 1950 mainly in relation to working of inventions and compulsory license/revocation. In 1957, the Government of India appointed Justice N. Rajagopala Ayyangar Committee to examine the question of revision of the Patent Law and advise government accordingly. The first part of the report described the evils the patent system and solution with recommendations in regards to the law. The committee recommended retention of the Patent System, despite its shortcomings. This report recommended major changes in the law which formed the basis of the introduction of the Patents Bill, 1965. This bill was introduced in the Lok Sabha on 21st September, 1965, which however lapsed. In 1967, again an amended bill was introduced which was referred to a Joint Parliamentary Committee and on the final recommendation of the Committee, the Patents Act, 1970 was passed. This Act repealed and replaced the 1911 Act so far as the patents law was concerned. However, the 1911 Act continued to be applicable to designs. Most of the provisions of the 1970 Act were brought into force on 20 th April 1972 with publication of the Patent Rules, 1972.

The Act was remained unchanged for almost 24 years without any change till December 1994 (post-economic liberalised period). Though in between two ordinances were issued, the major change was brought by the Patents (Amendment) Act, 1999 with retrospective effect from 1st January, 1995 providing provision for filing of applications for product patents in the areas of drugs, pharmaceuticals and agro chemicals though such patents were not allowed. However, such applications were to be examined only after 31-12-2004. Meanwhile, the applicants could be allowed Exclusive Marketing Rights (EMR) to sell or distribute these products in India, subject to fulfilment of certain conditions. Then subsequent amendment was brought as the Patents (Amendment) Act, 2002 which was effective from 20th May 2003 with the introduction of the new Patent Rules, 2003. The third amendment to the Patents Act 1970 was introduced through the Patents (Amendment) Ordinance, 2004 w.e.f. 1st January, 2005 and the ordinance was later replaced by the Patents (Amendment) Act 2005 brought into force from 1-1-2005.

The new patent regimen has led to the return of pharmaceutical multinationals, many of which had left India during 1970s. The multinational companies are now looking at India not only for its traditional strength in manufacturing but also as a highly attractive location for research and development, particularly in the conduct of clinical trials and other services.

The Patent Act as applicable to drugs and pharmaceuticals is only discussed. The Central Government is empowered to make rules for implementing the Act and regulating Patent Administration. Controller General of Patent Designs and Trademarks functioning under the Department of Industrial Policy and Promotions, Ministry of Commerce is the Administrative Authority for the Patent Act. The office of the Controller General of Patent Designs and Trademarks is located at Mumbai. There are four patent offices at present: Kolkata, Delhi, Chennai and Mumbai. The Kolkata office is the main patent office in the country.

A patent is a statutory right for an invention granted, by the Government to the inventor who has obtained the patent (known as patentee), in exchange of full disclosure of the invention, excluding others from making, using, selling, importing the patented product or process for producing that product without the patentee's consent. An invention relating either to a product or process is patentable if the invention meet the following criteria:

- It should be new (not published anywhere, not in public knowledge or public use, not claimed before in any specification),
- It should have inventive step or it must be non-obvious (technical advancement comparing to the existing knowledge, or have economic significance or both, or not obvious to persons skilled in the art),
- It should be capable of industrial application, and
- It should not fall under the categories of non-patentable items.

Though generally, patent filing is not allowed for the invention which has been published or publicly displayed, the Patent Act provides a grace period of 12 months for filing of patent application from the date of publication or public display or disclosure.

Even though the inventions comply with all requirements of patent like novelty, inventive step and utility criteria, **the following categories of inventions are not patentable under Patent Act:**

- Frivolous inventions or which claim anything obviously contrary to well-established natural laws (Machines that give more than 100% performance—perpetual motion machines).

- The primary use or commercial exploitation is contrary to law or morality or injurious to public health (gambling machine, house breaking device, beverage containing cancer producing substance even if it has good nutrition value).

- Mere discovery of scientific principles or the formulation of an abstract theory (Newton's Law, discovery of micro-organisms, discovery of natural gas). Genetically modified microorganisms are patentable.

- Mere discovery of a new form of a known substance which does not result in the enhancement of the known efficacy of that substance (Salts, esters, polymorphs, isomers, etc.). Salts, esters, ethers, polymorphs, metabolite, pure forms, particle size, isomers, complexes, combinations and derivatives of a known substance with enhanced efficacy are patentable. This provision falls under Section 3(d) of the Patent Act. The words 'enhanced efficacy' does not allow 'ever greening' of patents. The ever greening indicates extending the life of a patent beyond the 20 years by tweaking the molecule marginally, such as polymorph, crystalline, micronized, etc. This was a protecting clause and an interesting case related to this (Case of Glivec) is given in the box.

- Mere discovery of a new property; or mere new use for a known substance; or mere use of a known process machine unless such known process results in a new product form of a known substance which does not result in enhancement of known efficacy of that substance (new use of aspirin in heart ailments, new uses of neem).

- Substance obtained by mere admixture resulting only in the aggregation of the properties of the components thereof or a process for producing such substance (just combination of two medicines like paracetamol and ibuprofen). On the other hand, if combination is synergistic or if the formulation is unique like sustained release or novel drug delivery system are patentable.

- Mere arrangement and rearrangement or duplication of features of known devices, each functioning independently of one another in a known way (a clock and radio in a single cabinet).

- Method or process of testing during the process of manufacture for rendering the apparatus/machine more efficient (determination of chlorine content in production of chlorinated water).

- Method of agriculture or horticulture (producing new form of a known plant). Agriculture equipment is patentable.

- Process for medicinal, surgical, curative, prophylactic, diagnostic, therapeutic or other treatment of human beings or a similar treatment of animals to render them free of disease or to increase their economic value or that of their products (removal of cancer tumour, surgical process, method of vaccination). Surgical, therapeutic or diagnostic apparatus are patentable.

- Plants and animals in whole or any part thereof other than microorganisms, but including seeds, varieties and species and essentially biological process for production or propagation of plants and animals (Clones and new varieties of plants, a process for production of plants or animals if it consists entirely of natural phenomena such as crossing or selection).

- Mathematical method, business method, algorithms or computer programme per se. However, the new calculating machine is patentable.

- A literary, dramatic, musical or artistic work or any other aesthetic creation including cinematographic work and television productions: These subject matters fall under the copyright protection.

- Mere scheme or rule or method of performing mental act or method of playing game (method of teaching/learning). Novel apparatus for playing game or carrying out a scheme is patentable.

- Presentation of information (spoken words, visual display, power points).
- Topography of integrated circuits.
- Traditional knowledge or an aggregation or duplication of known properties of traditionally known component or components (Traditional Knowledge already in public domain—wound healing property of Haldi). Extraction of Azadirachtin from Neem can be patented—value addition leads to new process or product.
- Inventions relating to atomic energy (nuclear reactors, uranium).

The Story of Glivec Patent!

The Supreme Court's ruling on 1st April 2013 against challenge of the Swiss multinational pharmaceutical company, Novartis, is a public victory. Novartis has been challenging the provision of Indian Patent Act arguing for patent of its anti-cancer drug, Glivec. The Supreme Court dismissing the petition of Novartis upheld the public health provision of Indian Patent Act benefiting millions of patients not only in India but also around the globe.

While amending the Patent Act to comply with the obligations of World Trade Organization (WTO), the Indian Parliament kept a provision under Section 3(d) of the Act as a public health measure to safeguard the interest of poor patients against the misuse of patents. The Section 3(d) restricts patents for already known drugs unless the new claims are superior in efficacy. The pharma companies have been trying to extend the patent of their patented molecules by making slight and trivial changes to the existing original molecule. Glivec is chemically imatinib mesylate and is an excellent drug for leukemia, commonly called blood cancer. The imatinib mesylate is the salt form of the original molecule, imatinib. This is known as Gleevec in USA.

The Supreme Court observed that the original patent application filed in USA in 1994 had covered the imatinib mesylate as well as imatinib. In India, Novartis Pharma was trying to get patent for the beta crystalline variety of imatinib mesylate. Against the Novartis claim "Better physico-chemical qualities such as shape of the molecule, flowability, hygroscopicity and solubility satisfy the test for enhanced efficacy", the Supreme Court clarified "Physico-chemical properties of beta crystalline form of imatinib mesylate with improved flow properties, decreased hygroscopicity, and improved thermodynamic stability may be beneficial to the patients but they do not meet the standard of efficacy as required under Section 3(d). This new form of Glivec has patent in many countries including USA, Russia and China.

Novartis first patented imatinib in 1994. Once India signed WTO's Trade Related Intellectual Property Rights (TRIPS) agreement, it had applied for patent for mesylate salt form of imatinib in 1998 at Chennai Patent Office. The patent office rejected the application based on Section 3(d) of Patent (Amendment) Act 2005. Novartis then approached the Madras High Court challenging the decision of Chennai patent office and questioned the provision of the section. The Madras High Court rejected the Novartis challenge in 2007 but referred the case to the Intellectual Property Appellate Board (IPAB), which in turn rejected the application. The rejected Novartis finally approached Supreme Court of the country in 2009 and the Supreme Court finally dismissed Novartis's challenge. Dismissing the petition with cost the Supreme Court clarified that applicants of patent have to meet the standards of Section 3(d) of Indian Patent Act before they can get the patent under Indian Law".

At the time when Novartis got the patent in 1994 in USA, there was no product patent in India and hence, no patent was made available in India. This led to generic version of the molecule in the market reducing the treatment cost substantially. The generic products were made available at less than one-tenth of Novartis's price. The beta crystalline salt of the molecule is claimed to have improved bioavailability and such changes in old molecule is patentable in USA and Europe, often called ever greening patenting. Had the new beta crystalline form got a patent in India, the company's monopoly for marketing would be another 20 years and a big market as there would be no generic supply from India. Currently the cost of treatment of blood cancer with this generic version is Rs. 8000 per month while the cost with Novartis product would be Rs. 1.2 Lakh per month.

While the Supreme Court's judgment is welcomed worldwide, the critics have their own logic, but are unjustified. The critics say "India has killed medical innovation". Drug development is risky, requires enormous resources and progress comes step by step with one incremental innovation at a time. This incremental innovation too deserves patent. If no patent, no profit and no investment! No investment means no new drug. Without patent protection, an innovator company may not earn back the invested amount in Research and Development. It is also argued that this is not going to help the poor as more than 85% of Indian patients have been provided free Glivec.

But this was not just the case of Glivec alone and the judgment will have affect on many more drugs. This would facilitate early entry of generic medicines into the market for many other medicines. Earlier India rejected the patents of anti-HIV drugs on the grounds of mere modifications. Had Novartis won, it would have made provision for ever greening patents in India like USA and that would have provided patent for the new form with 20 years monopoly to market the medicine at a price of its choice. Now the judgment would prevent other companies approaching India for similar patents and India would continue to manufacture and supply low cost generic versions benefiting people worldwide.

[This is abstracted from author's write up in OrissaPost: Patent Medicine: Battle Finally Won! Dated 3rd April 2013]

Patenting procedure: The successive stages are:

- Filing patent application in prescribed form with the concerned patent office either with complete specification or with provisional specification along with prescribed fees. If filing with provisional specification, then complete specification is to be provided within 12 months.

- Formality checking by patent office and application number is given by the office.

- Publication in official journal after 18 months of secrecy (date of application, number, name and address of the applicant, and an abstract). Now the interested person gets the details on payment. When no secrecy is required, publication can be obtained within one month.

- Request for examination within 48 months of date of filing: The patent examiner within 1 to 3 months submits report to the patent controller on whether the claimed invention is not prohibited from grant of patent, whether the invention meets the criteria of patentability.

- First examination report containing gists of objections is issued within 6 months of filing of request.

- Response from the applicant: The applicant has to meet the requirements of the objections within 12 months.

- If objections are met, the grant of patent is approved by patent controller within 1 month.

- Pre-grant Opposition: After publication of grant of patent, an opposition can be filed within a period of 6 months. Opportunity of hearing the opponent is also available.

- Examination of pre-grant opposition: The opposition document is sent to the applicant. A period of 3 months is allowed for response. After examining the opposition and the submissions made during the hearing, Controller may
  - Either reject the opposition and grant the patent

- Or accept the opposition and modify/reject the patent application

  This is to be done within a period of 1 month from the date of completion of opposition proceedings.

- Grant of Patent: A certificate of patent is issued within 7 days. Then grant of patent is published in the official journal.

  Once a patent is granted, the patent can be kept in force for the full term by paying the prescribed fees. If patents are not renewed, it lapses and becomes public property. However, there is provision for restoration of a lapsed patent if applied for restoration within 18 months of lapse.

- Appeal and Appellate Board: The aggrieved person can appeal to the Appellate Board within 3 months of the decision of the controller of patents or the central government. The board may order amendment or revocation of patent.

Though applicant is free to file patent application on its own, there are patent agents whose services can be availed. The patent agents are registered persons with Indian Patent Office and are entitled to practice before the controller and to prepare all documents and transact all business. The patent agents are qualified with a degree in science, engineering or technology from the recognized universities and passed the qualifying examination prescribed for this purpose. They have the experience of not less than 10 years either as an examiner or discharged the functions of the controller.

Patent opposition: Like patenting system of other countries, Indian Patent System provides provision for opposition to patent application and patent grant: Pre-grant opposition and post-grant opposition. The salient points are given below:

Pre-grant Opposition

- Any person or third party or the government may challenge the application of grant of patent.
- Challenging in writing is to be done during the period: After publication of the patent application and before grant of patent (usually within six months of publication of patent application).
- The challenge is to be done under the following grounds:
  - Wrongfully obtaining invention
  - Anticipation by prior publication
  - Anticipation by prior date, prior claiming in India
  - Prior public knowledge or public use in India
  - Obviousness and lack of inventive step
  - Non-patentable subject matter
  - Insufficiency description of invention
  - Non-disclosure of information as per the requirement or providing materially false information
  - Patent application not filed within 12 months of filing the first application in a convention country
  - Non-disclosure or wrong mention of source of biological material
  - Invention anticipated with regard to traditional knowledge of any community anywhere in the world
- Authority: Controller General of Patents

Post-grant Opposition

- The person interested (person engaged in or in promoting research in the same field related to invention) can challenge.
- Challenging can be made at any time after the grant of patent but before the expiry of 12 months from the date of publication of grant of patent.

A Patent Case with Diverse Issues: The Story of Gilead's Sovaldi Patent—The patenting story of sovaldi is very interesting with diverse issues: Pre- and post-grant opposition, patent infringement and perhaps political compulsion too. Sovaldi is the brand name of Sofosbuvir and is a treatment for Hepatitis C. The cost of each tablet was $1000 in US requiring 12-week treatment ($84,000). A highly unaffordable treatment. Indian Patent Office granted a patent to Gilead Pharmasset in May 2016 which was

challenged in Delhi High Court. At this point of time (August 2017), the judgement is pending.

Gilead Science acquired the Pharmasset Limited, the company developed the drug and filed its first patent in 2003. Sofosbuvir is a pro-drug that is metabolized in the body to the active antiviral agent, 2'-deoxy-2'-α-fluoro-β-C-methyluridine-5'-mono-phosphate, a nucleotide analogue inhibitor of the HCV polymerase.

The Time Line of Activities

- The Gilead had filed the patent application in India in December 2005.
- The drug received regulatory approval from USFDA in 2013.
- Pre-grant opposition was filed by Delhi Network of Positive People (DNP+), US-based initiative for Medicine, Access and Knowledge (I-MAK) and Natco Pharma in 2013-2014.
- In 2014, Gilead entered into licence agreement with 13 Indian companies including Natco to manufacture and sell in countries identified in the licence. This was viewed as tactical move of Gilead to discourage further opposition. Natco withdrew its opposition to the patent application.
- In 2015, the patent office refused the granting of patent. The patent application did not prove the 'enhanced therapeutic efficacy' compared to its 'closest prior art' compound D1. This is requirement under Section 3(d). As the compound D1 was not marketed, the company did not show any comparative data.
- Gilead filed the writ petition before the Delhi High Court against the approval. The court observed that the Gilead was not given proper notice of objections and asked the patent office for a fresh hearing. The court permitted new pre-grant opposition too. Sankalp Rehabilitation Trust filed opposition against the patent application when freshly heard. Patent opponents argued that inventive step 'methyl (up) and fluro (down) at 2'

position of nucleoside' is a known art. It would be obvious to the person skilled in the art to do what the patent applicant had done.

- The Deputy Controller of Patents granted patent on 9th May 2016. The patent office observed that the patent application provides comparative activity and toxicity data in mice and monkey. Further, additional comparative activity data has been filed during the examination of the patent application. The Deputy Controller satisfied that the compound had enhanced efficacy.

The controversies here are: There is reversal of stand by the patent office on enhanced efficacy. The second issue was: The patent officer who rejected the patent earlier was kept out of fresh hearing—was it deliberate??

Merck alleged that Pharmasset developed the chemical, sofosbuvir, from Merck's patent that was filed in 2002. A Federal jury in March 2016, ordered Gilead to pay $200 million against the claim of $2 billion for infringing into the two patents of Merck.

- In May 2016, I-MAK and DNP + had filed an appeal with the Delhi High Court against the grant of patent. They claim that the patent officer had failed to assess the full scientific and legal evidence. "The base compound in sofosbuvir was developed with previously published technique". The analyst find the following flaws in the decision of the patent office:
  - Novelty: Existence of an inventive step and the present formulation is the result of extensive experimentation;
  - Enhanced layer of efficacy: Unsupported by the cogent chain of reasoning; and
  - Patent situation in other countries: Not permitted in China, Ukraine or Egypt.

The development of rejection and granting of patent is viewed by analyst as political compulsion. Gilead's application was rejected immediately before President Obama's visit to India, and its application was approved just before Prime Minister's schedule to travel to the US. This could be coincidence too.

Provision of Compulsory License: After the expiry of 3 years of granting of patent, compulsory license may be permissible on the following grounds:

- The reasonable requirements of the public with respect to the patented invention have not been satisfied; or
- That the patented invention is not available to the public at a reasonably affordable price; or
- That the patented invention is not worked in the territory of India.

This provision gives sweeping powers to the controller of patents to grant compulsory license. It offers powers to central government to take appropriate measures in the case of national emergency, circumstances of extreme urgency to revoke this compulsory license provision in national interest. The patent can be revoked after two years of first granting of compulsory license, if required.

Compulsory license is allowable for manufacture and export of patented pharmaceutical product to any country having insufficient or no manufacturing capacity in the pharmaceutical sector for the concerned product to address public health problems, provided compulsory license has been granted by such country allowed importation of the patented pharmaceutical products from India.

India so far issued only one CL (see the box). The patent office rejected the CL application of Lee Pharma against the Astra Zeneca's Saxagliptin in June 2016. Lee Pharma filed the application in June 2015 but failed to provide the evidence to satisfy the Controller of Patents on grounds required for CL (reasonable requirement of the public for saxagliptin, anti-diabetic drug). As the Indian Government is powerfully promoting the global initiative "MAKE IN INDIA", the provision of CL may have natural deaths. It would be extremely difficult to satisfy all the requirements of CL.

Patent protection is a territorial right and therefore, it is effective only within the territory of India. However, filing an application in India enables the applicant to file a corresponding application for same invention in convention countries, within or before the expiry of 12 months from the filing date in India. Separate patent for each country is required for getting protection for invention. There is no patent valid worldwide. The prior permission is necessary to file patent application abroad if the applicant is Indian and the invention is originated in India, applicant does not wish to file application in India prior to filing abroad, application is filed in India but six week period is not yet over, and the invention relates to atomic energy or defence purpose.

Patent infringement suits can be instituted in a district court. However, where counter claim for revocation is made, the suit is transferred to the High Court for decision.

The product patent refers the final product and it precludes others from manufacturing the product while the process patent covers only the method by which one makes the product. The process patent does not preclude others from entering the market with the same product as long as the individual or company is able to devise an alternate means of manufacture.

There are four other Acts related to Intellectual Property Rights:
- The Designs Act 2000.
- The Trademarks Act 1999.
- The Geographical Indications of Goods (Registration and Protection) Act 1999.
- The Copyrights Act 1957.

Government's IPR Policy

Justice Ayyangar Committee's report (1959) echoing "The existing patent law has failed in its main purpose to stimulate invention among Indians and to encourage the development and exploitation of new inventions for industrial purposes in the country so as to secure the benefits thereof to the largest section of the public" was the guiding force for bringing the Patent Act 1970. The inherited British formulated Act had a provision of strong patent protection and rights including product patent protection. This was in tune with universal Practice of European Countries at that period of time.

The Patent Act 1970 abolished product patent protection in pharmaceuticals in order to ensure that the medicines are available to the public at reasonable price. It offered only process patent for 5 years from grant or 7 years from filing. This gave the fruitful results. The Indian Generic Manufacturers were able to offer triple combination of anti-retrovirals (ARVs) at a fraction of the price being offered by patent holding multinational pharmaceutical companies.

India being a World Trade Organization (WTO) has no obligation to provide patent protection for any subject matter which has fallen into the public domain before the WTO came into being (01 January 1995). Thus any drug patent abroad before 1995 can continue to be manufactured and sold in India after 1995 even though these may be under patent protection in other countries. India has made full use of the 10 years transition period allowed to developing countries (that did not have product patent) to become fully compliant with WTO's requirements. With Patent Amendment Act 2005, India is completely in full complaint with WTO's requirements.

National Intellectual Property Rights Policy: The National Intellectual Property Rights Policy was approved by the Central Government on 12th May 2016. This is viewed as 'first of its kind' policy covering all forms of intellectual property in a single framework. DIPP has been made the nodal point to coordinate, guide, and oversee implementation and future development of IPRs in India. The policy will govern the following Acts: Patents, Trade Marks, Design, Geographical Indications of Goods, Copyright, Protection of Plant Varieties and Farmers' Rights, Semiconductor Integrated Circuits Layout Design and Biological Diversity. Its impact would reflect in all areas: Pharmaceuticals, software, electronics and communications, seeds, environmental goods, renewable energy, agriculture and health biotechnology, information and communication. The objectives of the policy are:

1. IPR Awareness—outreach and promotion— to create public awareness about the economic, social and cultural benefits of IPRs among all sections of society.

2. Generation of IPRs—to stimulate the generation of IPRs.

3. Legal and legislative framework—to have strong and effective IPR laws, which balance the interests of rights owners with larger public interest.

4. Administration and management—to modernize and strengthen service-oriented IPR administration.

5. Commercialization of IPRs—get value for IPRs through commercialization.

6. Enforcement and adjudication—to strengthen the enforcement and adjudicatory mechanisms for combating IPR infringements.

7. Human capital development—to strengthen and expand human resources, institutions and capacities for teaching, training, research and skill building in IPRs.

The apprehension is raised by the various section that the implementation of the policy may affect the access to new drugs. The provision like enhanced efficacy, compulsory licence may not find application in due course. However, the government has clarified that the policy is a balanced consideration of inventability, innovation and public health consideration. The policy will ensure that no changes are made in that Section (which prevents ever-greening of drug patents) and the patent-disabling Compulsory Licensing regime.

The GOI has initiated several strategies to promote innovation:

1. Establishment of new National Institutes of Sciences to promote basic sciences.

2. Development of National Biotechnology Strategies to include 100% biotechnology units funded by foreign direct investments, priority sector lending, tax credits for money spent on international patent filing, and creation of 10 biotechnology

parks with special economic zone status.

3. Initiating Department of Biotechnology's Mission Programme with theme "Science in the Service of Common Man". The programme is aimed at generating new vaccines, developing herbal products, and establishing mirror sites of genomic database in India.

4. Developing new generation vaccines and diagnostics vaccines for cholera, rabies, Japanese encephalitis, TB, Malaria and HIV.

5. Initiating Public–Private Partnership (PPP): The CSIR's PPP scheme aims to make India a global leader in the science and technology with a focus on bio-technology, bioinformatics, agriculture and plant biotechnology, drugs and pharmaceuticals.

6. Developing Golden Triangle: The integrated technology focussed on the development of Ayurvedic and traditional medical knowledge that synthesizes modern medicines, traditional medicines and modern science.

7. Promoting Innovation in Traditional Knowledge: The CSIR's initiative "Traditional Knowledge Digital Library (TKDL)" to prevent piracy and promote innovations through the use of Traditional Knowledge is an example.

8. Creating Department of Health Research: ICMR is being upgraded as Department of Health Research to ensure better coordination and promotions of National Health Programmes.

9. Small Business Innovation Research Initiative: The Department of Biotechnology aims to boost PPP with small and medium companies to support research and generating ideas.

10. Establishing National Innovation Foundation: As a unit of Department of Science and Technology (DST), it seeks to recognise, respect and reward grassroots technology innovators and traditional knowledge experts.

Milestone in Patent Legislation in India

1856 The first patent law was introduced by British to encourage inventions of new and useful manufactures and to induce inventions to disclose secret of their inventions.

1872 The earlier Act was consolidated to provide protection relating to designs and was renamed Patterns and Design Protection Act.

1888 The Indian Act was made in conformity with patent law of United Kingdom.

1911 The Indian Patent and Designs Act was enacted replacing all earlier Acts. The Patent Administration was brought under management of Controller of Patents.

1950 The Act amended relating to working of inventions and compulsory license/revocation.

1970 The Patent Act was enacted but came into effect only in 1972.

1971 The Uruguay Round Negotiations are ratified.

1994 India accepted WTO membership.

1994 Patent ordinance promulgated.

1995 The Uruguay Round agreements comes into effect.

1995 The Patent Amendment Bill is introduced in the Lok Sabha.

1996 The Patent Bill lapsed after the Rajya Sabha failed to clear.

1997 US complained to WTO that India is violating the TRIPS agreements.

1997 EU filed complaint with WTO on the failure of India to set up mailbox facilities.

1997 The WTO's dispute settlement body ruled against India.

1997 India appealed against the dispute settlement body's ruling.

1997 The WTO's Appellate Body rejected India's appeal.

1998 The WTO formally asked India to amend patent laws.

1998   India agreed to 15 months implementation period.

1998   The introduction of Amended Patent Act is deferred.

1998   India decided to accede to the Paris Convention.

1998   The dispute settlement body ruled against India on EU complaint.

1999   Deadline for complying with recommendations of dispute settlement body.

1999   First Amendment in Patent Act 1970— introduced mailbox system and set up a system of exclusive market rights (EMRs) to be retrospective from January 1, 1995 in conformity with TRIPS Agreement.

2001   Protection of plant varieties and Farmers Rights Act 2001 passed.

2002   Doha declaration on TRIPS agreement and Public Health.

2002   Second Patent Amendment Bill passed with several changes: The most important being the extension of patent term from 14 to 20 years and the reversal of burden of proof from patent holder to alleged infringer.

2002   The Biodiversity Bill passed in the Parliament.

2003   First Patent Ordinance.

2004   Second Patent Ordinance—complied with TRIPS Agreement in toto.

2005   The Patent (Amendment) Act 2005 and Patent (Amendment) Rules 2005 passed with effect from 01.01.2005.

2005   Published in gazette.

2014   Patent (Amendment) Rules 2014 (notifying the fees)

2014   Government constituted IP think tank.

2015   Think tank submitted final report.

2016   IPR policy approved by the Union Cabinet

The Strict Interpretations of Patentability Criteria in Rejecting Application for Critical AIDS Drug

New Delhi, 19 June 2008: The Indian Patent Office in New Delhi has rejected a patent application filed by the multinational pharmaceutical company Boehringer Ingelheim claiming a paediatric form of the anti-AIDS drug nevirapine. In May 2006, the Indian Network of People Living with HIV/AIDS (INP+) and the Positive Women's Network (PWN) had filed a pre-grant opposition against this application. The rejected patent application covers the syrup form of nevirapine, which is particularly important for children living with HIV who are unable to swallow tablets. This is the first decision from the Patent Offices on 13 patent oppositions filed by Indian civil society groups against HIV-related patent applications, and will set an important precedent for the others that are still pending.

The Indian Patents Act contains some important safeguards designed to ensure that frivolous patent applications are not granted at the cost of public health. These include Section 3(d) of the Patents Act, which prevents many "new forms" of known substances from being patented unless there is a significant improvement in efficacy, and Section 3(e) of the Act, which prevents "mere admixtures" of substances from being patented.

The opposition filed by INP+ and PWN had argued, among other things, that the particular application was not patentable under Indian law because the hemihydrate form of nevirapine was obvious to a person skilled in the art; that it was just a "new form" of an already known substance without any increased efficacy; and that the manufacture of nevirapine hemihydrate in an aqueous solution was just a "mere admixture" of ingredients that did not demonstrate any synergistic effects.

The Patent Office agreed with INP+ and PWN on all these grounds. In considering these arguments, the Patent Office considered as a "fact of law" the need to "give a strict interpretation of patentability criteria, as decision...thereof shall affect the fate of people suffering from HIV/AIDS for want of essential medicine." The Patent Office also cited approvingly to the Madras High Court's judgment in Novartis v. Union of India, which had observed that the "object which the [Patents (Amendment) Act, 2005] wanted to achieve [was] to...provide easy access to the citizens of this country to life saving drugs and to discharge their Constitutional obligation of providing good healthcare to its citizens."

PATENT LEGISLATIONS IN OTHER COUNTRIES

JAPAN: For more than 200 years (1616–1854), Japan followed the policy of isolation with government banning foreign contact except for a few limited contacts with only few countries. During this period Japan did not permit the import or utilize advance technologies developed in the USA and Europe. The manufacturing of new products based on technology developed in European countries and the USA was prohibited. The public were generally against proprietary inventions. The first patent law was enacted in 1871, known as Exclusive Right Law, but withdrawn one year later. In 1885, the new patent law was passed following the US and French Laws. Since then, it has been revised many times and since 1975, Patent Laws of Japan has been harmonized with major international legal instruments including World Intellectual Property Organization (WIPO).

The medical methods are out of patentability while pharmaceutical products are patentable.

USA: The modern American Patent System started with signing of first Patent Act 1790 by the President George Washington. However, during the period of economic depression in the 19th century, there had been increasing concern about the power of big business leading enactment of Sherman Antitrust Act in 1890. During this period, there had been increasing tendency of the courts to hold patents invalid. With

reviving economy, the patents regained the importance.

Prior to GATT, the drug patent period was only for 17 years from the date of issuance of patent and after GATT, the patent period begins on the date of issuance and valid for 20 years from the date of filing. The patent period is extendable for another five years in case of pre-marketing regulatory delay.

The US allows patent almost of any invention irrespective of the domain if the invention is novel, non-obvious and useful. The methods relating to medical activities and practices are generally patentable. However, a medical practitioner can use patented medical methods without risking infringement. [India has clearly excluded inventions which cannot be patented]

The US follows first to invent system meaning one who invents first have the rights on it. [India follows first to file system meaning it does not matter who invents first, it is the filer who gets the right over invention].

Pfizer Inc. won Vigra Patent Case: The Federal Court Ruled that Pfizer's Vigra (sildenafil) is valid and enforceable till October 2019 and generic version would infringe the patent. Teva Pharmaceutical Industries is now prevented from launching a generic version of vigra until October 2019. [Deccan Chronicle, Chennai, 16th August 2011]. There are several versions of this drug available in India.

A Case of Pre-grant Opposition: Madras High Court set aside the patent granted to F. Hoffman-La Roche AG (Roche) for valganciclovir (Patent No. 207232) for failure of the Indian patent office to comply with the patent law and remanded the matter back to the Patent Controller (*Source:* Ip-health Posting).

Valganciclovir is crucial for treatment of cytomegalovirus (CMV) retinitis, an opportunistic infection that affects persons living with HIV, and to prevent CMV infection in patients who have received organ transplants. This is a prodrug of an already known drug ganciclovir. This drug is at Roche's maximum retail price of over ₹ 1000 (approx USD 20; 1 USD = approx ₹ 50) per tablet, a patient who has to take a treatment course of approximately four months for CMV retinitis would have to pay about ₹ 250,000 (approx USD 5000). This puts the treatment out of reach for those who need them.

In July 2006, Indian Network for People Living with HIV/AIDS (INP+) and Tamil Nadu Networking People with HIV/AIDS (TNNP+) filed a pre-grant opposition before the Patent Office at Chennai objecting to the grant of a patent to Roche for valganciclovir and requested the Patent Office for a hearing. Under the Indian law, if an opponent requests a hearing, the Patent Office is required to hear the Opponent. The Patent Office sent the pre-grant opposition to Roche and received a reply from Roche. Satisfied that the objections raised by INP+ and TNNP+ had been met by Roche, the Patent Office went ahead and granted a patent without hearing INP+ and TNNP+. The grant of the patent was published in June 2007. After correspondence with the Patent Office failed to yield any result, INP+ and TNNP+ filed a petition in the Madras High Court in October 2008. They alleged that failure to grant them a hearing amounted to violation of the mandatory requirements of the patent and also a violation of the principles of natural justice. The Assistant Controller, who had granted the patent, filed a reply justifying the grant. Roche objected to the petition on the ground that INP+ and TNNP+ could take recourse to mechanisms such as post-grant opposition or revocation available under the patent law to challenge the grant of the patent.

The final hearings in the case took place in the third and fourth weeks of November 2008. It has been argued that the failure of the Indian patent office to hear the opponents amounted to a failure to comply with the mandatory provisions of the patent law and also violated the principles of natural justice. Reading from the affidavit filed by the Assistant Controller and other documents, it is shown how the Patent Office had considered the reply filed by Roche to the opposition before deciding to grant a patent. The petitioner informed the court that no order had been passed disposing off the pre-grant opposition. The counsel then referred the judges to the provisions of the patent law to show that even if an order was passed rejecting a pre-grant opposition, no appeal could be filed against such an order. It has been pointed out that were INP+ and TNNP+ to file a post-grant opposition or a revocation proceeding, it would amount to an admission of the grant of the patent. These proceedings, counsel argued, were separate causes of action and did not afford a remedy to INP+ and TNNP+ in this situation. It is thus pleaded that as the action of the Patent Office was illegal, the patent granted was void and without any legal effect and therefore the patent be set aside and the matter be sent back the Patent Office for a hearing.

The Counsel (appeared for Roche) argued that it was open to INP+ and TNNP+ to file a post-grant opposition or revocation proceeding. He said that a pre-grant opposition was in the nature of an administrative procedure and does not give rise to a dispute between the parties. He further argued that there was no need for the Controller to pass an order in a pre-grant opposition proceeding. Referring to an alleged delay in challenging the grant of the patent, he said that Roche would be prejudiced if the patent granted were set aside by the High Court and it would impact the infringement suit filed by Roche against Cipla before the Bombay High Court.

Rebutting the above arguments of Roche, counsel appearing on behalf of INP+ and TNNP+ said that a pre-grant opposition proceeding was a quasi-judicial proceeding (like a judicial proceeding) and it was a dispute between two parties. It is argued that when the grant of the patent itself was illegal from the outset, it was a continuing cause of action and there was no question of delay in approaching the court to set it aside. The counsel pointed out that if the patent was not set aside and the opposition filed by INP+ and TNNP+ was merely sent back to the Patent Office for a hearing, the proceeding would be akin to a post-grant opposition. It is further brought to the notice of the court that Roche could continue to import valganciclovir into India and sell it even if the patent were set aside.

In a landmark judgement delivered on 2 December 2008, the High Court set aside the grant of the patent and remanded the matter back to the Patent Office. The Court held that since the Petitioners represented public interest, there is no question of waiver of the principles of natural justice. Observing a bias in the affidavit filed by the Assistant Patent Controller, the High Court has directed that the opposition be heard by another patent official before 31 January 2009. The High Court also declined Roche's counsel's plea to stay the operative part of the order setting aside the patent until a certified copy of the order was issued to them to enable them to file an appeal.

India's first compulsory licence: The provision of CL intends to keep a balance of two conflicting objectives: Rewarding patentees for the invention and making the invention available for use when need arises. Though more than 50 countries had issued CL at various time, India has so far issued only one CL in March 2012 to Natco Pharma Limited for producing the generic version of Bayer Corporation's patent, Nexavar, a treatment of liver and kidney cancer.

- In 2011, Natco Pharma had applied for the country's first compulsory licence to sell a generic version of Bayer's patented medicine.
- Natco stated in its application that the German company's drug was unaffordable for the average Indian. Bayer's drug, Nexavar, costs about 2.85 lakh for a

month's course. Natco said it can sell its generic version, sorafenib tosylate, for just Rs. 8,900 for the same course.

- In December, Natco had sought a voluntary licence from Bayer for sorafenib tosylate that was refused. Indian laws allow a firm to apply for a compulsory licence only after the innovator company rejects the voluntary request.
- Although compulsory licensing allows a generic firm to legally make and sell the low-cost version, it has to pay some royalty, usually about 5% of sales.
- In 2012, the CL was issued. This was challenged subsequently. In March 2014, Intellectual Property Appellate Board (IPAB) upheld the CL issued on March 9, 2012.
- Finally, Supreme Court brought the legal issue of this CL to an end upholding the CL issued by the Patent Office.

Natco Pharma Files India's First Compulsory License Plea

(http://m.economictimes.com/PDAET/ articleshow/9462939.cms)

2 Aug, 2011, 2259 hrs IST, Khomba Singh, ET Bureau New Delhi: Natco Pharma has applied for the country's first compulsory license to sell a generic version of Bayer's patented medicine, a development whose outcome is expected to determine how global drug makers price their costly drugs in India.

In compulsory licensing, the government allows a generic firm to produce a patented product without the consent of the patent owner. It is one of the flexibilities on patent protection included in the WTO's agreement on intellectual property—TRIPS (Trade-Related aspects of Intellectual Property rights) Agreement.

Natco stated in its application that the German company's drug was unaffordable for the average Indian.

Bayer's drug, Nexavar, which is used to treat liver and kidney cancer, costs about 2.85 lakh for a month's course. Natco said it can sell its generic version, sorafenib tosylate, for just 8,900 for the same course.

Local drug firms and health activists are pushing for liberal use of compulsory licensing, saying that innovator companies charge exorbitantly high prices for their medicines. "A favourable decision for Natco will open the floodgates and encourage other local firms to apply for compulsory license for costly patented medicines," a senior industry said.

YK Sapru, chairman and CEO of Cancer Patients Aid Association (CPAA), said Natco's application, if approved, would be a big relief to those who can't afford Nexavar. There are an estimated 25 lakh cancer patients in India. In December, Natco had sought a voluntary license from Bayer for sorafenib tosylate that was refused. Indian laws allow a firm to apply for a compulsory license only after the innovator company rejects the voluntary request.

Experts say the face-off is going to be a long drawn, as the loser will invariably challenge the decision in court. There are at least two other voluntary license applications pending: Natco's with a GSK-Pfizer joint venture and Cipla's with US-based Merck and Co.

For Bayer, this is not the first challenge for Nexavar. Cipla has already launched its generic version without any permission and will have to pay penalty if the court rules in favour of Bayer in a pending patent case.

Although compulsory licensing allows a generic firm to legally make and sell the low-cost version, it has to pay some royalty, usually about 5% of sales. MNCs strongly oppose the use of this provision because it breaks their monopoly. They say such licensing is not a sustainable policy to address access of medicines as these products account for much less than 1% of Indian drug market.

Compulsory licensing provision has been used in countries such as Thailand, Brazil and South Africa.

In all these nations, the provision was used for HIV medicines, according to a commerce ministry discussion note on the use of such licenses. India spends an estimated $35 billion in healthcare cost. Unlike most other countries, where such costs are state-funded or insured, 90% of Indians pay from their own pocket.

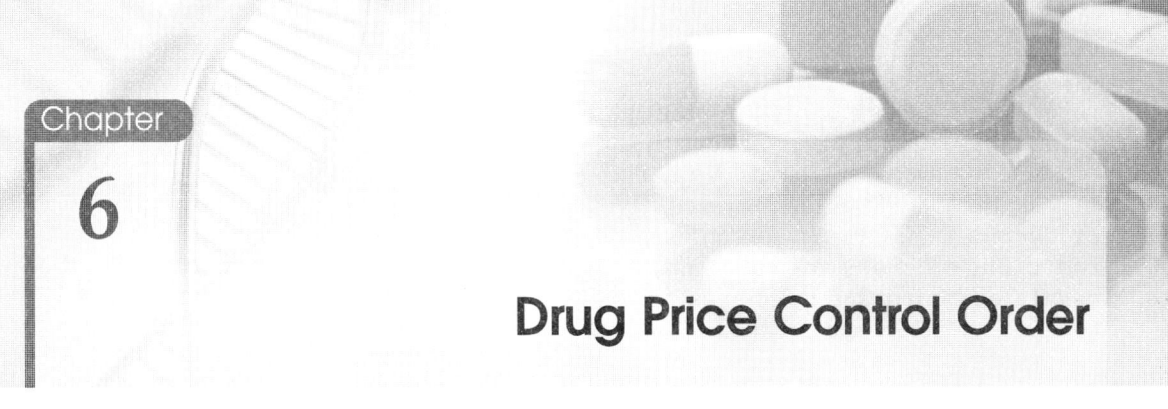

6

Drug Price Control Order

"Expensive medicines are always good: if not for the patient, at least for the druggist."

— *Russian Proverb*

After reading this chapter, you should be able to understand and appreciate

- The need of price control in medicines and how the pricing of medicines differ from other consumer goods
- Medicine price scenario in India
- Medicine price control mechanism in India including administrative provisions available for implementing price control order
- Medicine price control mechanism exist in other countries

Medicines (or, drugs used interchangeably) play a crucial role in saving lives, restoring health, and preventing diseases and epidemics. In many high income countries, over 70% of the medicines are publicly funded or have social insurance or other reimbursement scheme. In low and middle income countries including India, public medicine expenditure does not cover the basic medicine needs of the majority of the population. In these countries, the patients pay for 50–90% of the medicines from their own pocket. Study on drug expenditure pattern of state government showed wide variation that as low as 2% in case of Punjab to as high as 17% in Kerala during 2001–2002. Household drug expenditure has a sizeable share of household health expenditure in India. The 55th National Sample Survey Organization (NSSO) consumption expenditure survey revealed that the share of medicine in total outpatient treatment is extremely high. In rural India, spending on drugs accounts for 83% while it is 70% of the total treatment costs in urban areas. In fact, the share of medicine cost is as high as over 90% of total cost in states like Bihar, Himachal Pradesh, Jammu and Kashmir, and Orissa, etc.

The price of medicines often quoted as one of the lowest comparing with international price. The absolute price does not give the real picture of affordability, an essential requirement to improve access to essential medicine, a fundamental human right. The price needs to be compared using purchasing power parity of various countries. A case study reported the cost of 100 paracetamol tablets represents income from 8 working hours (one full day) of an unskilled worker in India, 1.3 hours in the USA and 1.5 hours in Switzerland. World Health Organization's estimate showed that only around one-third of the population in India have access to essential medicines against an world average of two-third.

It is assumed that market forces promote competition. In a free market the competition results in lowering and more important levelling the prices. This may be true in generic drug market, but not in proprietary market that exists in India. Besides this, the consumers or the patients have no/little choice in selecting medicines like other consumer products. The 5Cs (convince, confuse, coax, corrupt and cry) of pharmaceutical marketing clearly demonstrates the nexus of drug companies, doctors and chemists in maximizing profit at the cost of poor patients. The consumers are either at the mercy of doctors or chemists on medicines and the price they need to pay.

Medicine price de-regulation often led to abnormal price increase of essential medicines. In 1995, the price of a preparation for anaemia rose by 177% and the prices of anti-TB medicines rose by nearly 90%. A recent study reported that the price rise of medicines (not under price control) is around 10% per year while that of medicines (under price control) is just 1% over last decade.

The effective price control mechanism is a must failing which the medicines accessibility will become less and lesser as most of country men pay for medicines from their own pockets.

Drug Price Control in Other Countries

Across the globe the drug prices are controlled in one or other way. Such controls take the following forms in single or in combination of more than one instrument: ceiling on mark-up, fixed margin to wholesalers or pharmacists, price freeze, reimbursement, reference pricing, contributions to insurance premium, patient co-payments, generic substitutions, ceiling on promotional expenditure, differential value added tax on drugs, etc. To cite a few examples:

- All European Union countries have a form of price regulation.
- France regulates margin for wholesalers and pharmacists for reimbursable medicines. It sets prices in relation to relative cost.
- All reimbursable medicines in Italy are price controlled.
- Reimbursement drug prices are controlled by reference pricing system in Germany.

- UK has Pharmaceutical Price Regulation Scheme. Rate of return is fixed company by company through negotiations.
- The government fixes a specified discount for medicines sold to Medicaid programme, although drug prices are largely control free in the USA. The margin allowed for wholesalers is around 2% and pharmacies it is around 15% in the USA.
- Egypt fixes a maximum limit of 20% and 12% on profit to manufacturers of locally produced products and imported products respectively.

Drug Price Control System in India

In post independence era, during 1950s several commodities of day-to-day importance including medicines were on shortage. In order to tackle the situation, the Government of India promulgated Essential Commodities Act 1955 to prevent hoarding, black marketing, to ensure equitable distribution and exercise control over price. The Defence of India Act was invoked to curb the spiralling prices of medicines following Chinese aggression and declaration of emergency in 1962. The Drugs (Display of Prices) order 1962 and Drug (Control of Prices) Order 1963 were promulgated. Subsequently attempts were made to regulate prices further through Drugs Prices (Display and Control) Order 1966. Medicines being regarded as essential items, the Government of India first introduced Drug Price Control Order in 1970 under Essential Commodities Act 1955. This order captured 347 bulk drugs under its net. DPCO 1970 was more of a control on profitability of pharmaceutical industries. The government fixed the pre-tax profit of the company not to exceed 15% of its net sales. If the profit exceeds, the surplus was to be deposited to the government. Industries were free to decide the prices of the product subject to pre-tax profit limit. The pharmaceutical industries were predominantly multinationals and their subsidiaries. Individual product prices were not required approval and bureaucratic hurdles were very low. Taking advantage of process patents, the Indian pharmaceutical industries prospered from 1970 to 1979.

The next Drug Price Control was introduced in 1979 based Hathi Committee's recommendation and Drug Policy 1979. In this revision, DPCO stipulated ceiling prices for controlled categories of bulk drugs and their formulation. In fixing the price, the government continued to advocate profitability ceiling. Successive orders have been issued subsequently in 1987 and 1995. In 1987 order, the price control was just for 166 bulk drugs and which was further reduced to just 142 drugs. The DPCO 1995 further brought down the list of drugs under its purview to 76 and reduced again to 74. Subsequently government proposed New Pharmaceutical Policy in 2002 which sought to bring down the number of medicines to 35 under the price control mechanism. The policy was struck down by the Karnataka High Court. Subsequently, government approached Supreme Court (SC) and SC stayed the order of Karnataka High Court but ordered the government to formulate appropriate criteria to ensure that the essential and life-saving drugs do not fall out of price control.

Later, the government brought National Pharmaceutical Pricing Policy 2012 and a new Drug Price Control Order 2013. The purpose of the DPCO 2013 is to ensure affordability of the medicines to all sections of the society while preserving a rationale for ensuring a reasonable profit to manufacturers.

Drug Price Control Order 2013 (DPCO 2013)

The salient features are:

1. The government is empowered to direct the manufactures of bulk drugs and formulations to increase production and sell as required when situation warrants like emergency.
2. All strengths and dosage specified in NLEM are brought within the ambit of

Timeline on Drug Price Control in India [*Source*: Draft Pharmaceutical Policy 2017]	
1962	The Drugs (Display of Price) order 1962 under Defence of India Act 1915.
1963/April 1	The Drugs (Display of Price) order 1963 under Defence of India Act 1915. Price control for drugs introduced in the aftermath of India's war with China. Price of drugs were frozen.
1966	The Drug Prices (Display and Control) 1966. This is issued under Essential Commodities Act 1955. Drugs are declared as essential commodities. Prior approval for increase in prices introduced.
1968	The Drug Prices (Display and Control) 1966 amended. Drugs sold under pharmacopeial name were exempted from prior approval.
1970	DPCO 1970 introduced under Essential Commodities Act 1955.
1979	First comprehensive pricing mechanism introduced with DPCO 1979. 347 bulk drugs and their formulations were brought under the umbrella.
1986	List of controlled drugs are brought down to 142 bulk drugs and their formulations.
1995	DPCO 1995: Number of drugs and their formulations were brought down further to 74 bulk drugs.
1997	Establishment of NPPA
2002	Pharmaceutical policy sought to bring down the number of drugs under price control to 35. The policy is challenged in Karnataka High Court and stay order issued.
2003	Supreme Court struck down the High Court Order but directed the government to formulate appropriate criteria for ensuring that essential and life-saving drugs do not fall out of price control.
2012	National Pharmaceutical Pricing policy 2012 announced to regulate the price based on NLEM.
2013	DPCO 2013 introduced.

price control. These are called scheduled formulations. NLEM is dynamic in nature as periodically revised. DPCO 2013 initially covered the medicines of NLEM 2011 containing 348 items.

3. **Exemptions:** It does not cover the Homeopathic, Ayurvedic, Siddha and Unani medicines.

4. **Pricing calculation of scheduled formulation:** This is calculated using the following steps:

   a. **Step I:** Average Price to Retailer [P(s)] (Sum of prices to retailer of all the brands and generic versions of the medicine having market share more than or equal to one percent of the total market turnover on the basis of moving annual turnover of that medicine) ÷ (Total number of such brands and generic versions of the medicine having market share more than or equal to one percent of total market turnover on the basis of moving annual turnover for that medicine.)

   b. **Step II:** Ceiling price of the scheduled formulation [P(c)]:

   $$P(c) = P(s).(1 + M/100)$$

   where,

   P(s) = Average Price to Retailer for the same strength and dosage of the medicine as calculated in step 1 above.

   M = % Margin to retailer and its value = 16

   The ceiling price calculated above is applicable for imported medicines too.

5. **Retail price of a new drug for existing manufacturers of scheduled formulations:** The ceiling price for the drug available in the domestic market is to be calculated by the method mentioned above. But for the medicines which are not available in domestic market, the price is to be calculated based on the recommendation of Standing Committee and keeping 16% margin to the retailer.

6. **Ceiling price of a scheduled formulation in case of no reduction in price due to absence of competition:** This provision is applicable—(i) when the average price to the retailer calculated as above does not cause reduction in average price to retailer; or (ii) there are less than five manufacturer with one percent or more market share.

The ceiling price is to be calculated as:

(i) **in the event of other strengths or dosage forms of the same scheduled formulation as available in the list of scheduled formulation:**

   Step 1: First the Average Price to Retailer of such scheduled formulation, i.e. P(s) is calculated as under:

   $$P(s) = Pm \{1-(Pi1 + Pi2+...) \div (N*100)\}$$

   Where,

   Pm = Price to retailer of highest priced scheduled formulation under consideration.

   Pi = % reduction in average price to retailer of other strengths and dosage forms (calculated using formula given earlier for scheduled formulation with respect to the highest priced formulation taken for calculating the average price to retailer of such strengths and dosage forms.

   N = Number of such other strengths or dosage forms or both in the list of schedule formulations

   Step 2. The ceiling price of the scheduled formulation [P(c)] is to be calculated as under:

   $$P(c) = P(s) \times (1 + M/100)$$

   where

   P(s) = Average price to retailer of the scheduled formulation as calculated in step 1 hereinabove and

   M = % Margin to retailer and its value = 16

(ii) **In the event of other strengths or dosage forms of the scheduled formulation is not available in the schedule but there are other scheduled formulations in same sub-therapeutic category as that of the scheduled formulation,** then the ceiling price is to be calculated as under:

Step 1: First the Average Price to Retailer of such scheduled formulation [P(s)] is to be calculated as under:

$$P(s) = Pm \{1-(Pi1 + Pi2+...) \div (N*100)\},$$

Where,

Pm = Price of highest priced formulation taken for calculating the average price to retailer of the formulation under consideration.

Pi = % Reduction in average price to retailer of other schedule formulations (calculated as per the formula given for scheduled formulation) in same sub-therapeutic category as that of the scheduled formulation under consideration with respect to the highest priced formulation taken for calculating the average price to retailer.

N = Number of such other schedule formulations in same sub-therapeutic category as that of the scheduled formulation under consideration.

Step 2: The ceiling price of the scheduled formulation [P(c)] is to be calculated as under:

$$P(c) = P(s) \times (1 + M/100)$$

where,

P(s) = Average price to retailer of the scheduled formulation as calculated in step 1 above and

M = % Margin to retailer and its value = 16

Explanation: Where the scheduled formulation under consideration is coming under more than one sub-therapeutic category, the average price to retailer of the scheduled formulation shall be calculated after taking into consideration the percentage reduction in average price to retailer of other schedule formulations under all such sub-therapeutic categories and the lowest average price to retailer

shall be taken for calculating the ceiling price of the scheduled formulation under consideration;

(iii) **In case the other strengths or dosage forms of the scheduled formulation are not available in the schedule and there is no sub therapeutic category of the scheduled under consideration**, the ceiling price shall be calculated as under:

Step 1: First the Average Price to Retailer of such scheduled formulation [P(s)] is to be calculated as under:

$$P(s) = Pm \{1-(Pi1 + Pi2+...) \div (N*100)\}$$

Where,

Pm = Price of highest priced formulation taken for calculating the average price to retailer of the formulation under consideration.

Pi = % Reduction in average price to retailer of other schedule formulations (calculated as given earlier for scheduled formulation) in same therapeutic category as that of the scheduled formulation under consideration with respect to the highest priced formulation taken for calculating the average price to retailer.

N = Number of such other schedule formulations in same therapeutic category as that of the scheduled formulation under consideration.

Step 2. The ceiling price of the scheduled formulation [P(c)] is to be calculated as under:

$$P(c) = P(s) \times (1+M/100)$$

where

P(s) = Average price to retailer of the scheduled formulation as calculated in step 1 above and

M = % Margin to retailer and its value = 16

Explanation: Where the scheduled formulation under consideration is coming under more than one therapeutic category, the average price to retailer of the scheduled formulation shall be calculated after taking into consideration the percentage reduction in Average Price to Retailer of other schedule formulations under all such therapeutic categories and the lowest average price to retailer shall be taken for calculating the ceiling price of the scheduled formulation under consideration.

7. **Maximum retail price:**

Maximum retail price = Ceiling price + Local taxes (for scheduled formulation)

Maximum retail price = Retail price + Local taxes (for new drugs).

8. **Reference data and source of market based data:** The data available with IMS Health is used as the data for fixing the price. However, government may come out its own source in due course of time.

9. **Ceiling price or retail price of a pack:** The average price is fixed based on dosage unit: Per tablet, per capsule or per volume of injection. The ceiling price of pack is obtained by multiplying the same with the number or quantity in the pack.

When the unit of the dosage is not available in the schedule, lowest pack size of that category of medicine is taken as unit dosage.

10. **Price of formulations of NLEM:** The manufacturer is free to fix the price of the scheduled formulation equal to or below the ceiling price fixed.

11. **Overcharging:** When the manufacturer sells at a price higher than the ceiling price, the manufacturer is liable to deposit the over charge amount with interest.

The pharmaceutical companies have been overcharging many ways: Selling the scheduled medicines at a higher price than the ceiling price fixed by NPPA and increasing price at more than 10% for other medicines. Minister of State for Road Transport and Highways, Shipping and Chemicals and Fertilizers, Shri Mansukh Lal Mandaviya, while giving a written reply to a question in Lok Sabha on 25/7/2017, informed that, as on 30th June 2017, an amount of 238.84 crore has been recovered from the pharmaceutical companies against non-compliance of provisions of DPCO, 2013.

12. **Revision of ceiling price:** The Government is empowered to revise the ceiling price of scheduled formulation every year based on the wholesale price index (WPI) and the new price is scheduled to be announced on 1st April every year. The manufacturers can revise the price based on WPI and there is no need of prior approval from the government. The price may go down too if there is a decline in WPI.

13. **Revision of ceiling price based on moving annual turnover (MAT):** The ceiling prices are revised whenever the new NLEM is prepared or after five years of price fixing whichever are earlier.

14. **Monitoring the price of non-scheduled formulations:** The government monitors the price of such medicines to ensure that the annual increase is not more than 10 percent.

15. **Monitoring the availability of scheduled formulations:** The government monitors the production and availability of scheduled formulations and the respective active pharmaceutical ingredients in order to ensure their availability. Manufacturers are not allowed to discontinue the production at their will. The manufacturer intending to discontinue is required to give public notice and intimate the government in prescribed format at least six months prior to the intended date of discontinuation.

16. **Selling price:** No person is allowed to sell the medicines at higher price than the ceiling price or price labelled on the package.

17. **Maintenance of records:** The manufacturer has to maintain the record the sales of formulations and the active pharmaceutical ingredient.

18. **Power of entry, search and seizure:** The authorized gazetted officer of central or state government has the power to enter and search any place and seize any drug along with container and package in an attempt to ensure compliance of DPCO. The provision of Code of Criminal Procedure relating to search and seizure should be followed.

19. **Provision of review:** The aggrieved person who is not satisfied with price fixation or any other notification, may apply to the government (Department of Pharmaceuticals) within 30 days of the order for a review. Pending the decision of the government, the manufacturer is not permitted to sell the medicines at a price exceeding the ceiling price or retail price. Two review cases are discussed in the text box.

20. **Non-application of the provision in certain cases:** The DPCO is not applicable for a new patented drug (product/process), if developed through indigenous research and development, for a period of five years from the date of commencement of its commercial production. Similarly new drug with new delivery system is also exempted for five years.

Review Cases

Erroneous fixation of ORS price: M/S FDC Limited, the manufacturer of 'Electral' brand oral rehydration salts (ORS), filed a review petition. The company argued that while calculating the price to retailer, the NPPA has mistakenly included the company's health drink 'Enerzal' too. As Enerzal is only a food supplement and the manufacturing is done under a licence from Food Safety Standards Authority of India (FSSAI), this should not be clubbed with ORS, a life-saving drug. Company argued that ceiling price so fixed leads to huge loss for the company.

MRP of their Electral branded ORS pack of 21.8 g was Rs. 17.65 and after WPI reduction of 2.71% under the NPPA Notification S.O. 644(E) dated 2/3/16, it was

reduced to Rs. 17.17. If they apply the ceiling price Rs. 0.71 per g to their Electral branded ORS 21.8 g, the MRP works out to Rs. 16.25. It means MRP reduction from Rs. 17.17 to Rs. 16.25.

If the **Enerzal is removed, the number** of packs considered for price fixation will be reduced from 31 to 26. So also sum of PTR per unit (g) considered for price fixation will be reduced from Rs. 19.60 to Rs. 18.46. Accordingly, average PTR per g will increase from Rs. 0.63 to Rs. 0.71. After adding 16% retailer's margin, ceiling price (without local tax) per g would increase from Rs. 0.73 to Rs. 0.82. The current MRP of their Electral ORS pack of 21.8 g is Rs. 17.17 (i.e. after WPI reduction of 2.71% under the NPPA notification S.O. 644(E) dated 2/3/16). Therefore, if they apply correct and proper Price Rs. 0.82 per g to Electral 21.8 g ORS, MRP works out to Rs. 18.76 (inclusive of VAT 5%). Therefore, the company need not reduce MRP of their Electral ORS 21.8 g pack. **Government's Decision:** As the NPPA included a non-pharmaceutical substance in calculation for arriving a price to retailer; the government stayed the earlier order and advised the NPPA to fix the price afresh.

[Ref: No. 31015/30/2016-PI.I, Dated 14 September 2016, Department of Pharmaceuticals]

Review Petition Rejected by Government [Price Fixation of Effervescent Acetyl Salicylic Acid (ASA)]: Reckitt Benckiser (India) Limited filed a petition against the fixation of ceiling price of its product 'Colspirin' an effervescent ASA 100 mg tablet. The company argued that this product is different from plain ASA tablet as it has the composition (ASA + calcium carbonate) as active ingredient and anhydrous citric acid as excipient. NPPA viewed anhydrous citric acid as active ingredient as this is an ingredient of ORS. This formulation was earlier declared as FDC (Fixed Dose Combination) in 2008. But the company did not ask for price fixation as FDC as FDCs are treated as new drugs. New drug approval is tricky requires safety and

efficacy evaluation data. ASA effervescent tablets are in NLEM 2015. If the company wanted to be separately viewed, it should have applied as new drug for price fixation. The NLEM has effervescent tablet together with ASA tablet. In view of all these, the Department of Pharmaceuticals said "there is no separate provision for price fixation of ASA effervescent tablet" and thus the request of the company was rejected.
[Pharmabiz, November 3, 2016]

The DPCO 2013 was under scrutiny by many. Some of the points raised against the policy were:

- The simple average formula used for price fixing has no relation with its cost of production and may result in many price controlled medicines continue to be sold at high margins of 1000–3000%. Cost-based pricing would have been more rational.

- A civil society in its letter to the Prime Minister highlighted the discrepancy in pharma pricing. A drug of MRP Rs 315/- is offered to hospital at Rs 135/-. This example shows the profit margin of medicines. It has urged the government to take steps to ensure the difference between the actual price and MRP should not exceed 20%.

- In 2013, when the order was implemented, has effect for medicines in the NLEM 2011. The NLEM 2011 was under criticism as it failed to include many essential medicines including the medicines in WHO's list of essential medicines. The drugs like amikacin, cycloserin, glimepride

Items under DPCO	DPCO 1979	DPCO 1987	DPCO 1995	July 2006	DPCO 2013	2017
Number of drugs under price control	347	142	76	74	348 [National List of Essential Medicine 2011]	Many other drugs which are not in National List of Essential Medicines 2015 are also included. The cardiac stents are brought under price control.
Number of categories under which the above drugs are categorized	3	2	1	1	1	
MAPE percent allowed on normative or national ex-factory costs to meet post manufacturing expenses and to provide for margin to the manufacturer						
Category I	40	75	100	100		
Category II	55	100	Not Available	Not Available		
Category III	100	Not available	Not available	Not available		
Percentage of total domestic pharmaceutical sales covered under price control (approximate)	90	70	50	–		

Comparative chart of successive DPCO

were not the list and hence were outside the price control mechanism.

However, with revision of NLEM, these medicines are brought under price control.

- There were apprehensions that manufactures may stop the production of controlled drugs and switch to other drugs of the same category (not listed in schedule) or may go for different strengths. As the products developed under indigenous research and developments are exempted from price control for five years, the manufacturers may switch to different delivery system like sustained release delivery system.
- By simply combining one essential medicine with another non-essential medicine, the manufacturer can wriggle out of the ceiling price. Indian market is already flooded with FDCs.

With time, the government has not just restricted the controlling of the prices of medicines, but has fixed the ceiling prices for cardiac stents and orthopaedic implants. More details on cardiac stents are given in the box.

- **National pharmaceutical pricing authority (NPPA)** has been entrusted with the task of implementing the DPCO. NPPA was established on 29th August 1997 as an independent body of experts by Government of India (not as part of DPCO). The website of NPPA is http://nppaindia.nic.in. NPPA is now the body of the Department of Pharmaceuticals of Ministry of Chemicals and Fertilizers.

Lower Potency Product is Expensive than Higher Potency!

This sounds aberration. But true. Mr. Raj Vaidya, a community pharmacist of Goa, has found this in his practice. Three examples:

1. Amoxycillin and Potassium Clavulanate tablets IP [Augmentin 375]: MRP of 10 tablets is Rs 229.00; MRP of 10 tablets of Augmentin 625 is Rs 176.78.
2. Amoxycillin and Potassium Clavulanate tablets IP [Augpen 375]: MRP of 10 tablets is Rs 171.40; MRP of 10 tablets of Augpen 625 is Rs 169.45.

3. Atenolol tablets IP [Aten 25]: MRP of 15 tablets is Rs 30.10; MRP of 15 tablets of Aten 50 is Rs 25.40.

This raises several issues: Whether DPCO does not have provision to address these issues or it is the usual practice of companies to have such practice. Ironically, lower potency products [Amoxycillin and Potassium Clavulanate 375; and Atenolol 25] are not in the National List of Essential Medicines.

Authorities for Enforcement of Prices

NPPA, Drugs Controller of States/Food and Drug Administration, and Drug Inspectors are the enforcing authorities at national, state and district levels.

Functions of NPPA

The main functions of NPPA are to:

- Implement and enforce the provision of DPCO.
- Deal with legal matters arising out of decision of the authority.
- Monitor the availability of drugs, identify shortages if any, and to make remedial measures.
- Collect/maintain data on production, exports and imports, market share of individual companies, profitability of companies, etc. for bulk drugs and formulations.
- Undertake and/or sponsor relevant studies in respect of pricing of drugs and pharmaceuticals.
- Recruit or appoint the officers and other staff members of the authority.
- Render advice to the Government of India on changes/revisions in the drug policy.
- Render assistance to Government of India in the parliamentary matters relating to drug pricing.

Pricing of Medical Devices

Pricing of cardiac stents: In an attempt to make medical devices more affordable along with the life-saving drugs, NPPA capped the price of bare metal stents (BMS) at Rs 7260 [February 2017] and Drug Eluting Stent (DES) at Rs 29,600 [April 2017]. The prices are further revised and the current capping prices are: Rs 7400 and Rs 30,180 are for bare metal stents and DES respectively. This has slashed the price of cardiac stents by around 75%. The corresponding average MRPs before price control was at Rs 45,000 and Rs 1.21 lakh respectively.

Aggrieved with the price capping, one of the manufacturers, Boston Scientific, argued that the capped price was much lower than the import price of its product, Synergy. It requested for to raise the capping price to around Rs 75,000 ($1160). The company's request was rejected by the government citing "There is no major innovation". Before the price fixing the company was selling the Synergy stent at Rs 195,000 ($3000) in India. The government has decided one price for all DES on the basis that new generations of DES are not superior to earlier generations.

There is **no significant difference** between bio-absorbable vascular scaffolds (BVS) and DES. The DES releases a drug to prevent clotting as it clears blockage in an artery. The BVS is made up of organic material that dissolves in blood after cleaning the artery. BMS is a mesh-like tube of thin wire but does not release drug which are said to prevent clotting. BVS are considered to be more expensive and its price ranging up to Rs 2.5 lakh prior to capping. An article in Lancet reported "there is no difference between using DES and BVS stents. There is non-inferiority in terms of late luminal loss (restenosis) or superiority in vasomotor reactivity of the bio-resorbable vascular scaffolds compared with the drug-eluting stents" [Lancet Vol 389, 4th March 2017]. It further states that no significant differences between participants receiving drug-eluting stents and those receiving bare-metal stents in the composite outcome of death from any cause and non-fatal myocardial infarctions. Similarly another study involving 5000 patients published in New England Journal of Medicine claimed that there were no long-term differences in patient outcomes of BMS and DES [Daily News and Analysis of 04th March 2017]. Restenosis means renarrowing of arteries and upheaval vasomotor reactivity refers to artery going into spasm.

Violation of DPCO: NPPA found that there were around 200–300 cases of stent over pricing, hospital not giving the proper bills of stents. The NPPA directed the hospitals to bill stents separately to prevent overcharging of stents by the hospitals. Gujarat FDA reported the recovery of Rs 52 lakh of overcharged amount from around 20 hospitals [Pharmabiz, April 15, 2017).

In order to beat the price capping the companies have been using different ways like giving offer "Buying 10 and get 3 free". The multinational companies are reported to be fooling the people and government of India as far as price of the cardiac stents. These companies claim that selling the cardiac stents at the ceiling price is not commercially viable. But the truth is otherwise. These companies are reported to be selling these stents at far lower price in rich countries like

Stent type	India's price	Price in other countries
Abbot's bio-absorbable/ DES	Rs 1.9 lakh ($2900) Capped price approximately Rs 31,000 for DES	In Europe: DES or innovative DES costs from 40–100 Euro [Rs 2800 to 7000]. In US: The cost of DES ranges from Rs 62,000 ($950) to Rs 78,000 ($1200)
Bare metal stent	Capped price approximately Rs 7500	Rs 6300 in European countries

Source: ET Health world Dated May 15, 2017

Germany, UK and other European countries. The price is higher in US but lower than the pre-capping price. The given table gives a glance of it.

Companies like Abbot and Medtronic sought to withdraw their high priced products from Indian market citing unviability. However, the government invoked special power offered in the DPCO to prohibit the stent makers from withdrawing their products for next 6 months. This would ensure 'no problem in stent market'.

The government has not stopped at fixing the ceiling prices of cardiac stents. Recently it has fixed the ceiling price of orthopaedic implants.

The DPCO is a social measure to improve the access of medicines and other essential medical devices. Access to medicines has been accepted worldwide as a fundamental right.

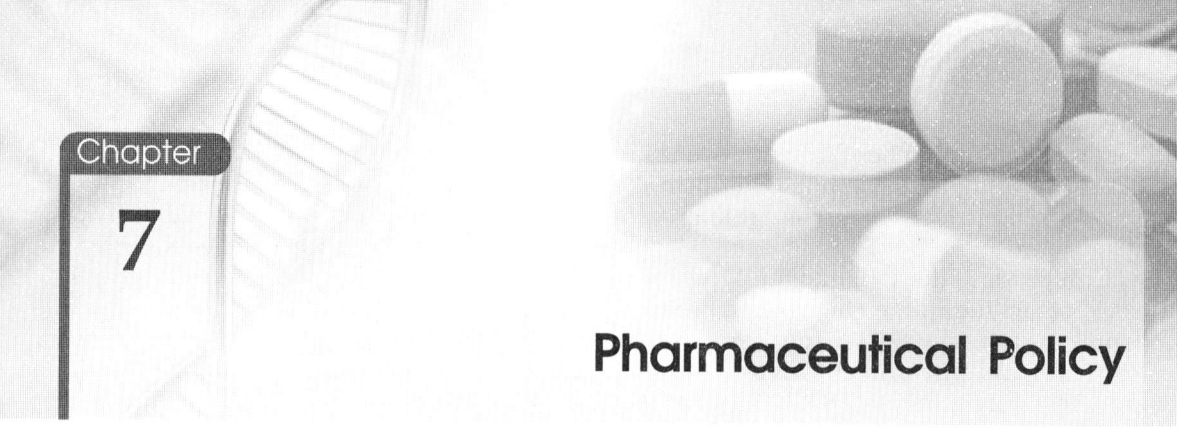

Pharmaceutical Policy

"The policy of being too cautious is the greatest risk of all."

— *Jawaharlal Nehru*

After reading this chapter, you should be able to understand and appreciate:
- Genesis of pharmaceutical policy
- Provisions of the policy
- Draft policy for revision of pharmaceutical policy

National Pharmaceutical (Drug) Policy is a commitment to a goal and guide for action. It is an official document of national government, which acts as a formal record of aspirations, aims, decisions, and commitments for solving problems associated with pharmaceuticals.

Tracing back to history it is found that the first drug policy was announced in 1978 mainly as a follow up of Hathi Committee Report and then after a gap of more than a decade in 1986. Both these initiatives were inspired by a concern with the industrial and commercial side of pharmaceuticals rather than by health related or medical considerations. The government intention was to develop indigenous industries and a broad technological base rather than to make the right quality of medicines available to the people at reasonable prices in response to their specific health need. Thereafter, the next policy was announced as Drug Policy 1994 (though just modified one) and till date this is the guiding principle for government decisions. One of the main objectives of the policy was "to ensure abundant availability of essential and life saving, and prophylactic medicines of good quality at reasonable prices". The results have

been encouraging. The price of medicines in this country is undoubtedly as one of the lowest in the world, but is in terms of absolute price. The price must be considered in terms of affordability.

Fortunately or unfortunately the announced policy, Pharmaceutical Policy 2002, could not be implemented. This was intended further liberalizing the price decontrol and more industry oriented than with health outlook. While keeping one of the objectives "ensuring abundant availability at reasonable price within the country of good quality essential pharmaceuticals of mass consumption", it proposed to bring down the medicines under price control mechanism from 74 drugs in 1995 to just around 35. Before the policy was implemented, it was stayed by the Karnataka High Court. Even the Supreme Court directed that ensuring essential and life saving drugs not to fall out of price control and to review the drugs which are essential and life saving in nature. Again the draft policy was announced in 2005, Pharmaceutical Policy 2006, which too did not get materialized. In view of Supreme Court's directions and subsequent other development in pharmaceutical scenario like product patent implementation, the government formulated just the National Pharmaceutical Pricing Policy (NPPP) 2012. Now, the government proposes to have a new policy and accordingly the Draft Pharmaceutical Policy is notified inviting public comments.

The competition stabilizes the price of consumer products where consumers have direct choice. But medicines are different types of commodities where real consumers have no choice but they pay for their medicines. Thus the philosophy of price stabilization through competition does not hold good.

The change of drug policy terminology to pharmaceutical policy is in consistent with international view. Internationally the term has been changed from drug to medicine and then to pharmaceutical.

The framing of Pharmaceutical Policy comes under the Department of Pharmaceuticals of the Ministry of Chemicals and Fertilizers of the Government of India. Perhaps, this is the reason of the policy proposals dominate the industrial aspects mainly promoting the drugs and pharmaceutical industries with little interest on health aspects.

The text limits its discussion to the Draft Pharmaceutical Policy 2017 and National Pharmaceutical Pricing Policy 2012. **Ideally, a Pharmaceutical Policy should address all the main four components: Access, Regulation, Quality and Use. But the draft policy is mostly focused on the first component: Access.** The access to medicines is influenced by both price and availability. This remains the main focus.

Time line of development of drug policy	
1978	First Policy called Drug Policy formulated
1986	Drug Policy of 1978 is revised
1994	Drug Policy is further revised: Industrial licensing abolished, only 5 drugs are reserved for Public Sector Units, foreign investment limit is raised to 51%, New drugs are exempted from price control, NPPA is created.
2002	Pharmaceutical Policy formulated based on the report of: Pharmaceutical Research and Development Committee [PRDC] and Drug Price Review Committee [DPRC]. Name changed from Drug Policy to Pharmaceutical Policy. Not implemented because of litigation.
2006	Revised Draft Pharmaceutical Policy. Not finalised.
2012	National Pharmaceutical Pricing Policy announced. Backbone of DPCO order 2013.
2017	Draft Pharmaceutical Policy announced inviting stakeholders suggestion/comments.

Draft Pharmaceutical Policy 2017

Key objectives: The draft policy's key objectives are:

- To make essential drugs accessible at affordable prices to the common masses.
- To provide a longer term stable policy environment for the pharmaceutical sector.
- To make India sufficiently self-reliant in end to end indigenous drug manufacturing;
- To ensure world class quality of drugs for domestic consumption and exports.
- To create an environment for R&D to produce innovator drugs.

The Important Policy Details with some Comments are Outlined

i. *Encouraging end to end indigenous manufacturing*: It is proposed that formulations produced from end to end (indigenously from API to product) will be given preference in government procurement. These products will be exempted from price control for five years. It is also proposed to create mega park for bulk drug production with common facilities like pollution control, effluent treatment.

ii. *Ensuring quality*: It is proposed to make Bioavailability and Bioequivalency (BA/ BE) tests mandatory for manufacturing of all drug products and for future renewal of licenses. While it is the best way to ensure quality not only among batches but also among the products of different manufacturers, there is apprehension that there are no enough facilities available in the country to take up the massive task—a few bio-availability/bioequivalency testing centres but a large number of products. The question also arises whether all the products require this testing. Biopharmaceutical Classification System (BCS) should be considered for making the test mandatory.

iii. *Ensuring compliance with international Standards*: All manufacturing units should adopt WHO's (World Health Organization) Good Manufacturing Practices (GMP) and Good Laboratory Practices (GLP). In order to encourage, it is proposed that the procurement under National Health Mission (NHM) both at central and state level would be only from GMP and GLP compliant units. The small scale industries would be given assistance to upgrade.

iv. *Accelerating the process of approval*: The decision on application of drug approval by central and state drugs authority should be conveyed within 3 months. The period may be extended by another 3 months but the author needs to record the reason for delay and communicate the same to the applicant.

v. *Brand Vs generic name*: It is proposed that only pharmacopoeia name or salt name should be used in the package of single ingredient products. Brand name is permissible only for patented drugs and fixed dose combinations. The principle is 'one company—one drug—one brand name—one price'. "This would not distinguish between innovation in generics and me—too drugs. That means this would discourage innovation", the critics believe.

vi. *Promoting generics*: E-prescription will be in operation where prescriptions will be computerized and drugs name will be picked up from dropdown menu containing generic name;

vii. *Trade margin*: The government proposes to fix the trade margin of drugs. Currently the government (NPPA) is in the process of fixing trade margin for medical devices like cardiac stents, orthopedic knee implants. There have been reports of unreasonable trade margin and bonus offers by various stockists, distributors and retailers.

viii. *Loan Licensing*: It is proposed to stop the loan licensing system except for biopharmaceuticals. There have been practice of P2P [Product to Product] manufacturing where one manufacturer manufactures one pharmacopeial drug in multiple brand names and given to the marketing companies to sell them at their chosen price. Both forms of loan licensing are to be stopped. With this many companies are likely to be affected as over 70% of MNCs and 50% of Indian brands are manufactured either in loan licensing or P2P model. The stopping of loan licensing may severely affect the availability of medicines.

ix. *Marketing practice*: The voluntary code of marketing practices would be made mandatory with penalty provision;

x. *Encouraging e-pharmacy*: It is proposed to introduce e-pharmacy with regulatory mechanism in place. This may encourage Foreign Direct Investment (FDI).

xi. *Developing database*: It is unfortunate that there is no database of drugs and products. It is proposed to create database. The Department of Pharmaceuticals in association with DCGI will develop database on manufacturer wise, brand wise products, product wise and brand wise manufacturer.

xii. *Introducing barcode system*: The compulsory barcode system with retail price is proposed. This would not only help in computerized billing but also help in preventing dispensing error.

xiii. *Skill development of pharmacists*: It is proposed to improve the skill of pharmacists to improve the service. The skill development should not be restricted to pharmacists but also to the assistants working in the pharmacy.

xiv. *Foreign direct investment*: The policy proposes series of measures to protect the domestic pharmaceutical companies against the acquisition by foreign investment. The government has already allowed up to 74% FDI through automatic route, but there is no mechanism to monitor the post-acquisition activities of the company. Indian domestic pharmas have state-of-the-art infrastructure and there have been apprehension that the foreign companies may acquire these firms. After acquisition, the firms may stop manufacturing drugs useful for India.

The policy proposes measures such as continuation of manufacturing essential medicines, expenditure on research & development, and technology transfer to seek approval of FDI;

xv. *National Institute of Pharmaceutical Education and Research*: The priority of strengthening the existing NIPERs than establishing new NIPER;

xvi. *Encouraging R&D*: The government proposes lower custom duty for imported products required for R&D. Novel Drug Delivery Systems are proposed to be treated as new drugs. It is also proposed to encourage gene and molecular level research through industryinstitute interaction. However, this looks to be too little;

xvii. *Price regulation Mechanism*:

a. *Basis of price regulation*: National List of Essential Medicines would be the basis of price control. But the government proposes that the list would be prepared by the Department of Pharmaceuticals (not by the Ministry of Health as done currently). There are possibilities that the health aspects may not get priority in developing the list of price control.

b. *Restructuring of NPPA*: The policy proposes to have a multimember advisory body consisting of doctors, pharmacists, other experts, civil societies, representative of industry, and government representative. The

advice of the body is recommendatory in nature and decision of NPPA is final. While modifying or rejecting the advice, the NPPA has to record the reason of not accepting or rejecting.

The NPPA would be made a multi-member body: Chairman, Member (Enforcement) and Member (Pricing). The decision would be taken by consensus. The authority will be assisted by the Member Secretary who would be appointed by the government.

The appeal against the NPPA would lie with the government and the appeal against the government would be decided by the judiciary.

The restructuring of NPPA is viewed as weakening the authority of NPPA: The power of deciding on drugs is proposed to be taken over by the government. The NPPA would have jurisdiction on fixing the ceiling price for the listed medicines given by the government, enforcing the implementation of ceiling price and adequate availability of these medicines. The multi-member authority too may weaken the body.

National Pharmaceutical Pricing Policy 2012 (NPPP 2012)

The NPPP 2012 was aimed at just as the principles for pricing of essential drugs as laid down in the National List of Essential Medicines 2011. It was only a temporary measure and a holistic policy proposed to be introduced later. [At present we see the Draft Pharmaceutical Policy 2017]. The NPPP 2012 is the continuation of Drugs Policy 1994. The key principles of price regulation under NPPP 2012 are:

- Essentiality of drugs
- Control of formulations price only
- Market-based pricing

The NPPP is slightly different from Drugs Policy of 1994. These differences are:

- The economic criteria or market share principle was used as criteria for bringing the drugs under price control in Drugs Policy 1994. The NPPP proposed essentiality as criteria for bringing the drugs under price control. All the Drugs under NLEM (as revised periodically) are brought under price control. The more details can be seen in Chapter-Drugs Price Control Order.

- It proposes to regulate the prices of formulations only. DPCO 1995 had 74 drugs under its basket. As the bulk drugs are difficult to be treated under the principles of essentiality, no bulk drugs are proposed to be controlled for price. The DPCO 2013 formulated under the NPPP controls the price of all formulations only.

It is proposed to use market-based pricing [while Drugs Policy 1994 was for cost based practice for fixing the ceiling price]. The methodology of fixing a ceiling price of NLEM medicines is by adopting the Simple Average Price of all the brands having market share (on the basis of Moving Annual Turnover) more than and equal to 1% of the total market turnover of that medicine, will be as per the formula below:

(Sum of prices of all the brands of the medicine having market share more than and equal to 1% of the total market turnover of that medicine) ÷ (Total number of manufacturers producing such brands of the medicine)

The civil societies have expressed their reservations on market based prices. It is argued that in each segment of drugs, the simple average price of all drugs with market share of minimum 1% may lead to price rise in many cases. They cited a few examples too. The cost based price of metformin was Rs. 14/- but market based price for the same would be Rs. 35/-. Similarly Atorvastatin price would go up from Rs. 17/- to Rs. 127/-.

The policy proposed to initiate measures for strengthening of the pharmaceutical industry in the following areas:

(a) Strengthening and rationalizing the drug regulatory system.

(b) Bringing on a common platform all the regulatory authorities related to drug standards, bio-pharmaceuticals, clinical trials and Pharmacopeia.

(c) Promotion of research and development in the pharmaceutical sector, directly through research institutions and universities, as well as through provision of seed capital, venture capital funding and subsidies to innovative drug companies.

(d) Enablement of domestic pharmaceutical companies to achieve international GMP/ GLP and GCP standards.

(e) Development of Human Resource, particularly in critical areas to meet the requirements of pharmaceutical industries.

(f) Rationalization of excise duties on pharmaceuticals.

(g) Setting up of common infrastructure through pharma development parks, pharma cluster schemes in order to strengthen and facilitate the smaller units in the pharmaceutical industries.

(h) Rationalization of pharma retail trade and strengthening of pharma supply chains.

PHARMACEUTICAL POLICY 2002

The basic objectives of Government's Policy relating to the drugs and pharmaceutical sector were enumerated in the Drug Policy of 1986. These basic objectives still remain largely valid. However, the drug and pharmaceutical industry in the country today faces new challenges on account of liberalization of the Indian economy, the globalization of the world economy and on account of new obligations undertaken by India under the WTO Agreements. These challenges require a change in emphasis in the current pharmaceutical policy and the need for new initiatives beyond those enumerated in the Drug Policy 1986, as modified in 1994, so that policy inputs are directed more towards promoting accelerated growth of the pharmaceutical industry and towards making it more internationally competitive. The need for radically improving the policy framework for knowledge-based industry has also been acknowledged by the Government. The Prime Minister's Advisory Council on Trade and Industry has made important recommendations regarding knowledge-based industry. The pharmaceutical industry has been identified as one of the most important knowledge-based industries in which India has a comparative advantage.

The process of liberalization set in motion in 1991, has considerably reduced the scope of industrial licensing and demolished many non-tariff barriers to imports. Important steps already taken in this regard are:

Industrial licensing for the manufacture of all drugs and pharmaceuticals has been abolished except for bulk drugs produced by the use of recombinant DNA technology, bulk drugs requiring *in vivo* use of nucleic acids, and specific cell/tissue targeted formulations.

Reservation of 5 drugs for manufacture by the public sector only was abolished in Feb. 1999, thus opening them up for manufacture by the private sector also. Foreign investment through automatic route was raised from 51% to 74% in March, 2000 and the same has been raised to 100%. Automatic approval for Foreign Technology Agreements is being given in the case of all bulk drugs, their intermediates and formulations except those produced by the use of recombinant DNA technology, for which the procedure prescribed by the Government would be followed.

Drugs and pharmaceuticals manufacturing units in the public sector are being allowed to face competition including competition from imports. Wherever possible, these units are being privatized. Extending the facility of weighted deductions of 150% of the expenditure on in-house research and development to cover as eligible expenditure, the expenditure on filing patents, obtaining regulatory approvals and clinical trials besides R&D in biotechnology. Introduction of the Patents (Second Amendment) bill in the Parliament provides for the extension in the life of a patent to 20 years.

The impact of the policies enunciated, from time to time, by the Government has been salutary. It has enabled the pharmaceutical industry to meet almost entirely the country's demand for formulations and substantially for bulk drugs. In the process, the pharmaceutical industry in India has achieved global recognition as a low-cost producer and supplier of quality bulk drugs and formulations to the world. In 1999–2000, drugs and pharmaceutical exports were ₹ 6631 crores out of a total production of ₹ 19,737 crores. However, two major issues have surfaced on account of globalization and implementation of our obligations under TRIPs which impact on long-term competitiveness of Indian industry. These have been addressed in the Pharmaceutical Policy-2002. A reorientation of the objectives of the current policy has also become necessary on account of these issues: The essentiality of improving incentives for research and development in the Indian pharmaceutical industry, to enable the industry to achieve sustainable growth particularly in view of anticipated changes in the Patent Law; and the need for reducing further the rigours of price control particularly in view of the ongoing process of liberalization.

It is against this backdrop that Pharmaceutical Policy-2002 is being enunciated.

Objectives

The main objectives of this policy are:

- Ensuring abundant availability at reasonable prices within the country of good quality essential pharmaceuticals of mass consumption.
- Strengthening the indigenous capability for cost effective quality production and exports of pharmaceuticals by reducing barriers to trade in the pharmaceutical sector.
- Strengthening the system of quality control over drug and pharmaceutical production and distribution to make quality an essential attribute of the Indian pharmaceutical industry and promoting rational use of pharmaceuticals.
- Encouraging R&D in the pharmaceutical sector in a manner compatible with the country's needs and with particular focus on diseases endemic or relevant to India by creating an environment conducive to channelising a higher level of investment into R&D in pharmaceuticals in India.
- Creating an incentive framework for the pharmaceutical industry which promotes

new investment into pharmaceutical industry and encourages the introduction of new technologies and new drugs.

Approach Adopted in the Review

In order to strengthen the pharmaceutical industry's research and development capabilities and to identify the support required by Indian pharmaceutical companies to undertake domestic R&D, a Committee was set up in 1999 by this Department by the name of Pharmaceutical Research and Development Committee (PRDC) under the Chairmanship of Director General of CSIR.

To qualify as R&D intensive company in India, the PRDC has suggested the following conditions (gold standards):

- Invest at least 5% of its turnover per annum in R&D,
- Invest at least ₹ 10 crore per annum in innovative research including new drug development, new delivery systems, etc. in India,
- Employ at least 100 research scientists in R&D in India, and has been granted at least 10 patents for research done in India,
- Own and operate manufacturing facilities in India.

The recommendations of the PRDC in so far as they relate to the Pharmaceutical Policy have been taken into account while formulating the proposals on pricing aspects.

The Pharmaceutical Research and Development Committee has recommended in its report, submitted inter alia, the setting up of a Drug Development Promotion Foundation (DDPF) and a Pharmaceutical Research and Development Support Fund (PRDSF). Necessary action in this regard has been initiated.

As far as the question of price control is concerned, the span of control has been gradually reduced since 1979. Presently, under DPCO, 1995 there are 74 bulk drugs and their formulations under price control covering approximately 40% of the total market. The functioning of the Drugs (Price Control) Order, 1995, has brought to light some problems in the administration of the price control mechanism for drugs and pharmaceuticals. In order to review the current drug price control mechanism, with the objective, inter alia, of reducing the rigours of price control, where they have become counter-productive, a committee, called the Drugs Price Control Review Committee (DPCRC), under the Chairmanship of Secretary, Department of Chemicals and Petrochemicals was set up in 1999, which has given its report. The recommendations of DPCRC have been examined and taken into account while formulating the "Pharmaceutical Policy 2002".

It has emerged that the domestic drugs and pharmaceuticals industry needs reorientation in order to meet the challenges and harness opportunities arising out of the liberalisation of the economy and the impending advent of the product patent regime. It has been decided that the span of price control over drugs and pharmaceuticals would be reduced substantially. However, keeping in view of interest of the weaker sections of the society, it is proposed that the government will retain the power to intervene comprehensively in cases where prices behave abnormally.

In view of the steps already taken and in the light of the approach indicated in the foregoing paragraphs, the decisions of the government are detailed below:

I. Industrial Licensing

Industrial licensing for all bulk drugs cleared by Drug Controller General (India), all their intermediates and formulations will be abolished, subject to stipulations laid down from time to time in the Industrial Policy, except in the cases of bulk drugs produced by the use of recombinant DNA technology, bulk drugs requiring *in vivo* use of nucleic acids as the active principles, and specific cell/tissue targetted formulations.

II. Foreign Investment

Foreign investment up to 100% will be permitted, subject to stipulations laid down from time to time in the Industrial Policy, through the automatic route in the case of all bulk drugs cleared by Drug Controller General (India), all their intermediates and formulations, except those, kept under industrial licensing.

III. Foreign Technology Agreements

Automatic approval for Foreign Technology Agreements will be available in the case of all bulk drugs cleared by Drug Controller General (India), all their intermediates and formulations, except those, kept under industrial licensing for which a special procedure prescribed by the government would be followed.

IV. Imports

Imports of drugs and pharmaceuticals will be as per EXIM (Export Import) policy in force. A centralized system of registration will be introduced under the Drugs and Cosmetics Act and Rules made thereunder. Ministry of Health and Family Welfare will enforce strict regulatory processes for import of bulk drugs and formulations.

V. Encouragement to Research and Development (R&D)

a. In principle approval to the establishment of the Pharmaceutical Research and Development Support Fund (PRDSF) under the administrative control of the Department of Science and Technology, which will also constitute a Drug Development Promotion Board (DDPB) on the lines of the Technology Development Board to administer the utilization of the PRDSF.

b. With a view to encouraging generation of intellectual property and facilitating indigenous endeavours in pharma R&D, appropriate fiscal incentives would be provided.

VI. Pricing

a. Span of Price Control

The guiding principle for identification of specific bulk drugs for price regulation should continue, as per DPCRC's recommendation, to be: (i) mass consumption nature of the drug and (ii) absence of

sufficient competition in such drugs. However, the DPCRC's recommendation regarding the new criteria for ascertaining the mass consumption nature of a bulk drug on the basis of the top selling brand is not acceptable as it gives rise to anomalies.

In this context, it may be noted that there is no tailor made data available for the purpose of ascertaining the mass consumption nature and absence of sufficient competition with reference to a particular bulk drug. There is only one source, namely "Retail Store Audit for Pharmaceutical Market in India" published by ORG-MARG, which lists out all major brands and their sale estimates on all India basis. This publication contains data for single ingredient as well as multiingredient formulations. However, it does not give complete description of all the ingredients of the pharmaceutical product listed therein.

Hence, there is need to obtain information in regard to composition of each brand, dosage formwise and packwise, from various other publications/sources, viz. Indian Pharmaceutical Guide (IPG), Current Index of Medical Specialities (CIMS), Monthly Index of Medical Specialities (MIMS), Drug Today, information provided by some manufacturers' label composition as indicated on market samples.

Though none of these sources can be said to be exhaustive and comprehensive in regard to market information, yet under the given circumstances, these are the best available. It has also been noted that the sale value of any combination formulation is not directly relatable to a single particular bulk drug forming part of the combination formulation. Combination formulations involve too many variables, viz. strength of a particular bulk drug and its proportion with respect to other bulk drugs used in the combination formulation, price difference between bulk drugs used in combination formulation, pack sizes, dosage forms, etc. In view of these facts, ORG-MARG sales data for combination formulation does not yield information in regard to mass consumption nature and the absence of sufficient competition with reference to a particular bulk drug. Also, it is to be borne in mind that processing of such data, which requires cross-checking with other publications and sources of information in regard to composition of each brand, dosage formwise and packwise may involve instances of omission/commission.

In view of the above, it would be logical to conclude that although ORG-MARG sale estimates available in regard to all single-ingredient formulations of a particular bulk drug would not yield the sale value of that bulk drug in the form of all its formulations, yet it would adequately reflect the mass consumption nature of that bulk drug in the form of single ingredient formulations, which may be used as a practical indicator for formulating the policy.

The Department through NPPA, with the help of NIPER, has developed the desired database for single ingredient formulations from the retail store audit data as published by ORG-MARG. On this basis, the Department proposes to undertake the exercise of identifying the bulk drugs of mass consumption nature and having absence of sufficient competition according to the following methodology:

The 279 items appearing in the alphabetical list of Essential Drugs in the National Essential Drug List (1996) of the Ministry of Health and Family Welfare and the 173 items, which are considered important by that Ministry from the point of view of their use in various Health Programmes, in emergency care, etc. with the exclusion, as in the past, therefrom of sera and vaccines, blood products, combinations, etc. should form the total basket out of which selection of bulk drugs be made for price regulation.

The ORG-MARG data of March 2001 would form the basis for determining the span of price control as suggested by DPCRC. The Moving Annual Total (MAT) value for any formulator in respect of any bulk drug will be arrived at by adding the MAT values of all his single-ingredient formulations of

that bulk drug, its salts, esters, stereo-isomers and derivatives, covering all the strengths, dosage forms and pack sizes listed against that formulator in all groups/categories of the ORG-MARG (March 2001). The MAT value for all the formulators, as specified, in respect of a particular bulk drug will be added to arrive at the total MAT value in the retail trade. The MAT value for an individual formulator, as specified, will be the basis for calculating the percentage share of that formulator in the total MAT value arrived in respect of that bulk drug.

Bulk Drugs will be kept under price regulation if:

a. The total MAT value, as derived, in respect of any particular bulk drug is more than ₹ 2500 lakhs (₹ 25 crore) and the percentage share, as specified, of any of the formulators is 50% or more.

b. The total MAT value, as arrived, in respect of any particular bulk drug is less than ₹ 2500 lakhs (₹ 25 crore) but more than ₹ 1000 lakhs (₹ 10 crore) and the percentage share, as defined, of any of the formulators is 90% or more.

All formulations containing a bulk drug as identified above, either individually or in combination with other bulk drugs, including those not identified for price control as bulk drug, will be under price control. The government shall, however, retain the following overriding power:

In cases of drugs/formulations listed by the Ministry of Health and Family Welfare, and those presently under price control, having significant MAT value as per ORG-MARG but not specified, as a result of this proposal, the NPPA would specially monitor intensively their price movement and consumption pattern. If any unusual movement of prices is observed or brought to the notice of the NPPA, the Authority would work out the price in accordance with the relevant provisions of the price control order.

c. Maximum Allowable Post-manufacturing Expenses (MAPE): Maximum Allowable

Post-manufacturing Expenses (MAPE) will be 100% for indigenously manu-factured formulations.

d. Margin for Imported Formulations: For imported formulations, the margin to cover selling and distribution expenses including interest and importer's profit shall not exceed fifty percent of the landed cost.

e. Pricing of Formulations

(i) For scheduled formulations, prices shall be determined as per the present practice. The timeframe for granting price approvals will be two months from the date of the receipt of the complete prescribed information.

(ii) The present stipulation that a manu-facturer, distributor or wholesaler shall sell a formulation to a retailer, unless otherwise permitted under the provi-sions of Drugs (Prices Control) Order or any other order made thereunder, at a price equal to the retail price, as specified by an order or notified by the government, (excluding excise duty, if any) minus sixteen percent thereof in case of scheduled drugs, will continue.

(iii) The present provision of limiting profi-tability of pharmaceutical companies, as per the Third schedule of the present Drugs (Prices Control) Order, 1995, would be done away with. How-ever, if necessary so to do in public interest, price of any formulation including a non-scheduled formu-lation would be fixed or revised by the government.

f. Ceiling prices: Ceiling prices may be fixed for any formulation, from time to time, and it would be obligatory for all, including small scale units or those marketing under generic name, to follow the price so fixed.

g. Exemptions

(i) A manufacturer producing a new drug patented under the Indian Patent Act, 1970, and not produced elsewhere, if developed through indigenous R&D, would be eligible for exemption from price control in respect of that drug for a period of 15 years from the date of the commencement of its commercial production in the country.

(ii) A manufacturer producing a drug in the country by a process developed through indigenous R&D and patented under the Indian Patent Act, 1970, would be eligible for exemption from price control in respect of that drug till the expiry of the patent from the date of the commencement of its commercial production in the country by the new patented process.

(iii) A formulation involving a new delivery system developed through indigenous R&D and patented under the Indian Patent Act, 1970, for process patent for formulation involving new delivery system would be eligible for exemption from price control in favour of the patent holder/formulator from the date of the commencement of its commercial production in the country till the expiry of the patent.

(iv) The DPCRC has suggested that the low-cost drugs measured in terms of "cost per day per medicine" may be taken out of price control. Any formulator can represent to NPPA with proof of per day cost to consumer-patient. NPPA will be authorised to exempt such formulation from price control if its cost to consumer-patient does not exceed ₹ 2/- per day, under intimation to the Government. All orders passed by the NPPA will be prospective in operation. Whenever the concerned formulator wishes to revise the price, he before effecting any change in price, would be bound to inform NPPA and seek fresh exemption and in case the cost to consumer-patient, on the basis of the proposed revised price, exceeds beyond the limit of ₹ 2/- per day, obtain the necessary price approval.

h. Pricing of Scheduled Bulk Drugs: For a scheduled bulk drug, the rate of return in case of basic manufacture would be higher by 4 percent over the existing 14 percent on net worth or 22 percent on capital employed. The timeframe for granting price approvals will be 4 months from the date of the receipt of the complete prescribed information. The government shall, however, retain the overriding power of fixing the maximum sale price of any bulk drug, in public interest.

i. Monitoring:

(i) The DPCRC's recommendations to have effective monitoring and enforcement system and to move away from the "controlled regime" to a "monitoring regime" is in the present context an extremely important recommendation as imports will increasingly compete with local drugs and pharmaceuticals in the domestic market. A new system based on solely market prices data is required to be evolved and controls applied selectively only to cases where, either profiteering, or monopoly profit seeking is noticed. The National Pharmaceutical Pricing Authority, set up in August, 1997, would need to be revamped and reoriented for this purpose. It will continue to be entrusted with the task of price fixation/price revision and other related matters, and would be empowered to take final decisions. It would also monitor the prices of decontrolled drugs and formulations and oversee the implementation of the drug prices control orders. The government would have the power of review of the price fixation/and price revision orders/notifications of NPPA.

(ii) Although the prices of some bulk drugs have been steadily decreasing, yet the same do not get reflected in the retail price of non-scheduled formulations. Also, there is need to check high margin/commission offered to the trade by printing high prices on the labels of medicines to the detriment of the consumers. It is, therefore, proposed to strengthen the National Pharmaceutical Pricing Authority by providing appropriate powers under the DPCO which would make it mandatory for the manufacturer to furnish all information as called for by NPPA and also to regulate such prices, wherever, required.

(iii) The other recommendations of DPCRC like giving powers to drug control authorities to dispose of small and petty offences, etc. will require an amendment to the Essential Commodities Act. This suggestion is considered not practicable. Monitoring price movement of drugs sold in the country as well as that of imported formulations will require developing appropriate mechanism in the NPPA.

j. Drug Price Equalization Account (DPEA): Provision would be made in the new Drugs (Prices Control) Order (DPCO) to ensure that amounts which have already accrued to the DPEA and those which are likely to accrue as a result of action in the past, are protected and used for the purpose stipulated in the existing DPCO.

VII. Quality Aspects

The Ministry of Health and Family Welfare would:

(i) Progressively benchmark the regulatory standards against the international standards for manufacturing,

(ii) Progressively harmonize standards for clinical testing with international practices,

(iii) Streamline the procedures and steps for quick evaluation and clearance of new drug applications, developed in India through indigenous R&D, and

(iv) Set up a world class Central Drug Standard Control Organisation (CDSCO) by modernizing, restructuring and reforming the existing system and establish an effective network of drugs standards enforcement administrations in the States with the CDSCO as a nodal center, to ensure high standards of quality, safety and efficacy of drugs and pharmaceuticals.

VIII. Pharmaceutical Education and Training

The National Institute of Pharmaceutical Education and Research (NIPER) has been set up by the Government of India as an institute of "national importance" to achieve excellence in pharmaceutical sciences and technologies, education and training. Through this institute, Government's endeavor will be to upgrade the standards of pharmacy education and R&D. Besides tackling problems of human resources development for academia and the indigenous pharmaceutical industry, the institute will make efforts to maximize collaborative research with the industry and other technical institutes in the area of drug discovery and pharma technology development.

Salient Features of Draft Policy 2006 (Excluding Price Control)

Objectives

1. To ensure availability at reasonable prices of good quality medicines within the country.
2. To improve accessibility of essential medicines for common man particularly the poorer section of the population.
3. To facilitate higher investment for increased production of good quality medicines.
4. To promote greater research and development in the pharmaceutical sector for providing suitable incentive in this regard.
5. To enable domestic pharmaceutical companies to become internationally competitive by implementing current Good Manufacturing Practices (GMP), Good Laboratory Practices (GLP), Good Clinical Practices (GCP) and other established international guidelines.
6. To facilitate higher growth in exports of Active Pharmaceutical Ingredients (APIs) and formulations by reducing the barriers to international trade in pharmaceutical sector.
7. To develop India as preferred global destination for pharma R&D and manufacturing.
8. To facilitate implementation of National Health Policy.

Policy Initiatives

1. Strengthening of Drug Regulatory System:
   a. Constitution of Independent and Autonomous body 'National Drug Authority' (NDA) replacing CDSCO.
   b. Amendment of Drugs and Cosmetics Act to make the penalties more deterrent for various offences in particular to spurious and substandard drugs.
   c. Long-term strategy: To merge NPPA and NDA to form National Authority on Drugs and Therapeutics (NADT).
2. Intellectual Property Rights (IPR) and Data Protection: Indian Laws and Policies pertaining to IPR to be fully compliant with the provisions of TRIPS.
   a. Modernization of patent offices.
   b. Setting up of Intellectual Property (IP) Cell in the Department of Chemicals and Petrochemicals to support innovator pharma small and medium enterprises.
   c. Establishment of expert group under the Chairmanship of Dr R A Mashelkar, Director General, Council for Scientific and Industrial Research.
3. Clinical Trials and Drug Development:
   a. Early decision on data protection.
   b. Improved regulatory infrastructure.
   c. Facilitate pre-clinical trials National Toxicology Centre set up in NIPER be made GLP compliant.
   d. Tax benefits available for R&D be extended to Clinical Trials.
   e. Exemption of import duty for clinical trial sample.
   f. To promote direct investment in clinical development and data management—exemption of service tax for 10 years up to 2015.
4. Public–Private Partnership (PPP) Programme for Anti-Cancer and Anti-HIV /

AIDS Medicines with concerned manufacturers and cancer hospitals:

a. Complete exemption of these drugs from all types of central, states and local taxes and levies.

b. To ask industry and trade to reduce profit margin.

c. To initiate subsidy scheme.

5. Price of drugs for other life threatening diseases: To bring under PPP model.

6. Patented Drugs: Mandatory price negotiations before granting marketing approval.

7. Trade margins.

8. Excise duty relief.

9. Maximum retail price inclusive of all taxes.

10. New DPCO.

11. Drugs and Therapeutics (Regulations) Act replacing existing DPCO.

12. NPPA: Strengthening.

13. Bulk procurement systems for drugs by government.

14. Lower prices for bulk purchases by government.

15. Promotion of generic drugs.

16. Control on pharmaceutical brands.

17. Quality Certification of Drugs.

18. Strengthening of pharma public sector undertakings (PSU).

19. Purchase preference to PSU.

20. Consumer awareness.

21. Schemes for providing accessibility of drugs to the poor (BPL families).

22. Health cess (2%) for funding schemes for poor in line of education cess.

23. Encouragement to community based organizations in the health sector.

24. Human resource development in pharmaceutical sector—establishment of NIPERs.

25. R&D fiscal incentives.

26. Development of Orphaned Drugs.

27. Schemes of interest subsidy for implementing Schedule M of Drugs and Cosmetics Rules (GMP).

28. Regulation of Drugs under Narcotic and Psychotropic Substances Act.

29. Establishment of Settlement Commission: To settle the issues relating to overcharging by pharma.

30. Drug Price Monitoring and Awareness fund.

31. Pharma Parks/SEZs (Special Economic Zones) for pharmaceutical industries.

32. Greater thrusts on Pharma Exports.

33. Pharmaceutical Distribution–Retailing.

34. Pharmaceutical Advisory Forum.

8

The Drugs and Magic Remedies (Objectionable Advertisements) Act
(Advertisements that Mislead are Act of Misdeed)

"Advertising is a racket like movies and brokerage business. You cannot be honest without admitting that its constructive contribution to the humanity is exactly minus zero".

— *Anonymous*

After reading this chapter, you should be able to understand and appreciate:
- The advertisements that are prohibited
- Misleading advertisement
- Administrative procedures for implementing the Act
- Regulatory situation of other countries
- Role of Advertising Standard Council of India

Advertising is all around us today. Advertising is a communication whose purpose is to inform the potential customers about products and services and how to use and obtain them. It attempts to persuade its audience to purchase goods or services. While advertising often is educative especially the Information, Education and Communication (IEC) materials distributed by government agencies, the information supplied by the promoter of medicines often is bias and misleading too. The critics are of the opinion that all advertising are inherently unethical. The public fall into the trap of such advertise-ment. This is really true for the suffering public who is desperate to try anything.

The unproven, usually ineffective, and sometimes dangerous medicines and treatment have been peddled throughout the human history. Such medicines may not have effective ingredients. The pamphlets of drugs with spurious claims were even the concern of the country as early as 1930 when Drug Enquiry Committee was constituted under the chairmanship of Col R N Chopra. In order to protect the interest of general innocent public, the Government of India brought the legislation "The Drugs and Magic Remedies (Objectionable Advertisements) Act" to prevent the false and misleading claims through advertisement. But it is not only out-dated but also ineffective in controlling such advertisements. There is rapid development in communication technology: It has grown from pamphlets or print media to radio to television to internet. The commercial message even started through SMS in mobile.

Today cures of questionable efficacy and gadgets of unproven value are being peddled through not only in the print, but also television and the internet. The internet has opened the doors for an unregulated market of quack cures, miraculous remedies for weight to sexual pleasure enhancement. There is proliferation of such advertisements making the suffering persons vulnerable. The New Indian Express in its editorial written "Saying exists in most Indian Languages that there are no cures for jealousy and baldness. Yet, advertisements often in newspapers and other media promoting medicines that can cure baldness. The medicines are usually prohibitively expensive and by the time the unwary consumer realises their uselessness, the drug sellers would have had their last laugh. This is one of the least implemented Acts. The advertisements appear in the mass media which the government is wary of touching that it would antagonise them. This is because review of the law has become urgent and unavoidable. It may even require enactment of new laws." The present Act is inadequate to deal with the present day situation. Further teething to the act is necessary. Some countries like New Zealand and the USA have completed the provision for Direct to Consumer Advertising (DTCA), it is not permissible in India.

Advertisements related to treatment of sex related and other incurable diseases have been common to certain drugs of Indian system of Medicines. In a meeting of state Directors of Indian System of Medicine and Homeopathy in December 1999, the central government impressed for strict enforcement of the Act.

The State Drugs Controller is the Authority for Implementation of the Act

The Parliamentary Standing Committee on Health and Family Welfare, GOI, in its 95th report noted that there has been recurring delay in amending DMR Act. The committee was critical on the misleading advertisements concerning AYUSH remedies over TV, Radio and other Print Media. It has noted the ineffectiveness of the DMR Act which is responsible for not been able to take stringent action against the misleading and exaggerated claims of efficacy of AYUSH medicines.

The central government has issued warning to TV channels against carrying advertisements with exaggerated or improper claims of ayurvedic, siddha, unani and homeopathic products and drugs. The channels should advertise only those products that have valid licenses, failure of which will attract action.

Advertising Standard Council of India (ASCI): ASCI, established in 1985, is a self-regulatory voluntary organization of the advertising industries. This has been regarded as 'advertising watchdog' and it has framed several guidelines. The public can complain to ASCI regarding any advertisement which they feel false or misleading, etc.

Once ASCI identifies a false claiming advertisement, it is expected to warn the advertiser to either remove the advertisement or modify. In case of non-compliance, it informs the state licensing authority for taking action. The Supreme Court too acknowledged the efforts of ASCI towards self-regulation of advertisements. ASCI has launched a mobile app 'ASCIonline' for the use by public. Some of the guidelines of ASCI are:

- That would help celebrities to perform due diligence on a product or brand they wish to endorse.

- Advertisements featuring celebrities need to doubly ensure that claims made in it are not misleading, false or sub-stantiated; so as not to harm the interest of the consumers.

- One of the code is that the advertisement should be truthful and honest. This is meant to safeguard against misleading advertisement. There should be special care and restraint with respect to advertisements addressed to those suffering from weakness, any real or perceived inadequacy of any physical attributes such as height or bust development, obesity, illness, impotence, infertility, baldness and the like to ensure that the claims or representations directly or by implications, do not exceed what is considered prudent by generally accepted standards or medical practice and actual efficacy of the product.

The Ministry of AYUSH has partnership with ASCI to co-regulate misleading advertisements in the AYUSH sector. The DCGI too has recognized self-regulations in advertising through ASCI's code.

Objective: To control the advertisement of drugs in certain cases, to prohibit the advertisement for certain purposes of remedies alleged to possess magic qualities and to provide for matters connected therewith.

The Act extends to the whole of India except the State of Jammu and Kashmir and applies to persons domiciled in the territories to which the Act extends who are outside the said territories. Though it has come into effect on 1st April 1955, the Act has been extended to some places at later dates. It has been extended to Pondicherry (now Pudducherry) on 01.10.1963, Dadra and Nagar Haveli on 01. 7. 1965 and Sikkim on 01.11.1989.

Prohibition of advertisement of certain drugs for treatment of certain diseases and disorders:

The following advertisements are prohibited which suggests the use of drugs or which may lead the use of drugs:

I. The procurement of miscarriage in women or prevention of conception in women; or

II. The maintenance or improvement of the capacity of human beings for sexual pleasure; or

III. The correction of menstrual disorders in women; or

IV. The diagnosis, cure, mitigation, treatment or prevention of any disease, disorder or condition specified in the schedule, or any disease, disorder or condition specified in the rules.

If the government deems fit, it can make rules for any disease, disorder or condition which requires timely consultation with a registered medical practitioner or for which no remedy exists and in consultation with DTAB or with other persons having special knowledge or practical experience in respect of Ayurvedic or Unani systems of medicine.

Prohibition of misleading advertisement relating to drugs:

The advertisements relating to drugs are prohibited if the advertisement contains any matter which:

I. Directly or indirectly gives a false impression about the true character of the drugs; or

II. Makes a false claim for the drug; or

III. Is false or misleading in any material.

The state government may authorize any person to scrutinize the misleading advertisements. If the person satisfied that the advertisement is contravening provision of misleading advertisements, he may direct the manufacturer, packer, distributor or seller to furnish the composition of the drug or ingredients or such information as required. The manufacturer, distributor, packer or seller is duty bound to comply the order of furnishing the necessary details. Failure to comply is treated contravention of the provision. Mere publication of advertisement will not be treated as contravention of the provision of the Act. But if the publisher or advertisement agency failed to comply with the order of furnishing details or the names and address of the manufacturer, packer, distributor or seller or advertisement agency who has asked the dissemination of such advertisements.

Prohibition of advertisement of magic remedies for certain diseases and disorders:

The publication of advertisement relating to magic remedies which directly or indirectly claims to be efficacious for disease or disorders mentioned under prohibition of advertisement of certain drugs for treatment of certain diseases or disorders by the persons purporting to carry on the profession of administering magic remedy is prohibited.

Prohibition of import or export of certain advertisements:

The document relating to prohibited advertisements described above in different categories are prohibited from importing or exporting into the territories to which the Act is effective. They are treated as goods of which import or export has been prohibited under Sea Customs Act 1878. If the custom collector has reasons to believe that any consignment contains documents pertaining to prohibition of import or export of advertisement, may detain the consignment and dispose it in accordance with Sea Custom Act 1878. He needs to inform his order to importer or exporter. When the importer or exporter is aggrieved by the decision of the custom collector, he can make representation to him within one week of the date of order and giving an undertaking not to dispose off the consignment without the consent of custom collector and return the consignment to the custom collector, the custom collector may issue order making over the consignment to the importer or exporter. The custom collector is required to consult the officer appointed by the central government for this purpose before issuing order of handing over the consignment. The importer or exporter who received the consignments after giving the undertaking should return the consignment or part of it as required within 10 days of receipt of notice.

Penalty

First conviction—imprisonment may extend to six months or with fine or both.

Subsequent conviction—imprisonment may extend to one year or with fine or both.

Power of Entry, Search, etc.

The gazetted officer authorized by state government has the power, within the local limits, to:

I. Enter and search any place at all reasonable times, with assistance, in which he has reason to believe that an offence has been or is being committed;

II. Seize any advertisement which he has reason to believe contravenes any provision of the Act;

III. Examine any record, register, document or any other material object found in any place which he has reason to believe that an offence has been or is being committed.

The Code of Criminal Procedure 1973 is to be followed in conducting any search or seizure and the seizure needs to be informed to a Magistrate and the custody of the seized materials be accepted based on Magistrate's order.

Offences

I. If the company contravenes any provision of the Act, every person in charge and was responsible for conduct of business of the company and the company shall be deemed to be guilty and shall be liable to be prosecuted. However, if he proves that the offence was committed without his knowledge or that he exercised all due diligence to prevent the commission of the offence, the person shall not be liable to any punishment.

II. If the offence under the Act is committed by a company with the consent or connivance of, or attributable to any neglect on the part of, any director or manager, secretary or other officer of company, such persons shall be deemed to be the guilty of the offence.

The offence punishable under the Act is cognizable. The offences can be tried in a court not inferior to that of Presidency Magistrate or a Magistrate of the first class.

When a person has been convicted by any court, the court may direct that any document, article or things that are seized are forfeited to the government.

No suit, prosecution or other legal proceedings lie against any person for anything if done in good faith.

Global Laws

USA: Federal Trade Commission (FTC) prescribes standards for endorsers of products. There are guidelines for endorsements by celebrities. "Good reason to believe" is a test to examine if the endorser actually uses or believes the features of the products. Celebrity endorsers are liable if they fail the test.

Europe: There is a voluntary self-imposed code which precludes celebrities from endorsing medicines, medical treatments, tobacco and alcohol.

UK: There is a control on medicine advertisements and the details are given in Blue Guide on advertising and promotion of medicines. Guideline lays down the requirements and restrictions for advertising. Advertisements of prescription only medicine to the public are prohibited.

Australia: There are industry self-regulating codes which govern the advertisements or promotion of therapeutic goods to the health professionals. Therapeutic Goods Advertising Code and Industry Code of Practice are the guiding force for promotion of therapeutic goods to the consumers. Therapeutic Goods Administration has the overall responsibility.

Exempted Advertisements

The following advertisements are exempted from the provision of the Act:

a. Any signboard or notice displayed by a registered medical practitioner on his premises indicating that treatment for any disease, disorder or condition specified in schedule (prohibition of advertisement of certain drugs for diagnosis, cure, mitigation, treatment or prevention of disease or disorder).

b. Any treatise or book dealing with any matter from a bonafide scientific or social standpoint.

c. Any advertisement relating to any drug sent confidentially to a registered medical practitioner by name, to a wholesale or retail chemist. Such documents should be sent by post where the address of such persons is given. The documents should have these words printed in indelible ink

The scheduled list of diseases for which advertisement of drugs prohibited

S. No.	Name of the disease or disorder or condition	S. No.	Name of the disease or disorder or condition
1	AIDS	30	Hydrocele
2	Asthma	31	Hysteria
3	Appendicitis	32	Infantile paralysis
4	Arteriosclerosis	33	Insanity
5	Blindness	34	Leprosy
6	Blood poisoning	35	Leucoderma
7	Bright's disease	36	Lockjaw
8	Cancer	37	Locomotor atoxia
9	Cataract	38	Lupus
10	Deafness	39	Nervous debility
11	Diabetes	40	Obesity
12	Disease and disorder of the brain	41	Paralysis
13	Disease and disorder of the optical system	42	Plague
14	Disease and disorders of the uterus	43	Pleurisy
15	Disorder of menstrual flow	44	Pneumonia
16	Disorder of nervous system	45	Rheumatism
17	Disorder of prostatic gland	46	Ruptures
18	Dropsy	47	Sexual impotence
19	Epilepsy	48	Smallpox
20	Female diseases in general	49	Stature of persons
21	Fevers (in general)	50	Sterility in women
22	Fits	51	Trachoma
23	Form and structure of the female bust	52	Tuberculosis
24	Gall stones, kidney stones and bladders stones	53	Tumors
25	Gangrene	54	Typhoid fever
26	Glaucoma	55	Ulcers of the gastrointestinal tract
27	Goitre	56	Venereal diseases including syphilis, gonorrhoea, soft chancre, venereal granuloma and lympho granuloma
28	Heart diseases		
29	High or low blood pressure		

on the top in a conspicuous manner "For the use of registered medical practitioner or a hospital or a laboratory".

d. Any advertisement relating to a drug printed or published by the government.

e. Any advertisement relating to a drug printed or published by any person with the previous sanction of the government granted prior to the commencement of Drugs and Magic Remedies (Objectionable Advertisement) Amendment Act 1963.

In the public interest the government has power to issue permission for advertisements relating to drug(s) by notifying in the official gazette. Such advertisements will not invite the provision of the Act.

The central government has power to make rules for carrying out the purpose of the Act by notification in the official gazette. Every rule made is required to be laid before each hose of parliament as soon as after it is made. When the houses agree in making modification or the houses agree that no such rule is needed, the rule will be modified or will be made of no effect. The rule made is known as Drugs and Magic Remedies (Objectionable Advertisements) Rules, 1955.

Some Examples

1. In *Hamdard Dawakhana v. Union of India*: Hamdard Dawakhana was asked to recall 40 drugs. But it choose to file a writ in Supreme Court in 1959 on the ground that their right to free speech and right to carry on trade or business were violated. Thus the Supreme Court was faced with the question as to whether the *Drug and Magic Remedies Act*, which put restrictions on the advertisements of drugs in certain cases and prohibited advertisements of drugs having magic qualities for curing diseases, was valid as it curbed the freedom of speech and expression of a person by imposing restrictions on advertisements. The Supreme Court held that, an advertisement is no doubt a form of speech and expression but every advertisement is not a matter dealing with the expression of ideas and hence advertisement of a commercial nature cannot fall within the concept of freedom of press.

2. Neeraj Clinic in Rishikesh: R K Gupta continued advertisements claiming that he was offering a sure cure for epilepsy. He was even declared as quack by Indian Medical Association when a committee found that he was giving his patients toxic drugs in high doses. Then in May 2003, following a complaint the Advertising Standard Council of India had held that the advertisement violated the *Drug and Magic Remedies Act*. Yet he continued with such advertisements and the authority failed to act resulting in thousands of consumers falling prey. Of course later, his clinic was raided.

3. Public Interest Litigation (PIL): Based on PIL by Salek Chand Jain, the Delhi High Court on 30 April 2003 has laid the state government of Delhi to act on the base of addresses and phone numbers given in advertisements and crack down on spiritual frauds. It was reported to have at least 200 self-styled miracle healers operating in Delhi and luring their victims with advertisements and wall paintings.

4. HIV/AIDS Cure: In 2006 a person promised that he could cure people of HIV/AIDS with coconut shell oil in Bangalore. Officials of Drugs Control Department raided his premises and confiscated medicines and pamphlets.

5. Divine mother claiming to have supernatural powers for curing many diseases: There was an advertisement in Newspaper in this regard. It was held that there was no indication of use of drugs and thus was construed to be an offence. The advertisement was published under the heading "Jyotish" meaning Astrology thus indicating of supernatural or spiritual or astrological solution. (Calcutta High court, 2003)

(*Source:* A Picture: http://www.thehindu.com/2006/06/17/stories/2006061724000500.htm)

Kerala DC raids Kunnath Pharma's factory, godown for violation of Drugs and Magic Remedies Act

(21/12/09)

Chennai, 21 Dec: An inspection team from Kerala Drugs Control Department with drug inspectors and intelligence wing officials seized bundles of an Ayurvedic drug, Musli Power Xtra, worth over ₹ 27 lakh from Kunnath Pharmaceuticals' factory in Moovattupuzha citing violation of the Drugs and Magic Remedies (Objectionable Advertisements) Act 1954. Simultaneous inspections were held in their godown in Thodupuzha and in the head office in Kochi. A case was registered against the drug company and the confiscated items were produced before the First Class Magistrate Court in Moovattupuzha. The case was initiated because the company has put on label the indication 'aphrodisiac' which is in violation of DMRA Act. This is the second time Kerala DC is taking action against the company for the violation of the Drug rules. In October last, the department had registered a case against the company for change of ingredient in the product which was gross violation of the Section 33 EE A (d) of Drugs and Cosmetics Act. The charge at that time was that the company has used Safed Musli in place of Nilappana. Last Friday, the surprise raids were conducted by the regulators and the intelligence wing of the department under the leadership of the Drugs Controller, M P George. The Drugs Controller said the enforcement officials have been getting complaints from across the country about the pharma company which was producing and marketing the Ayurvedic formulation, Musli Power Xtra, claiming that it would treat infertility problems in both men and women. He said, as part of the crack down on violations of drugs act in the state, the department had meticulously planned to conduct simultaneous raids in three places of the company in Idukki and Eranakulam districts to initiate stringent action against the violation. But the operation could not succeed as planned

because of disclosure of official secret, he said. "Even before the investigation teams could reach the sites, the company people somehow got wind of our move and they immediately shifted most of the parcels to safer places and put some bottles in place," the drugs controller said. He added that his plan was to confiscate all the products following continuous complaints and seal the premises. To a question whether the Ayurvedic department officials were aware of his move, he said most of the complaints received were about mixing up of allopathic ingredients in the medicine and the presence of allopathic drugs controllers are also required while collecting samples. So he sent a team of drug inspectors from both the divisions to all the three places for the raids. In Kerala both Allopathy and Ayurveda divisions comes under one drug controller. To another question, whether any action will be taken against the print and electronic media which have been releasing extensive advertisements for the product, the drugs controller did not answer. But he recalled his action against eleven newspapers in Kerala some years ago for violation of D&C Act, and the consequences he experienced during that period.

(*Source:* Pharmabiz)

FIR against Weight Loss Firm: Maharashtra FDA filed First Information Report (FIR) against Mumbai based weight loss firm, Dr Bhavana Shah's Fitness Highway Slimming Beauty and Wellness Private Limited, for publishing misleading advertisement in a reputed National Daily making a false claim. On receiving the show cause notice earlier, the firm stopped the advertisement but repeated again later.

The FDA officials raided the premises of the centre and enquired about the drug or treatment. It seems staff at the centre failed to give satisfactory answer which led to the FIR.

[Pharmabiz.com Dated May 06, 2014]

Medicinal and Toilet Preparations (Excise Duties) Act

"Like it or not, you have to pay your taxes. The trouble is that understanding taxation requires more than a genius mind."

— Albert Einstein

After reading this chapter, you should be able to understand and appreciate:
- Pharmaceutical products as dutiable goods
- Licensing procedure for manufacturing dutiable pharmaceutical products
- Interstate movement and export of dutiable pharmaceutical products
- Administrative procedures for implementing the Act

The Act empowers the central and state governments for the levy and collection of duties of excise on medicinal and toilet preparations containing alcohol, opium, Indian hemp or other narcotic drug or narcotics. The Act was passed in Parliament in 1955 but the Rules are made in 1956. The Act came into force on 01.4.1957 extending to whole of India. Excise Duty is a tax on manufacture or production of goods. Excise Duty on alcohol, alcoholic preparations, and narcotic substances is collected by the state government and is called "State Excise Duty". The Excise Duty on the rest of goods is called 'Central Excise' duty and is collected under Central Excise Act, 1944. The Sales Tax differs from Excise Duty as former is a tax on act of sale while the latter is a tax on the act of manufacture or production of goods. An Excise is described as an indirect tax levied and collected on goods manufactured in India.

Prior to the enactment of this Act, the duty on alcohol was different in different state as it was the state's subject. Single preparation was subjected to different duty: Compound Cardamom Tincture was subjected to the duty of ₹ 40/- in West Bengal and ₹ 5/- in Bihar for one London Proof Gallon of product. This was one of the reasons for interstate smuggling. The Medicinal and Toilet Preparations (Excise Duties) Act, 1955 replaced the state's Act. This provides a concessional rate of duty of alcohol for use in medicinal and toilet preparations in order to make these preparations affordable while the alcohol used as beverages are levied duty at a higher rate. Higher rate of duty levied at alcohol used for making beverage is because to make them costly indirectly discouraging people from drinking, a social evil. Thus the Act is meant for regulating medicinal and toilet preparations using alcohol and other narcotics so that they are not misused for drinking.

Goods and Services Tax (GST) is now implemented from July 1, 2017. GST is the biggest indirect tax reform in the history of independent India. This is a single indirect tax for the whole country which will make India further united making one India and one tax structure. The excise duties levied under Medicinal and Toilet Preparations (Excise Duties) Act are proposed to be engrossed under GST.

The Act Administration at Central comes under the Department of Revenue of Ministry of Finance and at state level under

the Department of Excise. [The Department of Excise in Tamil Nadu comes under the administrative control of Home, prohibition and excise department. The excise administration is done by the Commissioner of Prohibition and Excise. The District Collector supervises the excise administration at the district level]. Based on the way the Excise Duty is collected, the manufacture is divided into two types: Manufacture in Bond and Not Manufactured in Bond.

Dutiable Goods

The following medicinal and toilet preparations are treated as dutiable goods:

1. Allopathic medicinal preparations containing alcohol which are not capable of being consumed as ordinary alcohol beverages.
2. Medicinal preparations in Ayurvedic, Unani or other indigenous system of medicines containing self-generated alcohol (capable of being consumed/not capable of being consumed as ordinary alcohol beverages)/distilled or added alcohol/ containing narcotic drug or narcotic.
3. Homeopathic preparations containing alcohol.
4. Toilet preparations containing alcohol or narcotic drug or narcotic.

The manufacturer of such goods or the person who stores them in a warehouse has to pay the duty as leviable. The payment of duty is exempted on medicinal preparations containing alcohol manufactured in India and supplied direct from bonded manufactory or warehouse to the following institutions:

- Hospitals or dispensaries working under the supervision of central or state government.
- Hospital or dispensaries subsidized by central or state government.
- Charitable hospitals or dispensaries under the administrative control and management of a local body.
- Medical store deport of the central or state government.
- Other institutions certified by the principal medical officer of the district that the institution supply medicines free to the poor.

Payment of Duty

The dutiable goods are not permitted to be removed from manufacturing premises without payment of excise duty leviable. Such goods may be deposited without payment of duty in a warehouse or may be exported out of India under bond. The Excise Commissioner (EC) may permit the settlement of duty at intervals of not exceeding three months instead of each separate consignment of goods removed. The excess duty erroneously paid must be claimed within six months of such payment.

The exporter has to claim the rebate for duty from EC within one month of export and on production of duplicate application endorsed by the officer who examined the product at the site of export.

Rate of duty for medicinal and toilet preparations		
Sl. No.	Description	Rate of duty
1.	a. Allopathic medicinal preparations containing alcohol, narcotic drugs, or narcotic	16%
	b. Ayurvedic/Unani/Indigenous system medicinal preparations not containing alcohol but containing narcotic drug or narcotic	
	c. Toilet preparations containing alcohol, narcotic drug or narcotic	
2.	Ayurvedic/Unani/Indigenous system medicinal preparations containing alcohol which are prepared by distillation or to which alcohol has been added	6%
3.	a. Ayurvedic/Unani/Indigenous system medicinal preparations containing self-generated alcohol capable of consuming as ordinary alcohol beverage	
	b. Homeopathic preparations containing alcohol	4%
4.	a. Ayurvedic/Unani/Indigenous system medicinal preparations containing self-generated alcohol not capable of being consumed as ordinary alcohol beverage	Nil

Manufacturing Medicinal and Toilet Preparations

Two main types of license are issued under the Act to permit the manufacturing medicinal and toilet preparations:

- License to manufacture medicinal and toilet preparations under bond;
- License to manufacture medicinal and toilet preparations outside bond.

Salient Points of Licensing Procedure

- Licensing Authority: Excise Commissioner in case of Bonded Manufactory or warehouse; other officer as designated by the state government.
- Application for license is to be submitted at least 2 months before the commencement of the working of license.
- For renewal: Application is to be submitted at least one month before the commencement of the year for which it is required.
- If the license desires of transferring business to new premises, license should be suitably amended.
- The license can be suspended or revoked if the conditions of the medicinal and toilet preparations Act and the Rules are breached or convicted under Indian Penal Code after giving reasonable opportunity of show cause against the action proposed.
- The license fees paid is refundable if license is refused. However, the fees paid are not refundable on surrendering of license.

Documents to be submitted for seeking license: The applicant seeking license has to submit the following:

1. Application with name and address of the person/details of each member of the firm/Directors, Managers, etc. in case of company [True copy of the partnership deed, Memorandum of Association and the latest balance sheet]
2. The amount of capital proposed to be invested.
3. Name of the site and place of business.
4. Approximate date of commencing manufacturing.
5. The number and full description of apparatus and machines.
6. The maximum quantity of alcohol in London Proof Litre, Opium, Indian Hemp, or other narcotic drug or narcotic (in weight) likely to remain in the manufactory at one time.
7. Whether the proposed bonded manufactory requires the service of full time or part time excise officer.
8. License under the Drugs and Cosmetics Act.
9. List of all preparations proposed to be manufactured giving the percent or proportion of alcohol/opium/Indian hemp/ other narcotic drug or narcotic.
10. The plan of manufactory showing details like site, elevation plan of building, rooms, doors, windows, etc. including the quarter of the excise staff (if required). The state government is empowered to relax this norm for Hakims and Vaidyas who prepare and dispense medicinal preparations to their own patients (not for sale).

Requirements for License (Government of Maharashtra)

- Application to District Collector through Superintendent of State Excise of the District.
- Prescribed form with prescribed fees.
- Food and Drugs Administration's License and Plan.
- No dues of income tax and sales tax, solvency certificate.
- Antecedent report from police.

Procedure to be followed by the Licensing Authority: Before issuing license, the Licensing Authority needs to make enquiries relating to:

- Qualification and experience of technical personnel.
- Soundness of the applicant's financial position.
- The equipment of the bonded and non-bonded manufactory.
- Suitability of the proposed building.

The Licensing Authority fixes the security required to be furnished by the applicant either cash or interest-free securities (Government Promissory Notes, National Savings Certificates, Post Office Savings Bank Passbooks, or Post Office Cash Certificates, Fixed Deposit Receipts of State Bank of India or other approved bank).

Condition of the License

- License is to be exhibited in a conspicuous part of the business.
- The license is valid maximum for one year and expires on 31st March next.
- The business is to be conducted by the licensee personally or through authorized agent.
- The licensed premises and the concerned goods be allowed for inspection by the Excise Commissioner and other empowered officers.
- The licensee has to offer explanation with respect to management of premises as raised by the EC and other officers.
- The licensee has to allow the sampling of goods for analysis.
- The licensee has to maintain visit book paged and stamped where visiting officer would record remarks during inspection. The visit book is to be delivered to the authorized officer on the termination of license.
- In voices, each memorandum, permits and other related documents of the consignments for a period of one year.

Manufacturing

The provision of manufacturing medicinal and toilet preparations is divided into two types:

Manufacturing in Bond: In this case, alcohol on which duty is not paid is used under excise supervision. Manufacture outside bond: In this case, alcohol on which duty has already been paid is used. Rectified spirit for manufacture of medicinal and toilet preparations is ordinarily supplied from a distillery or a sprit warehouse of the state. However, the manufacturer is not precluded from obtaining rectified spirit from sources located outside the state.

Manufacture in Bond: The manufacturing of dutiable goods are permitted without payment of any duty of excise leviable in respect of alcohol, opium, Indian hemp, or other narcotic drug or narcotic which is to be used as an ingredient in the manufacture of dutiable goods. The salient points of such manufacturing are given below:

- The manufacturer has to give a bond with sufficient security to obtain rectified spirit without payment of duty.
- Construction and Specification for Bonded Manufactory:
  - Only one entrance to the branded manufactory and one door to each compartment is permissible. All doors should be secured with excise ticket lock during the absence of excise officer.
  - The manufactory must have :
    ○ One plain spirit store unless it is attached to distillery or rectified spirit warehouse.
    ○ At least one large room for manufacturing medicinal preparations.
    ○ One or more rooms for storing finished medicinal preparations.
    ○ Separate arrangement for manufacture of toilet preparations.
    ○ The storage of finished toilet preparations.
    ○ Accommodation with necessary furniture near bonded premises for officer in charge.
    ○ Malleable iron rods not less than 19 mm in thickness, set not more than 102 mm, embodied in brick work up to a depth of at least 51 mm and covered inside with strong wire netting or expanded metal of a mesh not exceeding 25 mm in diameter of length in every window of bonded premises.
    ○ A board on which the name of the room and a serial number are legibly painted in oil color on the outside of every room
    ○ All pipes from sinks or washbasins should discharge into closed drains forming part of general drainage system of the premise.

- All electric and gas connections should be fixed to admit the supply of electricity or gas being cut off and the regulators or switches being securely locked at the end of day's work.
- No alteration or addition can be made in bonded premises without the orders of Excise Commissioner.
  - The permanent vessels for storage of alcohol, opium, Indian hemp, and other narcotic drugs and narcotics and finished products should be secured with excise ticket locks.
  - All vessels intended to hold alcohol and liquid preparations are gauzed by the officer in charge.
- Receiving Rectified Spirit:
  - The licensee submits an indent in triplicate form countersigned by officer in charge and obtains rectified spirit from approved distillery or spirit warehouse. The original indent is sent to the distiller, the duplicate is sent through officer in charge to the distiller and the triplicate is retained as office copy. The distillery or warehouse officer, after receiving the duplicate copy of the indent, supplies the spirit. The licensee pays the cost price of the spirit.
  - The consignment of rectified spirit received is verified in volume and strength by the officer in charge and make necessary entry in the register. On verification, the rectified spirit is stored in one or more vessels in the spirit store.
- Issue of rectified spirit for use:
  - The required quantity of rectified spirit is issued on a requisition of the licensee from the spirit store for manufacturing. All rectified spirit so issued be used in the presence of the officer in charge. Rectified spirit should not be issued for any other purpose.
  - Finished medicinal and toilet preparations may be transferred from finished store to the laboratory of the manufactory for any other kind of preparations.

- Receiving and issuing opium, Indian hemp and other narcotic drugs and narcotics:
  - Indent for opium is to be made to the nearest sub-treasury or the Government Opium Factory, Ghazipur or to the warehouse or to the approved storage place.
  - Indian hemp and other narcotics are obtained from the nearest government warehouse.
  - On receipt of the above materials, they are verified and accounted for in the register. They are stored separately in the spirit store and secured by excise ticket locks.
  - They are issued for manufacturing purpose only.
- Manufacturing Dutiable Goods: Each preparation manufactured is to be registered and bear a distinctive serial number. Then they are removed to the finished product store and store in vessels after measurement. The issue of opium, Indian hemp, narcotic drugs and other narcotics are made under appropriate permit. The advice portion of such permit is to be sent to the officer in charge.
  - Every time the percolator or other vessels intended for alcohol is charged, it should be labelled with the following particulars:
    - The name and batch number of the preparation.
    - Description and quantity of alcohol placed in it from time to time.
    - The date of removal of the preparation and the quantity of such preparation removed.
  - On completion of production, the officer in charge permits the licensee to take free samples of 227 ml or such quantity as necessary for analysis in own laboratory and declaration of strength of alcohol and medicament.
  - The left over quantity after analysis is to be destroyed in the laboratory in the presence of officer in charge.
  - Separate account of the quantity used for analysis is to be maintained.

- Alcoholic strength of preparation as declared is entered in the register.
- Proper entry in register is necessary for removing these finished products.
- Officer in charge takes two samples from each batch of finished preparations for analysis and send one to chemical examiner. The second sample is intended for replacement of the original sample or repetition of analysis. The second sample is kept under excise ticket lock. These samples are supplied free and packaging and dispatching cost is borne by licensee.
- The duplicate sample should not be returned to the finished store: If the alcohol content declared by the chemical examiner is beyond the margin of 3% (unless the EC permits standardization of such substandard preparations) and spurious preparations.
- The report of the chemical examiner is to be shown to the licensee.
- Storage of finished products:
  - On completion of the production, they are stored in bulk jars or bottles each containing not less than 2273 ml.
  - Preparations ready for issue may be filled in bottles or containers of not less than 57 ml content.
  - Finished products containers should have label showing the name of the preparation, batch no., alcoholic strength and name of manufacturer.
  - Bulk containers should be labelled with actual contents in litre, its alcoholic strength and date of storage.
  - The containers are to be arranged appropriately to allow ready identification of each batch.
  - The products may be kept in store room for a period of 3 years or more as allowed. After this period, the licensee has to clear the products for consumption in the state or payment of excise duty or for removal to a bonded warehouse or for exportation.
  - Any deficiency with respect to bulk content of the finished product in store is to be recorded by the officer in charge. All such loss (in the absence of satisfactory explanation) invites penal rates of duty which should not be more than double of the prescribed. The EC is empowered to waive this duty if satisfied that the preparation has not gone into consumption.
- Disposal of substandard preparations: The substandard preparations with approval of EC are either destroyed in the presence of officer in charge or reprocessed. The excise duty is not leviable on the destroyed goods if EC believes that the deterioration occurred due to reasons beyond the control of the licensee.
- Disposal of recovered alcohol: The recovered alcohol in the course of production or distilled separately may be used in subsequent production if such alcohol is accounted for. If the recovered alcohol is unfit for use, it should be destroyed in the presence of officer in charge.
- Wastage in manufacture: The state government fixes the wastage permissible. Any wastage beyond this limit is charged with duty. If the alcoholic strength declared by chemical examiner exceed by 3 proof degrees than the highest allowable limit or to be below the lowest allowable limit, the issue from the bonded laboratory is with-held. The EC may allow the licensee to adjust the alcoholic strength or the medicament or ingredients provided the process does not impair the therapeutic or toiletry properties of the preparation. When the chemical examiner finds alcoholic strength in excess of more than 20 proof degrees, the excess duty is to be realized by the officer in charge. However, no refund of duty is permitted if the chemical examiner declares the strength lower than that of licensee.
- Issue from a bonded manufactory: The issue of the product may be made on payment of excise duty. The officer in charge on receiving the application allows the required quantities to be removed after issuing a permit. The duty leviable can be debited into the account of the

licensee. However, the transfer to another bonded warehouse can be made without payment of duty.

- **Role of Officer in Charge:**
  - Maintains account in prescribed form and ensures that the licensee too keeps the account. The two accounts are to be compared and reconciled before manufactory is closed at the end of the day's transaction.
  - Ensures that alcohol issued for certain preparations added to materials to make that preparation only. No portion of such alcohol is diverted for other purpose.
  - Ensures that only authorized persons enter into the manufactory premises during working hours.
  - Inspects the manufactory as assigned and collects duty.
  - Takes samples for analysis and sends to chemical examiner.

Manufacture Outside Bond: The salient points include:

- **Working hours:** The business of manufacture and sale is to be conducted between the hours of sunrise and sunset and on such days as fixed by the EC. The premises are to be kept closed from the hours of sunset to sunrise each day.
- **Building arrangement:**
  - The laboratory should be separated from the places used for other purposes.
  - The windows of the spirit store, laboratory and finished store should be fitted with malleable iron bars of not less than 19 mm in thickness, set at not more than 102 mm apart and fixed in the brick work to a depth of at least 51 mm at each end. On the inside of each window, there should be security fastened to the bars stout wire netting the aperture which should not exceed 25 mm in diameter.
  - There should be only one entry to the non-bonded manufactory and one door each to the laboratory, spirit store and finished store.

- All pipes from sinks and washbasins inside the manufactory premises should discharge into closed drains forming part of the general drainage system of the premise.
- All electric and gas connections with the licensed premises should be fixed as to admit the supply of electricity or gas being cut off and the regulators or switches being securely locked out at the end of day's work.
- There should be separate spirit store for the rectified spirit purchased at the duty of ₹ 1.10 paise, ₹ 3.85 paise and ₹ 15.50 paise per London Proof litre.
- There should be separate finished store for medicinal and toilet preparations.
- All alterations in arrangement of building and plant can be made only with previous sanction of EC.
- The conditions described above may be relaxed for:
  - Small manufacturers whose annual consumption of alcohol does not exceed 500 litres.
  - Persons who prepare for dispensing to their own patients (not for sale).

- **Receptacles:**
  - The permanent vessels for the storage of alcohol and finished preparations containing alcohol should be able to be gauzed accurately and tables should be computed to show the contents of every 20 mm and 2 mm of its depth.
  - The containers in the finished store should be made up of metal, porcelain, or glass as may be convenient and necessary.
  - Each permanent vessel should bear distinctive serial number, its full capacity and the purpose for which it is to be used, distinctly and indelibly marked on it. A record of these is to be kept in the register.
  - All receptacles containing alcohol and alcoholic preparations should have labels signed by manufacturer or his representative mentioning the batch no. the name of the preparation, and

the quantity of alcohol added in the receptacles during the course of manufacture.

- Label placed on macerators and percolators or carboys should show the quantity of proof spirit contained in them on each occasion and should be destroyed when they are emptied and cleaned.
- Labels on bottles filled for removal should show among other details, the alcoholic content in proof strength and the average percentage of absolute alcohol it contains.

- Receiving rectified spirit:
  - The licensee has to make indent in triplicate to obtain rectified spirit from any distillery or spirit warehouse approved by EC. The original copy goes to the distiller or spirit warehouse keeper. The duplicate is sent to the officer in charge of the distillery or spirit warehouse through the proper officer. The triplicate is kept as office copy.
  - If both the manufactory and distillery/spirit warehouse are located in the same state, the licensee of manufactory may authorize the owner of the distillery or warehouse to pay duty on his behalf.

- Receiving opium, Indian hemp and narcotic drugs and other narcotics:
  - Indent of opium should be made to the nearest sub-treasury or to the Government Opium Factory, Ghazipur, or to the warehouse or state approved place.
  - Indian hemp, narcotic drugs and other narcotics are to be obtained under permit.
  - On receipt they are verified in the non-bonded manufactory and accounted in the register. They (obtained free of duty) should be stored separately in the spirit store. Every time they are issued for use, should be accounted in the register.
  - The medicinal preparations containing alcohol capable of being consumed

should be manufactured only from rectified spirit on which duty of ₹ 3.85 or ₹ 15.50 per London Proof Litre has been paid depending on the type of preparation. They should not be manufactured with rectified spirit obtained at the duty of ₹ 1.10 per London Proof Litre.

- The quantity of rectified spirit in possession should not exceed the limit fixed.

- Manufacturing, storage and sale:
  - This should be carried out in the licensed premises only.
  - Each preparation manufactured is to be registered and should have serial number (batch number) recorded in the register. The register records the receipt and disposal of all rectified spirit, opium, Indian hemp and other narcotic drugs and narcotics drawn from the spirit store and the quantity of finished preparations manufactured.
  - The finished preparations are to be transferred from laboratory to finished store and are arranged to facilitate checking.
  - The finished preparations made from rectified spirit obtained at different rates of duty should be kept separately in the finished store.
  - The preparations stored in bulk should be measured to the nearest fluid ounce by the manufacturer and sealed.
  - When the contents are removed from bulk containers, this should be entered in the stock card with signature and date.

- Sampling:
  - The excise officer, in whose jurisdiction the manufactory located, without giving notice should take samples of not less than 13 percent and not more than 15 percent of the total number of medicinal and toilet preparations containing alcohol from the finished stocks at least once every month. The samples are forwarded to the chemical examiner for analysis and report

whether the alcoholic contents tally with the percentage of alcohol shown on the label affixed to the bottles.

– If the proof strength reported by the chemical examiner is more than 3% than shown on the label, the manufacturer is liable to a penalty at the rate of 10 times the difference in duty but not exceeding ₹ 2000/-. If such differences occur frequently, the EC may order cancellation of license.

– The excise officer has to take samples personally in the presence of manufacturer or his authorized agent. The EC and other officers authorized by EC are also authorized to take samples.

– The sample quantity should be 227 ml or quantity as fixed by EC.

– The sample should be in duplicate. The cork of the every bottle is to be fixed with officer's personal seal and manufacturer's seal (if desired by him). The label fixed to each bottle should state the name of the preparation and batch number.

– Out of two samples collected, one is to be sent for analysis. The sample is placed in a case and securely fastened with tape or wire to be supplied by the manufacturer. Then the sample should be sealed by the officer taking sample with personal seal and dispatched without delay to the chemical examiner at manufacturer's cost. The second sample is kept securely under lock and key in an almirah provided by the manufacturer until the result of analysis is obtained. This may be required by the chemical examiner for repeat analysis. If not required, the sample should be promptly returned to the manufacturer.

– The covering letter in duplicate advising the dispatch of samples should be sent to the chemical examiner containing facsimile of the seal and other information. The chemical examiner acknowledges the receipt of the samples in duplicate copy to the dispatching officer.

– No compensation is required to be paid to the manufacturer for samples taken for analysis.

• Maintenance of Records: The manufacturer has to maintain up to date, correct and proper accounts in the relevant register obtained from respective taluk office or excise officer. The account is to be delivered to the proper officer by 5th of each month. He has to furnish any other statement as required by EC.

• Employees: The manufacturer is required to furnish a list of employees who are required to enter non-bonded manufactory. Persons whose name is not in the list should not be allowed to enter without special permission of the officer. The manufacturer has to inform any change in the list of employees.

• Inspection:
   – The EC and excise officers may inspect the premises at all reasonable times.
   – The proper officer should inspect at least once in a month.
   – The state government may authorize any other officer of prohibition, land revenue, medical and public health department to inspect the non-bonded manufactory.

Classification of Medicinal and Toilet Preparations:

1. Allopathic Preparations:
   a. Official allopathic preparations: The preparations made based on latest edition (or, immediate preceding edition) of Pharmacopoeia and other official books of drug standards or formularies. The following pharmacopoeias and books of standards are recognized for this purpose: Indian Pharmacopoeia, National Formulary of India, and Official Pharmacopoeias of other countries, British Pharmaceutical Codex, National Formulary of USA, British Veterinary Codex, and Dental Formulary of USA.

   b. Non-official allopathic preparations: Preparations other than official allopathic preparations but conforming to the formulae displayed on the label.

Restricted list of preparations: List of medicinal preparations considered as capable of being misused as ordinary alcoholic beverage. For example, concentrated Peppermint water, concentrated distilled water and many other specified elixirs, spirits, etc. The central government may declare other unrestricted preparations as restricted preparations based on the request of state government and advice of the standing committee if such preparations are found to be widely used as ordinary alcoholic beverage.

Unofficial medicinal preparations manufactured for the first time after 01st April 1957 are usually presumed to be restricted preparations. However, the manufacturer intending to produce new alcoholic preparations may approach the state government for classification of his product [The state government forwards the request to the central government and the central government refers this to standing committee and finally based on recommendation of Standing Committee the central government declares as unrestricted preparation or otherwise].

2. Homeopathic preparations: The preparations based on Homeopathic Pharmacopoeia of India.
3. Preparations with narcotic ingredients: The rules relating to alcoholic medicinal and toilet preparations are applicable for preparations containing opium, Indian hemp, other narcotic drugs and narcotics.
4. Ayurvedic preparations: Asvas and Aristas are the principal types of Ayurvedic preparations in which alcoholic content is self generated and not added as such.
   a. Products containing self-generated alcohol: The preparations containing self-generated alcohol where alcohol content does not exceed 2% Proof Spirit do not warrant levy of duty. But if the alcohol content exceeds this limit, the duty is leviable.
   The Ayurvedic practitioners are allowed to manufacture and dispense these

preparations free of duty on the following conditions:
- The practitioner has license on payment of fee of ₹ 1/-.
- The preparations are used only for their patients and not for sale.
- The practitioner allows sampling by excise officer to ensure that they contain only self-generated alcohol.
- Daily account of manufacturing, dispensing and name and addresses of the patients are maintained.
   b. Preparations made by distillation or to which alcohol is added: They are treated as alcoholic preparations capable of being used as ordinary alcoholic beverage.

Standing Committee: The standing committee advises the central government on all matters connected with technical aspects of the administration of the Act and the Rules.

The standing committee is constituted with the following members:

i. The Drugs Controller of Government of India.
ii. The Chief Chemist, Central Revenue Control Laboratory.
iii. One Pharmacologist nominated by central government.
iv. The Adviser in Indigenous System of Medicine (AYUSH, Government of India).

The Drugs Controller, Chief Chemist and the Adviser may depute their immediate subordinate officers such as Deputy Drugs Controller, Deputy Chief Chemist and Deputy Adviser respectively to attend the meeting on their behalf.

The functions of the Standing Committee:

- To decide whether the particular preparation is entitled to be treated or continue to be treated as genuine medicinal and toilet preparation.
- To decide whether the genuine medicinal and toilet preparations should be treated or continue to be treated as restricted or unrestricted preparation. Before declaring as restricted preparation, the person is given an opportunity to express his views.

- Advising the central government on investigation: For this investigation four samples of each 227 ml or such other quantity as required should be taken.

Establishment of Bonded Warehouse: The manufacturers or dealers of dutiable goods are permitted to establish bonded warehouse anywhere in India. The duty paid goods and other goods are not permitted to be deposited in these warehouses. The salient points on warehousing are:

- A license from the Excise Commissioner is necessary for establishing private warehouse for storage of dutiable goods. The warehouse is to be secured by locks or fastening as directed by the Excise Commissioner.

- The license has to furnish a bond with surety or sufficient security to pay duty as the deposited goods and for the due and safe removal of such goods to another warehouse and for due observation of the provision of the Act and the Rules. In the event of the death, insolvency or insufficiency of surety, a fresh bond may be necessary.

- Receipt of goods: All goods brought for warehousing should be produced before the officer in charge of the warehouse or other officer and checked in his presence and assessed for duty prior to entry into the warehouse. The details of quantity and description of goods must be recorded. All goods received into the warehouse must be kept separate from other goods until the receipt account has been taken by the officer.

- Owner's power to deal with warehouse goods: The owner of goods is permitted, with sanction of officer, to sort, separate, pack and repack the goods and make alterations as may be necessary for pre-servations, sale or disposal. The officer may permit damaged goods remaining after such repacking to destroy them as per the guidelines given by the Excise Commissioner.

- Goods are not permitted to be removed except on payment of duty or for removal to any other bonded warehouse or for transport.

- Goods in warehouse may be deposited for a period of three years or such extended period as permitted by the Excise Commissioner. The owner has to remove goods remaining in the warehouse before this period of expiry: for consumption after payment of duty or to removal to other warehouse.

When the licensee intends to remove goods on payment of duty, he has to make an application in triplicate to the officer in charge at least 12 hours before the intended time of removal. On receiving the evidence of payment of the required amount into the treasury, the officer allows the clearance of goods.

- The Excise Commissioner is empowered to remit the duty for lost or destroyed goods.

- The licensee has to submit the monthly return to the Excise Commissioner showing the quantity of dutiable goods removed on payment of duty and other particulars as required by the state government.

- Offences: The following are treated as offences with respect to warehouse provisions:
  - Opening of any of the locks or doors except in the presence of the authorized officer.
  - Making alternation of the approved warehouse without the consent of the Excise Commissioner.
  - Removing the warehouse goods or privately concealing the goods either before or after warehousing.

Persons committing the offences are liable to a penalty extending to two thousand rupees and all such goods are liable to confiscation.

Inter-state Movement of Goods

- The movement of dutiable goods manufactured under bond or stored in a bonded warehouse is permitted from one state to the other after payment of duty.

- Movement to another bonded warehouse: The consigner and consignee have to enter into a bond with surety or sufficient security for the amount equal to double the duty chargeable. The bond is to be furnished to the officer of the warehouse of the removal and warehouse of destination.
- The Excise Commissioner may permit any person to remove warehouse goods from one to another by entering into a general agreement with surety or sufficient security. In the event of death, insolvency of the surety or the amount of bond is inadequate, a fresh bond may be necessary.
- Procedure for removal:
  - The application, in triplicate, for removal of goods is to be presented by the consigner to the officer in charge at least 24 hours before the intended removal.
  - The officer, after completing the removal certificate on all the copies of the application, sends the duplicate copy to the officer in charge of destination warehouse. He hands over the third copy of the application to the consigner for dispatching to consignee. The officer handover the transport permit too to the consigner.
  - On arrival of goods at the destination warehouse, the consignee has to present them together with the triplicate application and transport permit to the officer in charge. On verification, the officer completes re-warehousing certificate in duplicate and triplicate application. The duplicate copy of the application is returned to the officer in charge of the warehouse of removal and triplicate is to be given to the consignee to dispatch the consigner.
  - The consigner has to present the endorsed triplicate copy to the officer within 90 days of the date of issue of transport permit. When the consigner fails to submit the endorsed triplicate copy or the officer has not received the endorsed duplicate copy, the consigner is asked to pay the duty leviable within

10 days of demand notice. Failing this, no further removal of goods is permitted. Such duty paid is refunded later on presentation of endorsed triplicate copy of the application or on receipt of duplicate copy by the officer.
  - When the owner fails to pay the sum demanded, the goods may be detained to recover the dues. If the demand is not complied, the detained goods may be sold by public auction duly advertised in the official gazette. The net proceeds of the sales is adjusted against the amount due and the surplus should be returned to the owner.

Export of Dutiable Goods

The dutiable goods may be exported out of India, without payment of duty, from a warehouse or bonded manufactory. The exporter has to submit a bond with surety in prescribed format.

Procedure to be followed (in sequence):

1. Submission of separate application (in triplicate) for each consignment to the officer in charge [original is meant for custom officer/border examiner/postmaster; the duplicate is for the consigner and the triplicate is for keeping as office copy].
2. Examination of goods prior to dispatch:
   a. Goods under bond: The package should have the following information marked in ink or oil colour—progressive number commencing number for each year, owner's name, total quantity of dutiable goods with their alcoholic contents in London Proof Litre.
   b. Duty paid goods: The entire consignment is presented before the proper officer with 48 hours notice for supervising packing.
   c. The officer takes samples and ensures that the following particulars are noted in the body of each package: Name and address of the consignee, description of goods, alcoholic contents of the goods in London Proof Litre as declared by the manufacturer, gross weight of the package. Each package is fixed with

official seal in a manner that the package cannot be tempered without breaking the seal.

The sample drawn is sent to chemical examiner for analysis.

3. Examination at the place of export:

a. Export by post: The exporter has to present the sealed package along with the duplicate application to the post-master at the office of booking. The postmaster of the post office of final dispatch from India has to certify on the duplicate application that goods covered by application has been duly exported out of India and return the same to the postmaster of booking post office. The original application is returned to the officer in charge (who sent) after endorsement of certificate of export.

b. Export by other means: The goods are to be presented to the Custom Collector, Border Examiner, or any other authorized officer with the duplicate application. The goods are carefully examined including weighing, checking for intact seals and other particulars as mentioned on the duplicate application before allowing for export. After allowing export, the officer has to certify on duplicate copy of the application that goods have been duly exported (with the details like exports by sea or air, shipping bill number and date) and return to the exporter.

Entry, Search, Seizure and Investigation

- The Excise Commissioner authorized officers have free access to the licensed premises and to places where dutiable goods are manufactured, stored or kept for sale at all reasonable times with or without notice to the licensee. They can inspect the building, plant, machinery, stocks and accounts.

- If the licensee or his representative voluntarily obstructs or offers any resistance or willfully gives false or misleading information to the officer, they are liable to a penalty which may extend to five hundred rupees.

- The empowered excise officer may stop and detain any person found carrying or removing any dutiable good for transport and verify the documents.

- The excise officer (not below the rank of sub-inspector) may stop and search any vessel, car or other means of conveyance for dutiable goods and search at anytime, if there is reason to believe that dutiable goods are kept in contravention of the Act or Rules.

- The excise officers not below the rank of sub-inspector are empowered to seize and remove or detain any goods that are believed to have contravened the provision of Act or Rules.

- The officers in charge of police stations are authorized to keep seized articles in safe custody, pending the orders of Magistrate or Adjudging excise officer.

- Summons and notices:
  - The excise officer (not below the rank of sub-inspector) is empowered to summon any person to give evidence or produce documents or other things during enquiry.
  - Every summon or notice should be sent in writing in duplicate stating the purpose of its issue. It should be served to the concerned person. If not found, then the notice may be affixed on the conscious part of his house or business place.

- Disposal of seized articles: When materials are seized and subsequently released but not claimed by the owner within one month, they should be sold by public auction. The surplus amount if not claimed by the owner within three months, this is forfeited.

- The excise officer with minimum rank of sub-inspector is empowered to initiate prosecution. Such officers are also empowered to arrest persons believed to be liable for punishment. The arrested persons must be forwarded without delay to the nearest excise officer empowered to send the arrested persons to a Magistrate.

If no such excise office is available within a reasonable distance, the arrested persons must be forwarded to the officer-in-charge of the nearest police station. The officer-in-charge of the police station either admit him to bail or forward him without delay in custody to Magistrate.

- The code of Criminal Procedure is to be followed.

The Excise Commissioner is the adjudging officer. However, the state government may empower any excise officer to adjudge confiscation or penalty.

Appeals

- An appeal can be made to the Excise Commissioner against the orders of other officers.
- Appeal is to be made to the state government against the orders of Excise Commissioner.
- The appeal is to be filed against the order within three months of such order.
- The central government too receives the petition where there is no provision of appeal.
- Every appeal should accompany the order against whose the appeal is filed.

Offences and Penalties (Medicinal and Toilet Preparations (Excise Duties) Act)	
Type of offence	*Penalty prescribed*
Non-compliance with conditions of license	Imprisonment up to six months or fine up to two thousand rupees or both
Failure to pay duty	
Failure to pay duty as demanded	Detained goods are to be sold on public auction
Obstructing or giving false or misleading information	Extending to five hundred rupees
Accounting of stocks (deficiency of goods)	Ten times the duty chargeable or rupees two thousand, whichever is less
Accounting of stocks (failed to make necessary entry, false entry or tearing of the pages)	Up to two thousand rupees and registers and accounts are liable for confiscation
Waiting and measuring (refusal or neglect by the licensee)	Up to one thousand rupees
Destroying or breaking of locks, fastening etc.	Up to two thousand rupees
Goods sold except in prescribed containers bearing labels	Up to one thousand rupees
Willfully connives at any offence	Imprisonment up to six months or fine up to five hundred rupees or both
Vexatious search or seizure by excise officer	Up to two thousand rupees for every such offence
Officer disclosing information	Not exceeding one thousand rupees
Willfully giving false information leading to arrest or to search	Imprisonment up to two years or fine up to thousand rupees or both
Failure of excise officer on duty	Imprisonment up to three months or fine up to three months pay or both
Removal of dutiable goods without payment of duty	Extend to two thousand rupees and such goods are liable for confiscation
Failure to furnish the proof of export	Maximum of two thousand rupees extending to twice the amount of duty
Warehousing (Unauthorized Opening locks or doors, alteration of the approved warehouse, removing goods or privately concealing goods)	Extending to two thousand rupees and goods are liable for confiscation
Offence for which no penalty is specified (General penalty)	One thousand rupees with confiscation of goods

The Medicinal and Toilet Preparation (M&TP) branch of the Excise Department grants and renews various licenses for wholesale and retail sale of rectified spirit, denatured spirit, and manufacture and sale of medicines and toilet preparations containing alcohol and narcotics: opium, morphine, pathedine and Indian hemp, etc. certain permits for the import, export and transport of M&TP containing alcohol and narcotics.

The various types of licenses (purpose) include:

1. Manufacturing of medicines and cosmetics in bond.
2. Manufacturing of medicines, etc. out bond.
3. Manufacturing for use of narcotic drugs.
4. Retail sale of bhang and its admixture (on the basis of auction).
5. Wholesale supply of denatured spirit to retailers as well as to hospitals and others.
6. Wholesale supply of rectified spirit to manufacturer of medicines (in Bond), for research purpose to institutions and manufacturers of medicines.
7. Issuing of denatured spirit to hospitals, schools, painters and doctors for self consumption.
8. Retail sale of denatured spirit.
9. Issuing of rectified spirit to retailers for sale in the open market.
10. Issuing to doctors, schools, painters and households (Polishing) one time 5 litres limit.
11. Morphine and pathedine injection to doctors for self consumption.
12. Wholesale medicines containing narcotics.
13. Issuing of morphine and pathedine injection to chemists for possession and sale.
14. Issuing to hospitals and nursing homes.
15. Opium cards to addict of opium.

Fees Structure—Government of West Bengal, Department of Excise (website accessed on 14th August 2011)

Sl.	Category of license under the M&TP Act.	Fees payable at the time of grant of license	Renewal fees (in ₹)
	L-1 Allopathy		
1A	(1) PAC in alcohol consumed is less than 2250 lt. per annum	200.00	200.00
	(2) PAC in alcohol consumed is more than 2250 lt. per annum	400.00	400.00
1B	Medicinal and Toilet Preparations manufactured under bond not containing alcohol but containing opium , Indian hemp or other narcotic drug or narcotics.	20.00	20.00
1C	**L-1 Homoeopathy**		
	(1) PAC in alcohol consumed is less than 2250 lt. per annum	200.00	200.00
	(2) PAC in alcohol consumed is more than 2250 lt. per annum	400.00	400.00
1D	**L-1 Ayurveda**		
	Medicinal Preparations manufactured under bond in Ayurvedic, Unani, or other indigenous systems in medicines containing alcohol and which are prepared by distillation or to which alcohol has been added.	50.00	50.00
2A	**L-2 Allopathy**		
	(1) PAC in alcohol consumed is less than or equal to 70 lt. per annum.	20.00	20.00
	(2) PAC in alcohol consumed is more than 70 lt. but less than 280 lt. per annum.	50.00	50.00
	(3) PAC in alcohol consumed is more than 280 lt. per annum	400.00	400.00
2B	Medicinal and toilet preparations manufactured outside bond not containing alcohol but containing opium, Indian hemp, or other narcotic drugs or narcotics.	20.00	20.00

(Contd...)

(Contd...)

Sl.	Category of license under the M&TP Act.	Fees payable at the time of grant of license	Renewal fees (in ₹)
2C	**L-2 Homoeopathy**		
	(1) PAC in alcohol consumed is less than or equal to 70 lt. per annum.	20.00	20.00
	(2) PAC in alcohol consumed is more than 70 lt. but less than 280 lt. per annum.	50.00	50.00
	(3) PAC in alcohol consumed is more than 280 lt. per annum	400.00	400.00
2D	**L-2 Ayurveda**		
	Medicinal Preparations manufactured outside bond in Ayurvedic, Unani, or other indigenous systems in medicines containing alcohol and which are prepared by distillation or to which alcohol has been added.	50.00	50.00
3.	**Self-generated alcohol**		
	Manufacture of medicinal preparations containing self-generated alcohol in Ayurvedic or Unani or other indigenous systems of medicines by Ayurvedic or Unani practitioners for dispensing for use of their patients and not for sale to general public.	02.00	02.00
4.	Bonded warehouses	50.00	50.00
5.	Manufacture of medicinal preparations containing alcohol by hospitals, dispensaries and other charitable institutions which are eligible for exemption from duty under rule 7 and which are specifically authorized in this behalf by the state government or by the administration in the case of a Union Territory.	Nil	Nil

Chapter 10

The Medical Termination of Pregnancy Act

"Of course abortion is not right. But it is even less right to bring unwanted children into lifelong suffering. Making abortion illegal is not the way to prevent it."

— *Anonymous*

After reading this chapter, you should be able to understand and appreciate:

- The conditions under which a pregnancy can be terminated
- The persons who can perform such termination
- The place where such termination can be performed
- The procedure/protocol to be followed for termination
- The international scenario on abortion regulation

Throughout the world there are liberalized laws on abortion. There are about 8 percent of world's population lives in countries where law prevents abortion. Mortality and morbidity rates following illegal abortion are very high and often make the life of many women miserable. To reduce the colossal morbidity and mortality associated with abortion, Shantilal Shah Committee (1964) recommended liberalization of abortion laws in India in 1966. In 1969, Medical Termination of Pregnancy (MTP) Bill was introduced in Rajya Sabha and Lok Sabha which was later passed by the parliament in August 1971. It came into force from 1.4.1972 and extended to the whole of the country except the state of Jammu and Kashmir.

There is no fix trend on MTP. In 2008, there were 6.41 lakh abortions across 12,510 institutions approved to carryout MTP. India recorded 7.25 lakh MTPs in 2005, 7.21 lakh in 2006 and 6.82 lakh in 2007 and 7.01 lakh in 2014.

Abortion Laws Around the World

US: The abortion can be done at any stage by a woman even without the consent of spouse.

UK: Legally the abortion is permitted till 24 weeks of pregnancy under Abortion Act 1967. However, it can be done at any stage if doctors detect risk to mother's life or severe abnormalities in foetus.

Australia: Abortion is permitted at any stage of pregnancy in the capital territory. However, in other states, the rules allow termination between 14 and 28 weeks.

Canada: The termination of pregnancy is not permitted that has crossed 24-week period unless the experts are of opinion that continuation of pregnancy is a threat to life or foetus has severe abnormalities.

France: Abortion is permitted till 14 weeks of pregnancy. But it can be done at any stage if there is risk to other's life.

Japan: Abortion is permissible only if the pregnancy threatens woman's life or pregnancy caused by rape.

Brazil: Abortion is permissible only if woman's life is endangered by continuation of pregnancy. However, in 2012 Supreme Court allowed abortion if the foetus severely abnormal.

(*Source:* The Times of India, New Delhi, August 2, 2008, page 16.).

Prior to enactment of the legislation, the Indian Penal Code (Act No. 45 of 1860) permitted abortion only when it was justified for the good faith purpose of saving the life of the woman. The present act was intended to grant women freedom from unwanted pregnancies, especially when there was social censure or medical risk involved. Apart from these benefits, it also ensured the easy accessibility of abortion services. This can be viewed as path-breaking legislation which would eliminate unwanted or forced pregnancies, or going to quacks that resulted in postnatal trauma. It was for the first time that contraception failure was legally accepted as a valid reason for terminating pregnancy. MTP is one of the maternal healthcare measures to reduce maternal morbidity resulting from illegal abortion.

In a significant order while dismissing the plea of 10-year-old rape victim to abort her 32 weeks fetus as the medical report was against, the Supreme Court (SC) urged for setting up of permanent boards across the states so that the women especially child rape victims can receive expedient medical care. At present, women are forced to undertake the cumbersome process of approaching different courts, from district courts to high courts and finally the Supreme Court, for permission to medically terminate their pregnancies which are over 20 weeks.

In another judgement, SC Allowed 13-year-old rape survivor, a Mumbai-based seventh class student, to abort her 32-week-old fetus (6 September 2017). Based on medical board's report, SC directed to complete MTP

immediately. However, as the doctors found the fetus to be completely developed, they performed a cesarean operation and the girl delivered a boy.

World Health Organization Recommendations on Regulation, Policy and Human Rights Related to Abortion

- Laws and policies on abortion should protect women's health and their human rights.
- Regulatory, policy and programmatic barriers that hinder access to and timely provision of safe abortion care should be removed.
- An enabling regulatory and policy environment is needed to ensure that every woman who is legally eligible has ready access to safe abortion care.
- Policies should be geared for respecting, protecting and fulfilling the human rights of woman, to achieving positive health outcomes for women, to providing good quality contraceptive information and services, and to meeting the particular needs of poor women, adolescents, rape survivors and women living with HIV.

[*Source:* Bulletin of World Health Organization, 2017; 95, 542–544.]

Though the Act was intended to permit abortion on certain specified conditions, the general perception was that abortion is legalized. Unfortunately the act is often viewed as method of family planning or a method of reducing birth rate. The strong preference for sons under patriarchal traditions and the availability of inexpensive prenatal diagnostic techniques have resulted in an increased use of prenatal gender tests in India and selective abortion of girl child. In the name of contraceptive failure, MTP is continued resulting in sex selective abortion. This has caused the child sex ratio (0–6 years) plummeting from 874 girls for every 1,000 boys in 1991 to an abysmal 754 in 2001. The population census of 2011 reported the gender ratio at 940 females per 1000 males.

The MTP Act, 1971 was amended by the MTP (Amendment) Act, 2002. The main objective of the recent amendment to the MTP Act aimed at reducing the rate of unsafe abortions by making legal abortion more widely accessible. Lack of access to MTP services at the primary healthcare level is an important reason for the high rate of unsafe and illegal abortions. The amendment is aiming at decentralization of authority for approval and registration of MTP centres from the state to the district level.

Milestone in Abortion Legislation in India

- Indian Penal Code (Act No. 45 of 1860).
- Shah Committee Report, 1966.
- MTP Act, 1971.
- MTP Rules, 1975.
- MTP (Amendment) Act, 2002.
- MTP Rules, 2003.

The Act allows termination of certain pregnancies by the registered medical practitioners.

MTP Permissible

- Where the length of the pregnancy does not exceed twelve weeks; and if such medical practitioner is:
- Where the length of the pregnancy exceeds twelve weeks but does not exceed twenty weeks; if not less than two registered medical practitioners are:

of the opinion, formed in good faith, that,

  i. The continuance of the pregnancy would involve a risk to the life of the pregnant woman or of grave injury physical or mental health; or

  ii. There is a substantial risk that if the child were born, it would suffer from such physical or mental abnormalities as to be seriously handicapped.

Pregnancy caused by rape and the anguish caused by such pregnancy is presumed to constitute a grave injury to the mental health of the pregnant woman. Similarly the anguish caused by unwanted pregnancies as a result of contraceptive failure used for limiting the number of children is presumed to constitute a grave injury to the mental health of the pregnant woman.

- When length of pregnancy exceeds 20 weeks, if two registered medical practitioners are of the opinion that the continued pregnancy would endanger the women's life. It does not consider the condition of child to be born. It is legally not permissible.

The Nikita Mehta case (see box) has forced the authorities to review the act. It says "The Act has become old and a lot of new scientific and technological development have taken place since 1971. The Act needs to be concurrent with the present day ethics and social structure. It needs a review".

As long as the above conditions are fulfilled, the registered medical practitioners can terminate a pregnancy without the fear of being prosecuted.

In the event of abortion to save a woman's life the law makes exceptions: the doctor need not have stipulated experience or training but still needs to be allopathic doctor. A second opinion is not necessary for abortion beyond 12 weeks and the facility need not have prior certification.

The Government of India proposed for an Amendment of the Act, Draft Medical Termination of Pregnancy (Amendment) Bill 2014. This is yet to be passed by the Parliament. In recent time there have been many legal cases seeking permission from High Courts and Supreme Court for termination of pregnancy beyond 20 weeks. A few cases are cited in the box for readers' reference.

Women are Entitled to end Pregnancy Irrespective of Reason—Bombay High Court [September 19, 2016]

The court observed that:

- MTP Act should extend to the 'mental health' of the women and she should be allowed to opt out of an unwanted pregnancy irrespective of the reason. "Not allowing a woman to terminate her pregnancy amount to grave injury to her mental health". MTP should be allowed even if there is no risk to her physical health.

- The Act must be extended not just to married women, but also to those women who 'stay with their partners as married couples in live-in relationships'.

Pregnancy beyond 20 weeks

Bombay High Court denies abortion of 25 weeks foetus

A couple and a gynaecologist petitioned the Bombay high court (known as Nikita Mehta Case) with a request to permit an abortion beyond the legal 20 weeks on the grounds that the newborn's health may be at risk. The couple have asked to amend the provision to allow for an abortion "if the physical or mental health of the foetus is at risk. The court observed that the committee of medical experts should give a positive opinion on whether there is substantial risk that if the child is born, it will have serious mental or physical deformity for making a decision. The final report submitted by JJ Hospital Committee said "The committee is of the opinion that there are very least chances that the child will be born incapacitated and handicapped to survive". The High Court dismissed the plea to permit an abortion of 25 weeks foetus with a complete congenital heart blockage and malpositioned arteries that could, doctors say, require a pacemaker implantation soon after birth.

The justices observed "We can interpret the law and not make the law. The JJ report is clear that the child is not deformed. Once there is life, can you ask for it to be killed now? Is it any different from mercy killing?"

Rape Survivor can Terminate Pregnancy: Kerala High Court (November 15, 2016)

A woman from Kasaragod (Kerala) filed a petition seeking permission to terminate her pregnancy that had resulted from rape. Earlier her requests for termination were turned down by Kasaragod Government

Hospital and Kozhikode Medical College Hospital. She was in sexual relationship with a man who promised to marry her. She filed a police complaint of rape when the man did not keep his promise and married to another woman. On her petition, the High Court observed that a rape survivor is eligible for termination of pregnancy as unwanted pregnancy is a threat to her life.

The High Court ordered the Medical Superintendent of the Kozhikode Medical College Hospital to take necessary step for MTP.

Supreme court of India rejected the plea of HIV + Rape survivor to abort (9 May, 2017)

A 35-year-old destitute HIV+ woman facing complications in her 26 weeks pregnancy resulted from rape approached the Supreme Court seeking permission to abort her pregnancy. The apex court rejected her plea as the medical report prepared by AIIMS doctors said that her life might be in danger if MTP of foetus was done at such an advanced stage.

The court observed that this delay was due to fault of State Government and Patna Medical College Hospital. Earlier the State Government opposed her plea in High Court. The High Court refused to allow her abortion. By the time she approached the Supreme Court it was too late. However, the apex court ordered the State Government of Bihar to provide medical care at Patna and pay compensation of three lakh rupees under rape survivor scheme.

The Supreme Court during a hearing of a petition from Kolkata woman observed that law should be more meaningful and favours the amendment of the MTP Act to allow the MTP in case of terminally ill foetus beyond the current limits of 20 weeks.

Consent Required

- The pregnant woman's (attained 18 years of age) informed consent is required for MTP. No other person's consent is necessary.

- In case of pregnant minor: Written consent of guardian is necessary.
- In case of pregnant women (18 years and above) but of unsound mind, written consent of guardian is necessary.

It is important to note, in this section, that the consent of the woman is the essential factor for termination of her pregnancy. The husband's consent is irrelevant. Therefore, if the woman wants an abortion but her husband's objects to it, the abortion can still be done. However, if the woman does not want an abortion but her husband wants, it cannot be done.

No MTP without Consent even if Woman is Retarded

A rape victim, staying in a home for mentally challenged in Chandigarh, wanted to continue pregnancy till its full term and bear a child. As the said woman is assumed to be mentally incapable to making an informed decision, the Chandigarh High Court permitted MTP. On reversing the order of High Court, the Supreme Court in its final order observed "the MTP on a person found in a condition of borderline, mild or moderate mental retardation, is antidemocratic and violative of the guarantee of 'equal protection before the law' as laid down in Article 14 of our constitution.". The court also observed "There is no doubt that a woman's right to make reproductive choices is also a dimension of 'personal liberty' under Article 21.

"MTP cannot be done without the consent of the woman even if she is mentally retarded and not in a position to understand the consequences", the Supreme Court observed.
(*Source*: The Hindu, Tiruchirapalli, August 30, 2009.)

In case of pregnant minor, she may be advised to consult her parents, guardian, family members or friends before termination of pregnancy. However, if the minor decides not to consult them, she should still be allowed to go ahead with her decision to terminate pregnancy. The act also makes provisions for pregnant women who are unable to make a decision on account of illness: Severely mentally disabled, in a state of continuous unconsciousness.

Places for MTP

- A hospital established or maintained by government, or
- A place for the time being approved for the purpose of this Act by government or a district level committee constituted by the government with the chief medical officer or district health officer as chairperson of the committee.

However, exceptions are made for emergencies. A doctor may terminate a pregnancy if it is "immediately necessary to save the life of the pregnant woman". In such situations, the requisites relating to the length of pregnancy, the need for two medical opinions and the venue for operation do not apply.

Approval of Place for MTP

The approval process has been decentralized from the state level to district committee. The centralization of power for approval of places as MTP centres, from state to district level aims at enlarging the network of safe MTP centres. The non-government institutions may also take up abortions provided they obtain a license from Chief Medical Officer of the District. The Act provides punitive measures of 2–7 years imprisonment for individual provider or owner of facilities not approved or maintained by the government. To reduce the administrative delays, a timeframe has been defined for registration and mandates the district committee to inspect a facility within two months of receiving an application for registration and process the approval within next two months if no deficiency found, or within two months after rectification of any noted deficiency.

Requirements for Approval

- Safe and hygienic condition;
- Up to 12 weeks of pregnancy (first trimester): A gynecology/labor table, resuscitation and sterilization equipment, drugs and parenteral fluid, back-up

facilities for treatment of shock and facilities for transportation; and

- In case of second trimester (up to 20 weeks of pregnancy): An operation table and instruments for performing abdominal or gynecological surgery; anaesthetic equipment, resuscitation equipment and sterilization equipment, drugs and parenteral fluids and other requirements as notified by the government.

Composition and Terms of district committee:

- A gynecologist/surgeon/anaesthetist;
- Other members from local medical profession, non-government organization, and Panchayati Raj Institution of the district.
- One of the members of the committee must be a woman.
- Tenure of the committee is for two calendar years. Tenure of non-government members is for not more than two terms.

Approval Process

- Application for approval is to be addressed in prescribed form to the Chief Medical Officer of the District.
- Chief Medical Officer on verification of application inspects the place to satisfy himself that MTP can be performed under safe and hygienic condition.
- Chief Medical Officer would recommend the approval to the committee.
- The committee on consideration of application and recommendation of the Chief Medical Officer may issue a certificate of approval in prescribed form.

The certificate of approval should be conspicuously displayed at a place easily visible to the person visiting the place.

Inspection, Cancellation or Suspension of approval:

Chief Medical Officer may inspect the approved place as often as necessary to verify whether MTP is being performed under safe and hygienic condition. After inspection, if Chief Medical Officer satisfied that the facility is not maintained properly and MTP cannot be performed under safe and hygienic condition, may report the same to the committee giving details of the defects and deficiency. On satisfaction the committee may suspend or cancel the approval after the owner is given an opportunity to make presentation. Once the approval is cancelled or suspended, the owner may make addition or improvements in the place and may make application to the committee for approval. The aggrieved owner of the place may make an application to the government for review within a period of sixty days of such order. The government may condone the time delay, if required. After hearing the owner's view, the government may confirm, modify or reverse the order.

Experience and Training of registered Medical Practitioner for performing MTP:

The registered medical practitioner should have one or more of the following experience or training in gynecology and obstetrics:

- Registered medical practitioner (registered before the commencement of the Act)– minimum of three years of experience in the practice of gynecology and obstetrics;
- Registered Medical Practitioner completed six months of house surgery in gynecology and obstetrics; or experience at any hospital for a minimum period of one year in the practice of gynecology and obstetrics;
- Registered medical practitioner assisted in performing 25 MTP out of which at least five must have been performed independently. This training enables the medical practitioner to perform MTP for cases below 12 weeks.
- Registered Medical Practitioner holding a postgraduate degree or diploma in gynecology and obstetrics.

Maintenance of Records and Procedure followed:

The opinion of registered medical practitioners should be recorded in the prescribe form (Form I) and the registered medical practitioner who performs MTP should record such details within 3 hours of such MTP in Form I.

The consent recorded together with certified opinion of the registered medical practitioner(s) should be kept in envelope, sealed and kept in his/her custody until sent to the head of the hospital, owner of the approved place or chief medical officer. The serial number of the women in the admission register should be recorded in the envelope and such envelope should be marked as SECRET. Every envelope should have the name and address of the concerned registered medical practitioner.

On receipt of the envelope, the head of the hospital or owner of the approved place will keep them in safe custody. The owner of the approved place or head of the hospital is required to send the monthly statement on MTP to the Chief Medical Officer in Form II.

However, when MTP is performed in an unapproved place, every envelope should be sent by registered post to the chief medical officer of the state on the same day or in the following working day.

The head of the hospital or the owner of the approved place is required to maintain a register as prescribed in Form III recording the details of women admitted for MTP and the register is to be preserved for five years from the end of the calendar year. The entries in the admission register shall be made serially and a fresh serial shall be started at the commencement of each calendar year and the serial number of the particular year shall be distinguished from the serial number of other years by mentioning the year against the serial number, for example, serial number 5 of 1972 and serial number 5 of 1973 shall be mentioned as 5/1972 and 5/1973. Admission register is a secret document and the names and other particulars of the pregnant women will not be disclosed to any person. The admission register is to be kept in the safe custody by the head of the hospital or the owner of the approved place or by authorized person and will not be open for inspection except under the authority of law.

The registered medical practitioner may issue a certificate on the application of employed woman whose pregnancy is terminated in order to enable her to avail leave.

Such employer should not disclose such information.

Various Forms

Form I: Opinion and Record by Registered Medical Practitioner.

Form II: Monthly Statement

Form III: Admission Register.

Form A: Application for approval of place.

Form B: Certificate of approval of place.

Form C: Consent form.

Making Rules

The Central Government may, by notification in the official gazette, make rules to carry out the provisions of this Act with respect to the experience or training, or both, which a registered medical practitioner shall have if he intends to terminate any pregnancy under this Act or any other matter.

Every rule made by the Central Government under this Act is to be laid, as soon as may be after it is made, before each House of Parliament. If both Houses agree in making any modification in the rule or both Houses agree that the rule should not be made, the rule shall thereafter have effect only in such modified form or be of no effect.

Power to Make Regulations

The state government may make regulations for making provisions for taking opinion of registered medical practitioner(s), certification by registered medical practitioner, preservation or disposal of certificates; requiring registered medical practitioners to give intimation of termination, prohibiting the disclosure of such information in pursuance of regulations to unauthorized person.

Willful contravention or failure to comply with requirements of any regulation is punishable with fine which is extendable to one thousand rupees.

In a case of 10-year-old child rape victim, Chandigarh District Court has denied permission to abortion on the ground that the pregnancy is beyond 26 weeks (2017 case). The judgment raised several issues including call for revisiting the MTP Act. In this particular case, the victim's life is at risk either way: Whether in termination of pregnancy or in a delivery process that underage girl's body is not equipped to withstand. Besides, the legal process is often viewed as perversely long drawn leading to the pregnancy getting into advanced stage.

In the light of several cases of MTP reaching Supreme Court seeking permission beyond 20-week deadline because either their fetus was malformed or they were rape survivors, the demand 24-week abortion rising. This has another angle too. The underprivileged women are more impacted by this 20 week limit. There are overcrowding of government hospitals, the women find difficult to get appointment for ultrasound in the 18–20-week window when an anomaly scan requires to be performed. Even if a problem is detected, it takes another one or two weeks to get a confirmation and by this time, it crosses the legal limit of 20 weeks. Many cardiac anomalies can only be detected at 22–23 weeks only. Hence, the demand for 24 week abortion rising.

Draft Medical Termination of Pregnancy (Amendment) Bill, 2014

Realising the need of changing MTP conditions, the Ministry of Health and Welfare, proposed the amendment of the existing Act. Some notable features of the proposed Amendment are:

- In addition to registered medical practitioners the following categories of healthcare providers are also proposed for MTP:
  - Persons qualified with Ayurveda, Siddha, Unani, and Homeopathy and registered are also included;
  - Nurse or Auxiliary nurse.
- MTP is permissible beyond 20 weeks:
  - Pregnancy exceeds 20 weeks but not exceeding 24 weeks.
  - Length of pregnancy is insignificant (at any time MTP) if the diagnosis confirms substantial foetal abnormalities.

There has been news that this would not be pursued.

11

The Prevention of Cruelty to Animals Act

*"The greatness of a nation and its moral progress can be judged by the way its **animals** are treated. Vivisection is the blackest of all black crimes that the man is at present committing against God and His fair creation. It ill becomes us to invoke in our daily prayers the blessing of God, the Compassionate, if we in turn will not practice elementary compassion to our fellow creatures. And I abhor vivisection with my whole soul. All the scientific discoveries stained with the innocent blood I count as of no consequence".*

— *Mahatma Gandhi*

After reading this chapter, you should be able to understand and appreciate:

- Need of ethics in animal experimentation
- Obtaining Ethics Committee's approval
- Functions of Animal Welfare Board of India
- Constitution of the Committee for the Purpose of Control and Supervision of Experiments on Animals (CPCSEA)
- Mandates of CPCSEA
- Guiding Principles of Animal Experimentations

Animal experiments are widely used to develop new medicines and to test the safety of other products. The experiments are done to help decide whether the drug can be tested on human beings. Animal experiments eliminate some potential drugs as either ineffective or too dangerous to use on human beings. If a drug passes the animal test, it is then tested on a small human group before large-scale clinical trial. The animal toxicity data are required in the dossier for seeking permission for conducting clinical trials. Biologically humans are similar to mice and rats having the same set of genes. Their bodies' response to disease and treatments are similar to human beings. Today we have antibiotics, insulin, vaccines for polio and cervical cancer, organ transplantation, heart bypass surgery. All

these are developed and tested using animals, even the animals are used for manufacturing vaccines and sera.

On the other hand, while experiments on animals are done for scientific advancement for the benefit of mankind, the animals are often subjected to injury, pain, suffering and even deaths. In one study it is reported: Use of animals without health or genetic background knowledge (including strays and street dogs), animals leaving in filthy unhygienic condition, experiments being performed in unhygienic condition, sick and injured animals left unattended and animals denied post-operative care, etc. Often the question arises whether animal experimentations are justifiable! Counter arguments on animal experimentation say "some drugs that have been approved for through animal tests can cause serious and unexpected side effects for humans. A 2002 report in the Journal of American Medical Association (JAMA) found that in the last 25 years, more than 50 FDA approved drugs had to be taken off the market or relabelled because they caused adverse reactions". There is no guarantee that safety in animals will ensure similar safety in humans. When human gene information is available, why animals are used for experiments? Many alternative methods are being used by many researchers: Studies on cadavers, computer simulations, tissue culture, etc. It is possible now to test irritancy on egg membrane, produce vaccine from cell culture, and so on. The US FDA does not require the use of animals for safety testing of animals. There have been many prominent people fighting against the practice of vivisection. They include: Dr Annie Besant, Mahatma Gandhi, George Bernard Shaw and Menaka Gandhi.

With arguments and counter arguments going on, it is true that no one selects animal experimentation for fun and pleasure. Wherever alternative reliable methods are available, the scientists would switch over. The animal experimentations would continue in the field of biomedical research. In fact, animal research has contributed to 70% of Nobel prizes for physiology or medicine. But certainly there are ethical issues which require redressing.

There are no laws in the world which prohibits any animal experiment, no matter how painful or frivolous. In Great Britain, it is against the law for the medical students to practice surgery on animals. The Animal Welfare Act of the US is very weak and poorly enforced. It is basically a housekeeping Act that does not prohibit any type of animal experimentation. The Government of India enacted the legislation called 'The Prevention of Cruelty to Animals Act 1960' to prevent the infliction of unnecessary pain or suffering on animals. It extends to the whole of India except Jammu and Kashmir.

Though the Act covers several aspects of animal's cruelty, the present text restricts its domain to experimentation on animals.

Pamphlet (1966) by the Committee for the Purpose of Controlling and Supervising Experiments on Animals Chaired by Mr. Kamal Nayan Bajaj.

Vivisection, or animal experimentation, is one of the most inhuman cruelties against animals, which are being perpetrated in the world today. The object of these experiments is said to be in order to advance scientific knowledge, and to undertake research to save or prolong human or animal life and alleviating suffering. In the name of the science, however, animals are made to endure the most barbaric tortures ever invented by the human brain, often lasting over long periods and without any sort of anaesthetics.

Animal Welfare Board of India

The Government of India established Animal Welfare Board of India in 1962 with its head-quarter at Madras (now Chennai) for the promotion of animal welfare in general and for the purpose of protecting animals from being subjected to unnecessary pain or sufferings. It is an autonomous body working under the administrative control of the Ministry of Environment, Forests and Climate Changes. The board consists of 28 members representing Government of India, the veterinary profession, municipal bodies, practitioners of modern and indigenous systems of medicines, animal welfare organizations and humanitarians. Two members of Rajya Sabha and four members of Lok Sabha are on the board. The main functions of the board are:

- To keep the law in force in India for the prevention of cruelty to animals under constant study and advise the government on the amendments to be undertaken;

- To advise the central government on making rules with a view to prevent unnecessary pain or suffering;

- To advise the government or local authority or other persons on improvements in the design of vehicles so as to lessen the burden on draught animals;

- To take all such steps for amelioration of animals by encouraging or providing for the construction of sheds, water troughs and by providing veterinary assistance to animals;
- To advise the government or local authority or other persons in the design of slaughter house or in connection with slaughter of animals so the unnecessary mental or physical pain is eliminated and the animals are killed in as humane manner as possible;
- To take all such steps to ensure that unwanted animals are destroyed by local authorities;
- To encourage the formation of pinjra-poles, rescue homes, animal shelters, etc. through grant of financial assistance or otherwise;
- To cooperate and coordinate the work of associations or bodies established for the purpose of preventing unnecessary pain or suffering or protection of animals and birds;
- To give financial assistance to animal welfare organizations or to encourage their formation;
- To advise the government on the matter relating to medical care and attention to be provided to animal hospitals;
- To impart education in relation to the humane treatment of animals to encourage the formation of public opinion against the infliction of unnecessary pain or suffering to animals;
- To advise the government on any other matter related to either animal welfare or prevention of infliction of unnecessary pain or suffering of animals.

Committee for the Purpose of Control and Supervision of Experiments on Animals (CPCSEA)

Performance of experiments (including experiments involving operation) on animals for the purpose of the advancement by new discovery of physiological knowledge or of knowledge which would be useful for saving or prolonging life or alleviating suffering or for combating any disease in human being, animals, or plants is not unlawful. The central government constituted the Committee for the Purpose of Control and Supervision of Experiments on Animals (CPCSEA) in 1964, but the committee soon lapsed into inactivity. In February 1991, the CPCSEA was reconstituted. However, the committee again failed to address any of the very clear problems related to animal experimentation. In February 1996 a new CPCSEA was constituted, chaired by Smt. Maneka Gandhi (then a Member of Parliament). This revitalised CPCSEA introduced a draft of regulations in an attempt to regulate the industry and commenced an inspection programme to assess science and animal welfare.

Constitution of CPCSEA

1. Special Secretary [Ministry of Environment, Forest and Climate Change (MoEF&CC)]—Chairman.
2. Joint Secretary (Animal Welfare)—Vice Chairman.
3. Deputy Secretary (Animal Welfare)—Member Secretary.
4. Other members:
   a. Director, National Institute of Animal Welfare,
   b. Drugs Controller General of India,
   c. Experts or Officials from:
      i. Medical Council of India,
      ii. Veterinary Council of India,
      iii. Pharmacy Council of India,
      iv. University Grants Commission,
      v. Wildlife Institute of India,
      vi. Institutes under Department of Biotechnology,
      vii. Expert from Medical and Pharmacy Colleges,
      viii. Experts from Universities (Biotechnology, Zoology, Life Sciences, etc.)

Mandates of CPCSEA

The followings are the mandates of CPCSEA:
- Registration of establishments conducting experiments on animals.
- Registration of establishments engaged in breeding of laboratory animals.

- Constitution of Institutional Animal Ethics Committees (IAECs) in the establishment registered.
- Approval of Animal House Facilities of small and large animals.
- Permission for conducting experiments on large animals.
- Recommendation for import of animals for experimentations and breeding.
- Action against the establishments in case of violation of any legal norms/stipulations.

The CPCSEA issued guidelines for maintenance and conducting experiments involving all permitted species of animals for undertaking biomedical research. This is known as CPCSEA guidelines for Laboratory Animal Facility. The rules made by the committee are binding on individuals performing experiments outside institutions and on persons in charge of institutions in which experiments are performed. The committee may authorise any of its officers or any other person to inspect any institution or place where experiments are being carried out for the purpose of ensuring the compliance of the provisions of the Act and Rules. The officer or the person so authorised may:

- Enter at any reasonable time and inspect any institution or place in which experiments on animals are being carried out;
- Requires any person to produce any record kept by him with respect to experiments on animals.

If the committee is satisfied that the provisions of the Act or Rules are not complied, prohibit the person or institution from carrying on any such experiments either for a specified period or indefinitely, after giving an opportunity to the person or institution of being heard.

For performing experiments the approval of Institutional Ethics Committee (IEC) is necessary. The Pharmacy Council of India in its circular discourages the use of animals for experimentation.

The Rules under the Act made provision for establishing Society for Prevention of Cruelty in Animals (SPCA) in every district by the respective state governments. The managing committee of the society is appointed by the state government or local authority of the district.

Penalties: If any person contravenes any order by the committee with respect to prohibition of experiments or commits a breach of any condition imposed by the committee, he shall be punishable with fine which may extend to 200 rupees.

When the contravention or breach of condition has taken place in any institution, the person in charge of the institution is deemed to be guilty of offence and shall be punishable accordingly.

Suffering of Animals during Experiments

Evidence gathered by the CPCSEA during the course of inspection of 467 laboratories showed a horrifying picture of state of research inside animal experimentation facilities. There were deplorable standards of animal care in majority of the facilities inspected. The findings include:

- Use of animals without health or genetic background knowledge (including strays-street dogs).
- Animals living in filthy, unhygienic conditions.
- Experiments being performed in similar unhygienic conditions.
- Sick and injured animals left unattended and the animals denied post-operative care.
- Some institutions had been without a veterinary officer in attendance for years.
- Rats and mice infected with disease, and infested with mite and tapeworms.
- Horses with their hooves infested with maggots.
- Rats being blinded during orbital bleed procedure.
- Hot irons used to brand horses.
- Inadequate and often wholly unsuitable facilities: Lacking appropriate ventilation or even a water supply.
- A lack of consistency of standards between the facilities, ranging from

derelict buildings being used to house experimental cattle, to a variety of rusting cages for other animals.

- Animals severely restricted in their movements, and overcrowded in small, dirty cages.
- Animals self-mutilating and performing abnormal, repetitive and stereotype behaviours.
- Inadequate provision of food and water.
- Brutal procedures such as drilling holes in the skull of conscious sheep and then injecting rabies virus into the brain for a discredited vaccine.
- Placing live and conscious frogs in refrigerators in order to freeze them.
- Failure to identify or utilise non-animal methods when they are available.

(Animal Experimentation in Animals in India, Animal Defenders International and National Anti-Vivisection Society, 2003.)

CPCSEA suspended the licence: The committee for the Purpose of Control and Supervision of Experiments on Animals had temporarily suspended the license of Mediclone Biotech Private limited to conduct experiments on animals. The company extracts large volumes of blood from horses and other animals to make anti-toxins anti-venoms. The inspection conducted by the People for Ethical Treatment of Animals (PeTA) and Animal Welfare Board of India (AWBI) reported exploiting horses while denying the veterinary care for painful conditions. The findings includes company breeding horses without authorization.

The company failed to improve the facilities and hence this suspension of licence.

[Pharma Web, Issue No. 34, April-June 2017].

The rules made in 1998 by the committee for Control and Supervision of Experiments on Animals has laid down the constitution of Institutional Animal ethics Committee. The committee consist of a biological scientist, two scientists from different biological disciplines, a veterinarian involved in care of animals, the scientist in charge of the animal facility of the institute, a scientist from outside the institute, a non-scientist from outside the institute and a representative or nominee of the Central Committee (CPSSEA). There is provision for co-option of a specialist while reviewing special projects.

Functions of Animal Ethics Committee

- To review and approve projects involving animal experimentations.
- To ensure that the minimum number of animals of appropriate species and quality are being employed and that they do not undergo unnecessary sufferings during experimentations.
- To review the skills of the scientists and technicians conducting the experiments and confirms its adequacy.
- To ensure use of appropriate anaesthetic, sedative or analgesic and, if indicated, use of an acceptable method of euthanasia at the termination of study and appropriate method of disposal.
- To ensure that the animals are provided proper husbandry, appropriate living condition and veterinary care.
- To conduct periodic review of ongoing projects and to terminate a study if there is unnecessary suffering to the animals or if generated data does not warrant further study.

Guiding Principles for Animal Experimentations

1. 4 Rs:
   a. Replacements—methods which avoid or replace the use of animals in research should be given priority. Replacement alternatives should be given due and full consideration before switching to animal experimentation;
   b. Reduction—use of methods that enable researchers to have comparable levels of information from fewer animals; or

to obtain more information in same number of animals is encouraged;

c. Refinement—use of methods that alleviate or minimize potential pain, suffering or distress and enhance animal welfare is encouraged;

d. Reuse and rehabilitation—after completion of an experiment, the use of same animal for other experiments is encouraged. Appropriate after care (rehabilitation) of the animals exposed to experiments should be ensured until the point of natural death.

2. The animal lowest on the phylogenetic scale which may give scientifically valid results should be first considered.

3. The experiment should be designed with the minimum number of animals to give statistically valid results at 95% degree of confidence.

4. Wherever possible, computational modeling, simulations or *in silico* analysis should be carried out. The *in vitro* assays with cell line or tissue culture should be encouraged. The *ex vivo* studies with organs collected from slaughter house or culling animals may be used wherever feasible.

Proposed Animal Welfare Act 2011 (Salient Points) (To replace the Prevention of Cruelty to Animals Act 1960)

- Proposes the setting up of a committee for the purpose of control and supervision of experiments on animals to ensure that the experiments are performed with due care and humanity.

- The committee is to take measures necessary to ensure that the animals are not subjected to unnecessary trauma, pain or suffering before, during or after the performance of experiments on them.

- The committee consists of a number of officials and non-officials and representatives from Central Zoo Authority, the Veterinary Council of India and members of animal welfare organizations.

- Those who commit cruelty towards animals will face punishments including imprisonment and heavy penalties.

- It is proposed to prevent repetitive experiments. The committee is empowered to ask the institutions to maintain records of various experiments performed by it and to maintain details of various available non-animal alternatives.

- Where the experiments are performed in any institution, the responsibility for such experiments would be on the person in charge of the institution.

- The experiments involving operations are performed under the influence of an anaesthetic of sufficient potency to prevent the animals from feeling pain.

- The hospitals including undergraduate medical colleges, pharmacy colleges, zoology and other degree, diploma colleges and universities should avoid experiments and dissections of the animals.

12

The Clinical Establishments (Registration and Regulation) Act

"A Hospital Bed is a Parked Taxi with Meter Running"

— *Groucho Marx*

After reading this chapter, you should be able to understand and appreciate:

- The purpose of the Act
- Authorities for Administration of the Act
- Role of Central and State Governments
- Offences and Penalties

The constitution of India mandates that the government should take initiative for improving public health. India's health system is far from satisfactory. The study shows that nearly 80% of outpatient care and about 60% of inpatient care are provided by the private care providers. 40% of the private care are likely to be provided by informal unqualified persons. The out of pocket expenditure is very high: About 70% of total health spending. There were reports of exploitation of the patients by the private healthcare providers. There are no standardized care too. Healthcare in India suffers from under-regulation subjecting the populace to poor quality of treatment, quackery menace and high costs. There has been expectation of the people that the government should bring improvement in our health care system through bringing legislation in order to ensure minimum standard of care and prevent exploitation of the general public. With this background in mind, the Clinical Establishment Act 2010 was enacted. The Act was passed in Parliament on 17th August 2010 and the Rules were made in 2012. The Act came into force on 1st March 2012. In short, the Act can be viewed as a 'Tool to Improve Health Care'.

The Act is administered by the Ministry of Health and Family Welfare at central level and by the Department of Health at state level. The Act is applicable to all kinds of clinical establishments from public and private sectors, of all recognized systems of medicine including single doctor clinics. However, establishments run by the Armed forces are exempted from the provision of the Act.

High Court pulls up government on Clinical Establishment Act: In case of May 2015, a medical student is alleged to have died of over dose of anaesthesia during hair transplant. The Madras High Court is reported to have serious questions to the central and state governments with respect to CEA. The court has asked the governments to enact appropriate legislation to regulate the new types of clinics like hair transplant centres, beauty clinics, studios, and spas.

Source: http://medicaldialogues.in/chennai-hc-court-pulls-up-government-on-clinical-establishment-act/, Accessed on 03rd November 2017)

Aim and Objectives of the Act: The Act aims to register and regulate clinical establishments based on minimum standards in order to improve quality of public health care in the country. The objectives of the Act are:

i. To establish digital registry of Clinical Establishments at National, State and District levels.

ii. To prevent quackery by unqualified practitioners by introducing registration system, which is mandatory.

iii. To improve quality of health care through standardization of health care facilities by prescribing minimum standards of facilities and services for all categories of health care establishments (except teaching hospitals) and ensuring compliance of other conditions of registration like compliance to standard treatment guidelines, stabilization of emergency medical condition, display of range of rates to be charged, maintenance of records, etc.

Global Scenario: The minimum standards for hospitals in USA was developed as early as in 1917 by the American College of Surgeons. Health Quality Services of UK is the oldest accreditation service in Europe.

In China, the central government sets broad policy guidelines but leaves the implementation details to local governments. The Malaysia has Malaysian Society for Quality in Health (MSQH) and was formed by combined efforts of the Ministry of Health Malaysia and Association of Private Hospitals of Malaysia. Thailand introduced universal coverage reforms in 2001.

The salient points of the act are:

* The Act:
  - Assists in generation of reliable and comprehensive database (or registry) for all types of clinical establishments in the country at district, state and national level.
  - Helps classifying various types of clinical establishments into categories and determine category wise basic minimum standards.
  - Defines basic minimum standards for operation, using participatory and consultative approach to ensure uniformity across all establishments. The minimum standards indicate basic standards which are mandatory and certain standards which are desirable.
  - Assists Government in obtaining information and data required from clinical establishments for public health interventions including outbreak and disaster management.

* It establishes the multi-stakeholder bodies: National Council for Clinical Establishments, State Council for Clinical Establishments, District Registration Authority.

* The Act allows for two-step process of registration—provisional and permanent registration. Provisional registration is done through a process of self-declaration, without any inquiry or inspection. Permanent registration would be undertaken after categorization, classification and notification of category wise minimum standards.

* The Act places the entire process of registration and the data of clinical establishments in the public domain which ensures transparency.

* Details of charges, facilities available would be prominently displayed at a conspicuous place at each establishment

* Registry of clinical establishments would aid in policy formulation and resource allocation.

* Cancellation of registration would occur at any time, if conditions for registration are not complied with.

* Clinical Establishment is to provide emergency medical treatment within staff and facilities available.

* The Act may control or act as deterrent against quackery by introducing registration which is applicable only to clinical establishments of recognized systems of medicine and no one can run a clinical establishment without registration.

- It lays down provisions for healthcare providers to maintain records and reporting as prescribed and provide information and statistics that may be asked for by the authority.

The State Council for Clinical Establishment and District Registration Authority are the implementing authorities for the Act.

Classification of Clinical Establishments: The clinical establishments are classified based on different principles such as facilities, location, ownership, system of medicine, etc. Here the classification as done for the hospital is only given.

I. Based on Facilities

The allopathic hospitals are categorised into four levels:

Type	Facilities and Examples	
Hospital Level 1	1(A)	General Medical Services with indoor admission facilities; Support System like pharmacy, laboratory, etc. Ex: Primary health centre, government and private hospitals, nursing homes.
	1(B)	Facilities as in 1(A) + at least one basic speciality services like general medicine, general surgery, paediatrics, obstetrics and gynaecology and dentistry, providing indoor and OPD services. Support system like pharmacy, laboratory, etc. Ex: General hospital, single/ multiple basic medical specialties provided at community health centre, sub-divisional hospital.
Hospital Level 2 (non-teaching)		Facilities in 1(A) and 1(B) + other medical specialities. Support system like pharmacy, laboratory, imaging facilities, operation theatre, etc. Ex: District hospital, corporate hospitals, referral hospital, regional/state hospital, nursing home and private hospital

(Contd...)

(Contd...)

Type	Facilities and Examples
Hospital Level 3 (non-teaching) Super-specialty services	Facilities in 1(A), 1(B) and 2 + at least one super-speciality. Support system like pharmacy, laboratory, imaging facilities, operation theatre, etc. Ex: Corporate hospitals, referral hospitals, regional/state hospital, nursing home and private hospital
Hospital Level 4 (teaching)	Facilities of Level 2 and may have facilities of Level 3; Medical Council of India recognition as teaching institution. Ex: Medical College Hospital

II. Other Classification System

- **Location:**
  - Rural
  - Urban
  - Metro
  - Notified/inaccessible areas (including hilly or tribal areas)
- **Ownership:**
  - Government/Public
    - Central government
    - State government
    - Local government (Municipality, Zilla parishad, etc.)
    - Public sector undertaking
    - Other ministries and departments (Railways, Police, etc.)
    - Employee State Insurance Corporation
    - Autonomous organization under government
  - Non-government/private
    - Individual proprietorship
    - Partnership
    - Registered companies (registered under central/provincial/state Act)
    - Society/trust (Registered a central/ provincial/state Act)
- **System of medicine**
  - Allopathy (modern medicine)
  - AYUSH
- **Type/size**
  - *Clinics (outpatient)*: Single practitioner or polyclinic
  - Day care facility

- Hospitals including Nursing Homes
- Dental Clinics and Dental Hospitals
- Diagnostic Centres.

Role of Governments

Central Government's Responsibilities	State Government's Responsibilities
• Notification of the Act	• Notification of State Rules
• Notification of the National Council and Rules for the functioning	• Constitute and notify the State/Union Territory Council of Clinical Establishments
• Classification and Categorization of the Clinical Establishments by Central Government based on the recommendations of the National Council	• Constitute and notify District Registration Authorities in all districts
	• Begin the process of provisional registration
• Establish Minimum Standards for the different categories of Clinical Establishments based on the recommendations of the National Council.	• Identification and notification of Registrars of Clinical Establishment at State Level (Director of Health Services) and District level (District Health Officer)
• Develop and pre-scribe the form and manner in which the registry (National, State and District level) is to be maintained.	• Disseminate information about the Act and Rules at various levels and among stakeholders
• Provide oversight and assistance to the States and UTs for the imple-mentation of the CEA 2010 including capacity building.	
• Assistance for the drafting of Rules of the Act. Draft of Model Rules circulated to all implementing States/UTs.	

(Contd...)

(Contd...)

Central Government's Responsibilities	State Government's Responsibilities
• Assist States and UTs in adoption of the proposed web-based registration system and offline registration systems.	
• Assistance to the State and UTs Councils for any other matter that may be required.	

Authorities

National Council for Clinical Establishments

Constitution

National Council is a 20-member body under ex-officio Chairman Director General of Health Services, GoI. Officer of rank of Joint Secretary of Ministry of Health and Family Welfare dealing with the subject of Clinical Establishments Act shall be ex-officio Secretary of National Council. The National Council has elected members from regulatory councils for allopathic Doctors (MCI, DCI), Pharmacy, Nursing, Indian systems of Medicine (Ayurveda, Siddha, Unani), Homoeopathy, Indian Medical Association (IMA) and nominated representatives of Bureau of Indian Standards (BIS), Zonal Council, North Eastern Council other paramedical systems, consumer groups and association of Indian System of Medicine.

Functions

- Compile and publish a National Register of clinical establishments within two years from the date of the commencement of this Act.
- Classify the clinical establishments into different categories.
- Develop the minimum standards and their periodic review.
- Determine within a period of two years from its establishment, the first set of standards for ensuring proper healthcare by the clinical establishments.

- Collect the statistics in respect of clinical establishments.
- Perform any other function determined by the Central Government from time to time.

Health being a state subject, the implementation of the Act is dependent on enacting the Act or similar Act at state level. All states have not yet adopted the Act. The state is at liberty to make its legislation. The West Bengal Government passed its Act, The West Bengal Clinical Establishment (Registration, Regulation and Transparency) Act 2017. It has established Clinical Establishment Regulatory Commission as the Authority. The commission is empowered to monitor, regulate and supervise the functions of private hospitals and enforce transparency in these establishments. The commission has the power to fix the rates of treatments including diagnostics. It can also award compensation to the victims of negligent treatments not exceeding 50 lakh rupees.

Civil courts would have no jurisdiction over action taken by the Commission and aggrieved parties can only seek redress at High Courts or the Supreme Court.

State Council for Clinical Establishments

Composition

- Secretary, Health ex-officio—Chairman;
- Director of Health Services—ex-officio member-secretary;
- Directors of different streams of Indian Systems of Medicine—ex-officio members;
- One representative each to be elected by the executive committee of
  - State Medical Council of India
  - State Dental Council of India
  - State Nursing Council of India
  - State Pharmacy Council of India
- Three representatives to be elected by the Executive of the State Council or Union Territory Council, as the case may be, of Indian Medicine representing the Ayurveda, Siddha and Unani systems of medicines;

- One representative to be elected by the State Council of the Indian Medical Association;
- One representative from the line of paramedical systems
- Two representatives from the State level consumer groups or reputed non-governmental organizations working in the field of health.

Functions

- Compiling and updating the State Registers of Clinical Establishment;
- Sending monthly returns for updating the National Register;
- Representing the State in the National Council;
- Hearing of appeals against the orders of the authority;
- Publication on annual basis a report on the state of implementation of standards within their respective States.

District Registering Authority

Composition

- District Collector/District Magistrate: Chairman;
- District Chief Medical Officer/District Health Officer: Convenor;
- Three members nominated by District Magistrate:
  - City Police Commissioner/SSP/SP or nominee
  - Senior officer of local self-government at district level
  - Professional Medical Association/Body.

Functions

- Grant/renew provisional (within 10 days)/permanent registration
- Publish:
  a. List of provisionally registered (within 45 days after grant),
  b. Clinical Establishments who submit evidence for permanent registration and invite objections if any (30 days),
  c. Expired Registrations

- May issue a notice to Clinical Establishment to show cause within 3 months, if condition(s) of registration are not met
- To enter and search unregistered CE (after due notice)
- Inspection and inquiry of registered clinical establishments through multi-member inspection team inform the deficiency and actions to be taken by clinical establishment
- May cancel registration (after giving reasonable opportunity) and giving reasons
- After cancelling registration, immediately restrain clinical establishment if imminent danger to the health and safety of patients
- Recover penalties
- Maintain district register of clinical establishments.

Registration of Clinical Establishments

Conditions for Registration and Renewal: The clinical establishment organization needs to comply with:

- The minimum standards of facilities and services as may be prescribed;
- The minimum requirements of personnel as may be prescribed;
- Provisions for maintenance of records and reporting as may be prescribed;
- The clinical establishment shall undertake to provide within the staff and facilities available such medical examination and treatment as may be required to stabilize the emergency medical condition of any individual who comes or is brought to such clinical establishment.
- Display the Registration Certificate at a prominent place.
- Display the rates charged for each type of service provided and facilities available, for the benefit of patient at a conspicuous place in local language and in English.
- Charge the rates for each type of procedures and services within the range of rates determined and issued by the central government from time to time, in consultation with the state governments.

- Ensure compliance with Standard Treatment Guidelines as may be determined and issued by the central government or state governments, as the case may be, from time to time.
- Maintain and provide electronic medical/health records of every patient, as may be determined and issued by the central government or state government, as the case may be, from time to time.
- Maintain and provide information and statistics in accordance with all other applicable laws that are in force and rules made thereunder.

Registration Procedure

There are two types of registration: Provisional and permanent. Provisional registration is granted on application within 10 days by the Chief Medical officer of the District. But the permanent registration is granted only if the establishment conforms to the notified minimum standards. The application can be made by visiting the office, by sending the application by post or submitting the application on line at clinical establishment portal.

Offences and Penalties

Offence	Penalty in Rupees upto		
	first offence	Second offence	Subsequent offence
Running clinical establishment without registration	50000	200000	500000
Contravention of any other provision of the Act	10000	50000	500000
Whoever knowingly serves in an unregistered clinical establishment	25000		
Minor deficiencies which do not pose imminent danger	10000		

There is no imprisonment provision under the Act.

The Act can be viewed as a tool to regulate the vast and heterogeneous private sector, to improve quality, reduce direct and indirect costs of the care, promote transparency and keep patients informed about the quality of care. Some stakeholders raised reservations against some provisions like cumbersome procedures of obtaining 'No Objection Certificate' from different regulatory agencies for setting up a clinical establishment. There are issues with the clause of emergency patient stabilization. As per the regulation, the clinical establishments will be expected to intervene to stabilize the patients with an emergency medical condition (Heart attack or Appendicitis) before transferring them. Though rule says "the intervention should be made within the staff and facilities available". But the interpretation is always a matter of dispute!

Karnataka Private Medical Establishments Bill 2017: As an Amendments to the Karnataka Private Medical Establishments Act 2007, the Government proposes this bill. The significant features of the bill are: Regulation of costs in private hospitals, prohibiting the hospitals from levying any additional costs from those set by the government, setting up of grievance redressal committee to look into the complaints against private hospitals and penalizing the doctors for negligence. The bill proposes the penalty of imprisonment up to three years and fine of Rs 5 lakh.

Some stakeholders are opposing the bill stating that this would be a 'draconian' law.

[*Source*: https://health.economictimes.indiatimes.com/news/hospitals/40000-private-hospitals-clinics-closed-in-karnataka/61485393 Accessed on 5th November 2017]

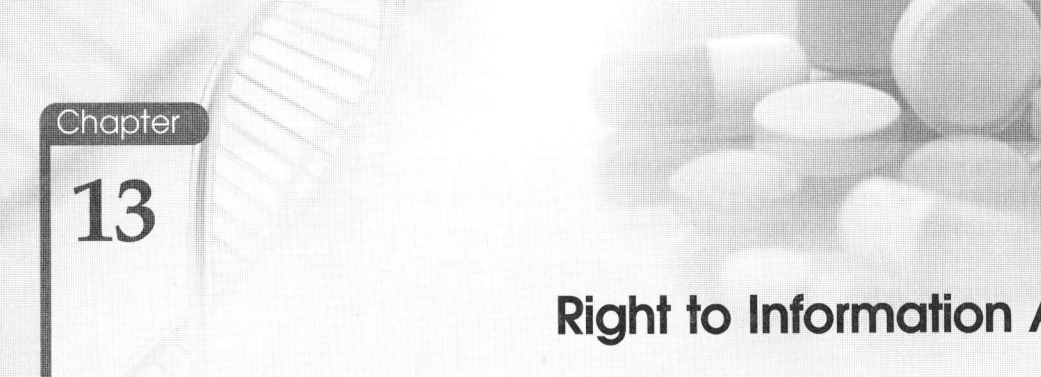

Right to Information Act

"Right to know is like right to live."

— *Anonymous*

After reading this chapter, you should be able to understand and appreciate:
- Importance of right to information
- What information can be obtained
- What information cannot be disclosed
- Procedure for obtaining information
- Administrative procedure for implementing the Act

Everyone of us has several questions in mind. When we all pay several types of tax to the government, what the government does with the revenue it generates. Even the beggar pays tax when he or she purchases commodities. Why do we have such concerns? This is because we find no medicines in hospitals; we find our roads are not repaired for a long time; people die of starvation and so on. Can we question the government? Yes, now we have right to question government through Right to Information (RTI) Act.

The Parliament of India has passed Right to Information Laws, which empower citizens to question the government, inspect their files, take copies of government documents and also to inspect government works. The Right to Information Act 2005 provides effective access to information for citizens of India, which is under the control of the public authorities. It promotes transparency and accountability in the working of every public authority. It extends to the whole of India except the state of Jammu and Kashmir. In order to ensure greater and more effective access to information, it was decided to repeal the Freedom of Information Act, 2002 and

enact another law for providing an effective framework. To achieve this object, the Right to Information Bill was introduced in the Parliament and was passed by the Lok Sabha on 11th May, 2005 and by the Rajya Sabha on 12th May, 2005 and it received the assent on 15th June, 2005. It came on the Statute Book as The Right to Information Act, 2005.

The Department of Personnel and Training, Ministry of Personnel, Public Grievances and Pensions to provide a RTI Portal Gateway to the citizens for quick search of information on the details of first Appellate Authorities, Public Information Officer (PIOs), etc. amongst others, besides access to RTI related information/disclosures published on the web by various Public Authorities under the Government of India as well as the state governments. This is the nodal department for implementing the provision of the Act at central level.

The RTI covers all central, state and local government bodies. Information is the currency that every citizen requires to participate in the life and governance of society. The greater the access of the citizens to information, the greater would be the responsiveness of the governments to the community needs. Though some state governments had enacted laws in one or other form to provide access to public information prior to central RTI Act, enactment of central law brought several innovations at state level.

The provision of the Act is not applicable to the intelligence and security organisations specified in the Second Schedule: Intelligence Bureau, Research and Analysis Wing of the Cabinet Secretariat, Directorate of Revenue Intelligence, Central Economic Intelligence Bureau, Directorate of Enforcement, Narcotics Control Bureau, Aviation Research Centre, Special Frontier Force, Border Security Force, Central Reserve Police Force, Indo-Tibetan Border Police, Central Industrial Security Force, National Security Guards, Assam Rifles, Special Service Bureau, Special Branch (CID), Andaman and Nicobar, Crime Branch-CID-CB, Dadra and Nagar Haveli and Special Branch, Lakshadweep Police. However, information pertaining to the allegations of corruption and human rights violations is not excluded.

There are a few significant rulings or judgements in recent times. These are:

- The Central Information Commission ruled that the Union and State Cabinets are "Public Authorities". They are liable to answer public questions addressed to them under RTI Act.

- The office of the Chief Justice of India and Governors are not covered under the ambit of the Act.

- In a notification issued in 2015, the central government asked the Public Information Officers to issue the documents or records as 'Certified' whenever requested. This makes the documents received to have legal sanctity. Earlier, the Kerala High Court ruled that should bear the certification that they were issued under RTI Act.

- The Central Information Commissioner has said "The citizens have no right to repeat the same or similar or slightly altered information request under the RTI Act for which he already got a response". The CIC said that the filing of repeated RTI applications by an applicant seeking similar information shall be reasonable ground for rejecting the plea for which reply has been given.

The patients do have right to their medical records: The patient's record were refused by the Institute of Human Behaviour and Allied Sciences to a former official of Research and Analysis Wing. The institute cited Section 8(1)(h) of RTI Act which allows an authority to withhold information which would impede an investigation. However, the CIC rejected the contention and ruled that the patients have the right to their medical records under Articles 19 and 21 of the Constitution. The CIC ruled that hospitals, government or private, have a duty to provide information of patients under RTI Act, Consumer Protection Act, the Medical Council Act, World Medical ethics and Constitutional Rights.

Background of Enactment of Right to Information Act

The RTI Act was first successfully enacted by the State Government of Tamil Nadu in 1997. Many other states followed: Goa (1997), Rajasthan (2000), Karnataka (2000) and Delhi (2001). The first movement of RTI in India was initiated by Mazdoor Kisaan Shakti Sangathan (Organization for the Empowerment of Workers and Peasants) (MKSS) in Rajasthan. Initially the movement was just meant for justice in wages, livelihoods and land. The public hearings (Jan Sunwais) organized by MKSS evoked wide response that even led to the organization of National Workshop of Officials and Activists at Lal Bahadur Shastri National Academy of Administration, Mussori, in October 1995. At the same time, the Chief Minister of Rajasthan announced in legislature that it would provide free photocopies of all official documents related to local development works. However, this was never followed up. The struggle continued, spreaded to other places.

The Indian Parliament had enacted the "Freedom of Information Act, 2002" in order to promote transparency and accountability in administration. Later as a part of the National Common Minimum Program of the Government planned to have more meaningful "Freedom of Information Act" which would be more "progressive, participatory and meaningful". Based on this philosophy the new legislation "RTI Act" was enacted repealing "Freedom of Information Act, 2002".

RTI at International Level: At International Level, RTI has been recognized as one of the human rights. In 2004, the free expression rapporteurs of the United Nations (UN), Organizations of American States and Organization of Security and Cooperation in Europe issued a Joint Declaration on International Mechanisms for promoting Freedom of Expression and affirmed that the right to access to information as 'fundamental human right'. The Governments should respect by enacting laws 'based on principles of maximum disclosure'. The African Charter on Human and People's Rights, 1981 states that every individual should have the right to receive information.

Exposing Corruption in Medicine Procurement at Public Sector Unit

Applicants belonging to Anuppur, Madhya Pradesh and Koria district of Chhattisgarh filed RTI applications with the PIO of South Eastern Coal Fields Ltd. (SECL) situated at its head office in Bilaspur during the months of February–April 2006. They sought the following information:

1. Names of all medicines procured by SECL for distribution through its primary health centres and its OPD clinics in the Hasdev coal mines area during the financial year 2005–06. (They cater exclusively to the employees of SECL and their families).
2. Quantity of medicines procured during the same period.
3. Supply price of each item.
4. Copies of all purchase orders issued by SECL for these medicines.

5. Name and contact details of suppliers who bagged the purchase order.

All three applicants received the requested information within the 30 days deadline stipulated in the RTI Act. Armed with these documents, applicants worked for several weeks crosschecking the data along with a team of about 25 committed volunteers. Based on the research it was found out that fictitious companies were shown as suppliers of luxury items in the name of procurement of medical supplies.

Next, the volunteers crosschecked the rates at which the medicines had been supplied only to find that the retail outlets sold the same items a lot cheaper.

These details were published in local magazine popular in the coal mining belt of Madhya Pradesh and Chhattisgarh. Thereafter, the Vigilance unit instituted a formal investigation and action against the concerned officials was initiated.

(*Source:* Price water house Coopers' (PwC) Understanding the "Key Issues and Constraints" in implementing the RTI Act June 2009.)

Right to Information and Obligations of Public Authorities

1. Every public authority needs to:
   a. Maintain all its records duly catalogued and indexed in a manner and the form which facilitates the right to information and ensure that all records (that are appropriate to be computerised) are computerised and connected through a network all over the country to facilitate their access;
   b. Publish within one hundred and twenty days from the enactment of this Act:
      i. The particulars of its organisation, functions and duties;
      ii. The powers and duties of its officers and employees;
      iii. The procedure followed in the decision-making process, including channels of supervision and accountability;

iv. The norms set by it for the discharge of its functions;

v. The rules, regulations, instructions, manuals and records, held by it or under its control or used by its employees for discharging its functions;

vi. A statement of the categories of documents that are held by it or under its control;

vii. The particulars of any arrangement that exists for consultation with, or representation by, the members of the public in relation to the formulation of its policy or implementation thereof;

viii. A statement of the boards, councils, committees and other bodies consisting of two or more persons constituted as its part or for the purpose of its advice, and as to whether meetings of those boards, councils, committees and other bodies are open to the public, or the minutes of such meetings are accessible for public;

ix. A directory of its officers and employees;

x. The monthly remuneration received by each of its officers and employees, including the system of compensation as provided in its regulations;

xi. The budget allocated to each of its agency, indicating the particulars of all plans, proposed expenditures and reports on disbursements made;

xii. The manner of execution of subsidy programmes, including the amounts allocated and the details of beneficiaries of such programmes;

xiii. Particulars of recipients of concessions, permits or authorisations granted by it;

xiv. Details in respect of the information, available to or held by it, reduced in an electronic form;

xv. The particulars of facilities available to citizens for obtaining information, including the working hours of a library or reading room, if maintained for public use;

xvi. The names, designations and other particulars of the Public Information Officers;

xvii. Such other information as may be prescribed and thereafter update these publications every year.

c. Publish all relevant facts while formulating important policies or announcing the decisions which affect public;

d. Provide reasons for its administrative or quasi-judicial decisions to affected persons.

2. The public authority should take steps to provide as much information suo motu to the public at regular intervals through various means of communications, including internet, so that the public have minimum resort to the use of this Act to obtain information.

3. Every information should be disseminated widely and in such form and manner which is easily accessible to the public.

4. All materials should be disseminated in cost effective manner and in local language. The information should be accessible to the Central Public Information Officer or State Public Information Officer as far as possible in electronic format.

5. Every public authority has to designate as many officers as the Central Public Information Officers or State Public Information Officers in all administrative units or offices. He is also responsible to designate as a Central Assistant Public Information Officer or a State Assistant Public Information Officer at each sub-divisional level or other sub-district level. These officers would receive the RTI application or appeal and forward them to the respective Public Information Officer. The Central Public Information Officer or State Public Information Officer should deal with requests from persons seeking

information and render reasonable assistance to the persons seeking such information. They may seek the assistance of any other officer necessary for the proper discharge of duties. Any officer, whose assistance has been sought, has to render all assistance to the Central Public Information Officer or State Public Information Officer.

6. **Submitting Application for Information:** The person desiring to seek information has to apply in writing or through electronic means to the Central Public Information Officer (or, Central Assistant Public Information Officer) or State Public Information Officer (or, State Assistant Public Information Officer) with prescribed fees. And specifying the details of information sought.

When the request cannot be made in writing, the Central Public Information Officer or State Public Information Officer should render all reasonable assistance to the person making the request orally to reduce the same in writing.

No reason or the other details of the person is to be specified for seeking information except the contact details.

When the information sought is available or dealt with by other public authority, the application is to be transferred to the authority concerned within five days of receipt of application under intimation to the applicant seeking information.

7. **Processing of RTI Applications:** On receipt of application requesting for information, Central Public Information Officer or State Public Information Officer, as expeditiously as possible, and in any case within thirty days of the receipt of the request, either provide the information on payment of prescribed fee or reject the request. When the information sought for concerns the life or liberty of a person, the same has to be provided within forty-eight hours of the receipt of the request. When the officers fail to submit the request within 30 days, it is deemed that they have refused to give the information.

When further fees are required to be paid by the person requested for information, the same is to be intimated giving the details of calculation for the fees charged with a request to remit the amount. The person concerned is also informed of the appellate authority and other details for readdress against the decision of the officer on fees.

Sensorily disable persons should be provided special assistance to access information. The applicants are charged for providing information in print or electronic form. However, the persons below the poverty line are not to be charged. If the information is not provided within the time period of 30 days, then the information provided later would be free of charge.

When the application is rejected, the Central or State Public Information Officer should inform the applicant with: Reasons for rejection, the period within which appeal may be preferred, and the appellate authority.

8. **Exemption from Disclosure (information not to provided):** The following information need not be provided:

- Information, disclosure of which would prejudicially affect the sovereignty and integrity of India, the security, strategic, scientific or economic interests of the State, relation with foreign State or lead to incitement of an offence;

- Information which has been expressly forbidden to be published by any court of law or tribunal or the disclosure of which may constitute contempt of court;

- Information, the disclosure of which would cause a breach of privilege of Parliament or the State Legislature;

- Information available to a person in his fiduciary relationship, unless the competent authority is satisfied that the larger public interest warrants the disclosure of such information;

- Information received in confidence from foreign government;

- Information, the disclosure of which would endanger the life or physical safety of any person or identify the source of information or assistance given in confidence for law enforcement or security purposes;

- Information which would impede the process of investigation or apprehension or prosecution of offenders;
- Cabinet papers including records of deliberations of the Council of Ministers, Secretaries and other officers;
- Personal information: The disclosure of which has no relationship to any public activity or interest, or which would cause unwarranted invasion of the privacy of the individual. The information which cannot be denied to the Parliament or Assembly of Legislators cannot be denied to persons. Notwithstanding anything under Official Secrets Act, the public authority may allow access to information, if public interest in disclosure outweighs the harm to the protected interests. The information relating to any occurrence, event or matter which has taken place, occurred or happened twenty years before the date on which any request is made should be provided.
- Request for information is rejected if it involves an infringement of copyright subsisting in a person other than the State.

Clinical Trial Related Information are Exempted from RTI: With a view to protect patient-related information and preserve exclusive intellectual property rights of the pharmaceutical companies, the Central Information Commission (CIC) passed a decision acknowledging exemption from disclosure of information on clinical trials under RTI Act.

A RTI application was filed seeking information on post-licensure HPV Vaccination and usage of certain drugs: Gardasil and Cervatrix, in age group outside the age group on whom they were tested. The applicants' intention was to verify whether the licensing authorities had verified the data prior to approving the same. It was contended by them that for the transparency and accountability purposes in biomedical research, disclosure of information was essential.

CIC while passing its decision said that transparency is essential in biomedical research. However, such information may not be divulged in the public domain as it includes several substantial strategic, scientific data along with patient-related information.

The decision states "The problem would persist wherein data are interlinked and segregation is not possible making it a contesting issue for disclosure of information. However, with regard to clinical trials, patient related data and trade secrets and intellectual property of the pharmaceutical companies may not be disclosed."

(*Source:* Pharmabiz.com dated June 18, 2011.)

9. **Partial Information to be provided:** When request for information is rejected as it is exempted from disclosure, access may be provided to that part of the record which does not contain any information which is exempt from disclosure. However, when access is granted to part of the record, the Central or State Public Information Officer has to inform the applicant with the following details: Only part of the request is provided, reason for such decision, the name and designation of person giving the decision, details of fees and the applicant's right to get review the decision with senior officer or with Central or State Information Commission.

10. **Information from third party:** When the information sought is related to/has been supplied by third party who treats the information as confidential, Central or State Public Information Officer issues notice to the third party of its intention of disclosure and invite the third party to make a submission in writing or orally, regarding whether the information should be disclosed. The third party's reply should be taken into consideration before

providing the information. Except in the case of trade or commercial secrets protected by law, disclosure may be allowed if the public interest in disclosure outweighs in importance any possible harm or injury to the interests of such third party.

On receipt of notice from the Central or State Public Information Officer, the third party may make representation, if any, within 10 days of receiving notice. The officer has to make a decision on disclosure within 40 days of the receiving request for information. The third party is given an opportunity to appeal against the decision on disclosure.

Central Information Commission (CIC)

Composition: The central government is empowered to appoint Central Information Commission with the following members to exercise powers and to perform functions as assigned under the Act:

1. The Chief Information Commissioner; and
2. Such number of Central Information Commissioners, not exceeding ten.

The Chief Information Commissioner and Information Commissioners are appointed by the President on the recommendation of a committee consisting of—the Prime Minister, who shall be the Chairperson of the committee; the Leader of Opposition in the Lok Sabha; and a Union Cabinet Minister to be nominated by the Prime Minister. Where the Leader of Opposition in the House of the People has not been recognised, the Leader of the single largest group in opposition of the government in the House of the People shall be deemed to be the Leader of Opposition.

The general superintendence, direction and management of the affairs of the Central Information Commission vest in the Chief Information Commissioner who is assisted by the Information Commissioners. The Head Office of the Central Information Commission is located at Delhi.

- **Eligibility:** The Chief Information Commissioner and Information Commissioners should be persons of eminence in public life with wide knowledge and experience in law, science and technology, social service, management, journalism, mass media or administration and governance. They should not be the Member of Parliament or Member of the Legislature of any State or Union territory, as the case may be, or hold any other office of profit or connected with any political party or carrying on any business or pursuing any profession.

- **Office:** The Chief Information Commissioner holds office for a term of five years from the date on which he enters upon his office or 65 years of age whichever is earlier. He or she is not eligible for reappointment. Every Information Commissioner too holds office for a term of five years or till he attains the age of sixty-five years, whichever is earlier, and is not be eligible for reappointment. Every Information Commissioner is eligible after vacating office for appointment as the Chief Information Commissioner. In cases, where Information Commissioner is appointed as Chief Information Commissioner, the total period should not exceed five years. They may resign from the office by writing the President. The salary and allowances of Chief Information Commissioner and Commissioners are the same as that are paid to the Chief Election Commissioner and Election Commissioners respectively. The central government provides the necessary officers and other staff for efficient functioning of Central Information Commission.

- **Removal from office:** The Chief Information Commissioner or any Information Commissioner can be removed from office only by order of the President on the ground of proved misbehaviour or incapacity after obtaining the enquiry report of the Supreme Court, on a reference made to it by the President. The President may suspend them from office, and if deem necessary prohibit also from attending the office during inquiry, the Chief Information Commissioner or Information Commissioner in respect of whom a reference has been made to the Supreme Court. The President may order removal from office, if the Chief Information Commissioner or Information Commissioner is adjudged an insolvent; or: has been convicted of an offence which, in the opinion of the President, involves moral turpitude; or engages during his term of office in any paid employment outside the duties of his office; or is, in the opinion of the President, unfit to continue in office by reason of infirmity of mind or body; or has acquired such financial or other interest as is likely to affect prejudicially his functions as the Chief Information Commissioner or Information Commissioner.

Losing Right to Seek Information

The State Information Commission of Punjab forfeited the Rights of Mr. Amarjit Singh Dhamotia to seek information from the local civic body under RTI Act. The commission observed that Mr. Dhamotia has been seeking 'inane and voluminous information and has already filed more than 500 applications". This has drastically hampered the routine work of civic corporations as many of its officers are busy all the day securing information sought by him. This act of Mr. Dhamotia has been viewed as blatant misuse of RTI Act. The Information Commissioner observing his application as "misuse of the RTI Act with an unsavory motive" directed the public authority to ignore Mr. Dhamotia's application in future.

[Appeal Case Nos. 217, 218, 219 and 220 of 2017 and order of 05 April 2017.]

State Information Commission (SIC)

- **Constitution:** Every state government constitutes a body known as (name of the state) Information Commission consisting of the State Chief Information Commissioner, and such number of State Information Commissioners, not exceeding ten. The State Chief Information Commissioner and the State Information Commissioners are appointed by the Governor on the recommendation of a committee consisting of the Chief Minister, who shall

be the Chairperson of the committee; the Leader of Opposition in the Legislative Assembly; and a Cabinet Minister nominated by the Chief Minister. Where the Leader of Opposition in the Legislative Assembly has not been recognised, the Leader of the single largest group in opposition of the Government in the Legislative Assembly is deemed to be the Leader of Opposition. *The Tamil Nadu Information Commission consists of one State Chief Information Commissioner and six Information Commissioners.*

The general superintendence, direction and management of the affairs of the State Information Commission vest on the State Chief Information Commissioner who is assisted by the State Information Commissioners. The headquarters of the State Information Commission is established in a place in the state as the state government decides. *The headquarter of Tamil Nadu Information Commission is located at No. 2 Sir Theagaraya Salai, Near Aalai Amman Koil, Teynampet, Chennai - 600018.*

- **Eligibility:** The State Chief Information Commissioner and the State Information Commissioners should be persons of eminence in public life with wide knowledge and experience in law, science and technology, social service, management, journalism, mass media or administration and governance. They should not be the Member of Parliament or Member of the Legislature of any State or Union territory, or hold any other office of profit or connected with any political party or carrying on any business or pursuing any profession.

- **Office:** The State Chief Information Commissioner holds office for a term of five years or 65 years of age whichever is earlier. He or she is not eligible for reappointment. Every Information Commissioner too holds office for a term of five years or till he attains the age of sixty-five years, whichever is earlier, and is not be eligible for reappointment. Every Information Commissioner is eligible after vacating office for appointment as the State Chief Information Commissioner.

In case, where Information Commissioner is appointed as State Chief Information Commissioner, the total period should not exceed five years. They may resign from the office by writing the Governor. The salary and allowances of State Chief Information Commissioner is on par with that of Election Commissioner and the salary and allowances of Information Commissioners would be on par with the Chief Secretary of the State. The state government provides the necessary officers and other staff for efficient functioning of State Information Commission.

- **Removal from office:** The Chief Information Commissioner or any Information Commissioner can be removed from office only by the order of the Governor on the ground of proved misbehaviour or incapacity after obtaining the enquiry report of the Supreme Court, on a reference made to it by the Governor. The Governor may suspend them from office, and if deem necessary prohibit also from attending the office during inquiry, the State Chief Information Commissioner or Information Commissioner in respect of whom a reference has been made to the Supreme Court. The Governor may order removal from office, if the Chief Information Commissioner or Information Commissioner is adjudged an insolvent; or has been convicted of an offence which, in the opinion of the Governor, involves moral turpitude; or engages during his term of office in any paid employment outside the duties of his office; or is in the opinion of the Governor, unfit to continue in office by reason of infirmity of mind or body; or has acquired such financial or other interest as is likely to affect prejudicially his functions as the State Chief Information Commissioner or Information Commissioner.

Power and Functions of Information Commission

The Central or State Information Commission has the duty to receive and enquire into the complaint from any person:

- Who has been unable to submit a request for information either for reasons that the officers are not appointed or his/her application is not accepted for forwarding to the Central Public Information Officer or State Public Information Officer as applicable;
- Who has been refused access to any information;
- Who has not been given the response within the time limit;
- Who has been required to pay an unreasonable amount as fees;
- Who believes that the given information is incomplete, misleading or false.

The information commission has the same powers as are vested in a civil court while trying a suit under the Code of Civil Procedure, 1908, in respect of the following matters:

- Summoning and enforcing the attendance of persons and compel them to give oral or written evidence on oath and to produce the documents or things;
- Requiring the discovery and inspection of documents;
- Receiving evidence on affidavit;
- Requisitioning any public record or copies thereof from any court or office; and
- Issuing summons for examination of witnesses or documents.

During enquiry, the Commission examines any record to which this Act applies which is under the control of the public authority, and no such record may be withheld from it on any ground.

The Central Information Commission or State Information Commission has the power to:

- Require the public authority to take any such step as may be necessary to secure compliance with the provisions of this Act: Providing access to information, if so requested, in a particular form; by appointing a Central Public Information Officer or State Public Information Officer; by publishing certain information or categories of information; by making necessary changes to its practices in relation to the maintenance, management and destruction of records; and by enhancing the provision of training on the right to information for its officials.

- Require the public authority to compensate the complainant for any loss or other detriment suffered;
- Impose any of the penalties provided under this Act;
- Reject the application.

Appeal: The person, who does not receive the decision within the time limit, is aggrieved by the decision of Central or State Public Information Officer may prefer appeal within 30 days of the order to the senior officer to the rank of Central or State Public Information Officer respectively. Such officer may admit the appeal even after the expiry of 30 days if he/she believes that appellant was prevented from filing an appeal on time.

A second appeal against the decision can be filed within ninety days from the date on which the decision should have been made or

RTI Authorities and Fees Structure (Medicine Regulation)

Parameters	Central information commission	Tamil Nadu state information commission
Public information officers (CDSCO)	On Technical Matter: Mr. Jayant Kumar Asst. Drugs Controller (India), Phone : 23216367 - Ext - 216/208	Deputy Director of Drugs Control Office of the Director of Drugs Control, No.359, Anna Salai, Teynampet, Chennai-6
Appellate Authorities (CDSCO)	Dr. G. N. Singh, Drugs Controller General (I) Phones: 91-11-23236965 (D) Fax: 91-11-23236973.	Director of Drugs Control Office of the Director of Drugs Control, No.359, Anna Salai, Teynampet, Chennai-6
Public Information Officers (Pharmacy Council of India)	Smt. Archna Mudgal, Registrar-cum-SecretaryPharmacy Council of India Combined Councils' Building, Kotla Road, Aiwan-E-Ghalib Marg, New Delhi - 110 002	–
Appellate Authorities (Pharmacy Council of India)	Prof. M.D.Karvekar# 1449, Sector 7, 4th Main1st Cross, H.S.R. Lay Out Bangalore - 560 102 (Karnataka)	–
Application Fees:	₹ 10/- in the form of demand draft/ bankers' cheque or postal order or by cash. No fees will be charged from people living below the poverty line. (www.cdsco.nic.in accessed on 25 September 2011)	₹ 10/- can be paid as demand draft/bankers' cheque or postal money order or paid to government treasury or by fixing non-judicial court stamp or paid in cash. No fees will be charged from people living below the poverty line.
Other Fees	• ₹ 2/- per page of A4/A3 sizes. • Actual charges for larger paper. • Actual cost for samples or models. • For inspection, ₹ 5/- per hour or part thereof after the first hour which is free. • ₹ 50/- per floppy. • Actual cost of books or ₹ 2/- per page of photocopy for extracts from publication. No fees will be charged from people living below the poverty line. (www.cdsco.nic.in accessed on 25 September 2011)	• ₹ 2/- per page of A4/A3 sizes. • Actual charges for larger paper. • Actual cost for samples or models. • For inspection, ₹ 5/- per hour or part thereof after the first hour which is free. • ₹ 50/- per floppy. • Actual cost of books and other printed matter. No fees will be charged from people living below the poverty line.

Time limit for disposing RTI application

Situation	Time limit for disposing off applications
1 Supply of information in normal course	30 days
2 Supply of information if it concerns the life or liberty of a person.	48 hours
3 Supply of information if the application is received through APIO	05 days shall be added to the time period indicated at Sr. No. 1 and 2.
4 Supply of information if application/request is received after transfer from another public authority: (a) In normal course (b) In case the information concerns the life or liberty of a person.	(a) Within 30 days of the receipt of the application by the concerned public authority. (b) Within 48 hours of receipt of the application by the concerned public authority
5 Supply of information by organizations specified in the Second Schedule: (a) If information relates to allegations of violation of human rights. (b) In case information relates to allegations of corruption.	(a) 45 days from the receipt of application. (b) Within 30 days of the receipt of application.
6 Supply of information if it relates to third party and the third party has treated it as confidential.	Should be provided after following the procedure given in para 23 to 28 of this part of the document.
7 Supply of information where the applicant is asked to pay additional fee.	The period intervening between informing the applicant about additional fee and the payment of fee by the applicant shall be excluded for calculating the period reply.

was actually received, with the Central Information Commission or the State Information Commission. Regarding disclosure of information of the third party, third party may file appeal within thirty days from the date of the order.

An appeal has to be disposed off within thirty days of the receipt of the appeal or within such extended period not exceeding a total of forty-five days from the date of filing. The decision of the Central Information Commission or State Information Commission is binding.

Penalty: Where the Central Information Commission or the State Information Commission, deciding any complaint or appeal is of the opinion that the Central Public Information Officer or the State Public Information Officer has, without any reasonable cause, refused to receive an application for information or has not furnished information within the time specified or malafidely denied the request for information or knowingly given incorrect, incomplete or misleading information or destroyed information which was the subject of the request or obstructed in any manner in furnishing the information, it may impose a penalty of two hundred and fifty rupees each day till application is received or information is furnished, so however, the total amount of such penalty shall not exceed twenty-five thousand rupees.

Pharmaceutical Ethics

"Ethics is not definable, is not implementable, because it is not conscious, it involves not only our thinking, but also our feeling."

— *Valdemar W Setzer*

After reading this chapter, you should be able to understand and appreciate:
- The value of ethics and professional behavior of pharmacists
- Procedure to be followed while the pharmacists:
  1. Handling with prescriptions and medicines
  2. Dealing with medical profession, public, apprentice pharmacists, and fellow professionals
- New Code of Ethics as described under Pharmacy Practice Regulation
- Basis of International Scenario on Pharmaceutical Ethics.

In the society, every individual's conduct is subject to a lot of scrutiny by others. In this context, one talks about a code of conduct and a code of ethics. Such a code is all about standard of public behavior, dealing with others, about duties and responsibilities, about work ethics, about what is acceptable or unacceptable, and about a set of dos and don'ts, etc. All these elements in the code of conduct are dictated and shaped by the prevalent value system(s), social and societal expectations and of course the ground realities.

Ethical behavior helps us to decide the tricky situation we face: What is right and what is wrong, what is good and what is bad, what is fair and what is unfair. Ethics is a requirement for human life. Without it, our action would be random and aimless. The codes of ethics do not provide ready solutions to all situations but such codes do facilitate in taking appropriate decisions. The code of professional ethics lays down the standards of integrity, professionalism and confidentiality which all members of the profession shall be bound to respect in their work. The ethical behavior of a professional is guided by two major parameters: Systemic knowledge of the profession and skills to perform, and performance influenced by individual and situational variables. Truly, a professional may fail but ethical behavior never fails.

Ethics is considered as a science of morality. Morality explains what is right and what is wrong. Ethics had evolved over a period of time and is greatly influenced by the political, geographical, religious and cultural forces. It is also dependent on peoples' education and reasoning power. Ethics and Law are independent but overlays with each other. Ethics and Integrity probably always go together and both are non-negotiable always. What is ethical need not necessarily be a law and what is law need not be ethical.

Unfortunately, everyday we unearth the open secret that all 'codes' and rules and regulation of all kinds in today's India are violated than followed. Those following and complying with codes/rules are mere minorities in the societies. What is necessary is the determined and persistence launch of campaign to sensitize the professionals on their code of conduct and need of compliance. Strict adherence to code of ethics would make the professionals feel proud of their actions. In this chapter the code of ethics as adopted by the Pharmacy Council of India is narrated.

CODE OF PHARMACEUTICAL ETHICS

General Introduction

The profession of pharmacy is noble in its ideals and pious in its character. Apart from being a career for earning livelihood, it has inherent in it the attitude of service and sacrifice in the interests of the suffering humanity. In handling, selling, distributing, compounding and dispensing medical substances including poisons and potent drugs a pharmacist is, in collaboration with medical men and others, charged with the onerous responsibility of safeguarding the health of people, as such he has to uphold the interests of his patrons above all things. The lofty ideals set up by Charaka, the ancient Philosopher Physician and Pharmacist in his erunciation : "Even if your own life be in danger you should not betray or neglect the interests of your patients" should be fondly cherished by all Pharmacist. Government restricts the practice of Pharmacy to those who qualify under regulatory requirements and grant them privileges necessarily denied to others. In return Government expects the Pharmacist to recognise his responsibilities and to fulfill his professional obligations honorably and with due regard for the well being of Society.

Standards of professional conduct for pharmacy are necessary in the public interest to ensure an efficient pharmaceutical service. Every pharmacist should not only be willing to play his part in giving such a service but should also avoid any act or omission which would prejudice the giving of the services or impair confidence in any respect for pharmacists as a body. The nature of pharmaceutical practice is such that its demands may be beyond the capacity of the individual to carry out as quickly or as efficiently as the needs of the public. There should, therefore at all times, be a readiness to assist colleagues with information or advice. A Pharmacist must, above all, be a good citizen and must uphold and defend the laws of the state and the Nation.

Pharmacists in Relation to his Job (Scope of Pharmaceutical Services)

When premises are registered under statutory requirements and opened as a pharmacy, a reasonably comprehensive pharmaceutical service should be provided. This involves the supply of commonly required medicines of this nature without undue delay. It also involves willingness to furnish emergency supplies at all times.

The condition in a pharmacy should be such as to preclude avoidable risk or error or of accidental contamination in the preparation, dispensing and supply of medicines.

The appearance of the premises should reflect the professional character of the pharmacy. It should be clear to the public that the practice of pharmacy is carried out in the establishment. Signs, notices, descriptions, wording on business, stationary and related indications, should be restrained in size, design and terms. Descriptions which denote or imply pharmaceutical qualifications should be limited to those of which the use is restricted by law and should not draw invidious distinction between pharmacists. A notice stating that dispensing under Employees State Insurance Scheme (ESIS) or any such other schemes sponsored by government is carried out may be exhibited at the premises. In every pharmacy there should be a pharmacist in personal control of the pharmacy who will be regarded as primarily responsible for the observance of proper standards of conduct in connection with it. Any obstruction of the pharmacist in the execution of his duty by the owner will be regarded as a failure on the part of the owner to observe the standards in question.

Handling of Prescriptions

When a prescription is presented for dispensing, it should be received by a pharmacist without any discussion or comment over it regarding the merits and demerits of its therapeutic efficiency. The Pharmacist should not show any physiognomic expression of alarm or astonishment upon the receipt of a prescription; as such things may cause anxiety in patients or their agents and may even shake their faith in their physician. Any question on a prescription should be answered with every caution and care; it should neither offend a patron nor should it disclose any information, which might have been intentionally, withheld from him.

It is not within the privilege of a Pharmacist to add, omit or substitute any ingredient or alter the composition of a prescription without the consent of the prescriber, unless the change is emergent or is demanded purely by the technique of the pharmaceutical art and does not cause any alteration in the therapeutic action of the recipe. In case of any obvious error in it due to any ommission, incompatibility or overdosage, the prescription should be referred back to the prescriber for correction or approval of the change suggested. While such an act is imperative in the best interest of the patient, in no case should it be done in a manner, which may jeopardize the reputation of the prescriber concerned.

In matter of refilling prescriptions a pharmacist should solely be guided by the instructions of the prescriber and he should advise patients to use medicines or remedies strictly in accordance with the intention of the physician as noted on the prescription.

Handling of Drugs

All possible care should be taken to dispense a prescription correctly by weighing and measuring all ingredients in correct proportions by the help of scale and measures: visual estimations must be avoided. Further, a Pharmacist should always use drugs and medicinal preparations of standard quality available. He should never fill his prescriptions with spurious, sub-standard and unethical preparations.

A pharmacist should be very judicious in dealing with drugs and medicinal preparations known to be judicious or to be used for addiction or any other abusive purposes.

Such drugs and preparations should not be supplied to anyone if there is reason to suppose that it is required for such purpose.

Apprentice Pharmacists

While in-charge of a dispensary, drugstore or hospital pharmacy where apprentice pharmacists are admitted for practical training, a pharmacist should see that the trainees are given full facilities for their work so that on the completion of their training they have acquired sufficient technique and skill to make themselves dependable pharmacists. No certificate or credentials should be granted unless the above criterion is attained and the recipient has proved himself worthy of the same.

Pharmacists in Relation to his Trade Price Structure

Prices charged from customers should be fair and in keeping with the quality and quantity of commodity supplied and the labour and skill required in making it ready for use, so as to ensure an adequate remuneration to the pharmacist taking into consideration his knowledge, skill, the time consumed and the great responsibility involved, but at the same time without unduly taxing the purchaser.

Fair Trade Practices

No attempt should be made to capture the business of a contemporary by cut-throat competition, that is, by offering any sort of prizes or gifts or any kind of allurement to patronizers or by knowingly charging lower prices for medical commodities than those charged by fellow pharmacist if they reasonable. In case any order or prescription genuinely intended to be served by some dispensary is brought by mistake to another, the latter should refuse to accept it and should direct the customer to the right place. Labels, trademarks and other signs and symbols of contemporaries should not be imitated or copied.

Purchase of Drugs

Drugs should always be purchased from genuine and reputable sources and a pharmacist should always be on his guard not to aid or abet, directly or indirectly the manufacture, possession, distribution and sale of spurious or sub-standard drugs.

Hawking of Drugs

Hawking of drugs and medicinal should not be encouraged nor should any attempt be made to solicit orders for such substances from door to door. 'Self-service' method of operating pharmacies and drug-stores should not be used as this practice may lead to the distribution of therapeutic substances without an expert supervision and thus would encourage self-medication, which is highly undesirable.

Advertising and Displays

No display material either on the premises, in the press or elsewhere should be used by a pharmacist in connection with the sale to the public of medicines or medical appliances which is undignified in style or which contains:

(a) Any wording design or illustration reflecting unfavourably on pharmacists collectivity or upon any group or individual.

(b) A disparaging reference, direct or by implication to other suppliers.

(c) Misleading, or exaggerated statements or claims.

(d) The word "Cure" in reference to an ailment or symptoms of ill-health.

(e) A guarantee of therapeutic efficacy.

(f) An appeal to fear.

(g) An offer to refund money paid.

(h) A prize, competition or similar scheme.

(i) Any reference to a medical practitioner or a hospital or the use of the terms "Doctor" or "Dr." or "Nurse" in connection with the name of the preparation not already established.

(j) A reference to sexual weakness, premature ageing or loss of virility.

(k) A reference to complaints of sexual nature in terms which lack the reticence proper to the subject.

No article or preparation advertised to the public by means of display material of a kind mentioned above should be exhibited in a pharmacy if it is known or could reasonably be known that the article or preparation is so advertised.

Contraceptive preparations and appliances or their illustrations should not be exhibited except a notice approved by regulations or bearing the words "Family Planning Requisites". Under no circumstances should lustful obscene and indecent publications of any kind or description be sold or distributed, as this practice is highly detrimental to the moral welfare of the Nation.

Pharmacists in Relation to Medical Profession Limitation of Professional Activity

Whereas it is expected that medical practitioners in general would not take to the practice of pharmacy by owing drug stores, as this ultimately leads to coded prescriptions and monopolistic practices detrimental to the pharmaceutical profession and also to the interest of patients, it should be made a general rule that pharmacists under no circumstances take to medical practice, that is to diagnosing diseases and prescribing remedies therefore even if requested by patrons to do so. In cases of accidents and emergencies a pharmacist may, however, render First Aid to the victim.

No pharmacist should recommend particular medical practitioner unless specifically asked to do so.

Clandestine Arrangements

No pharmacist should enter into any secret arrangements or contract with a physician to offer him any commission or any advantage of any description in return for his favour of patronage by recommending his dispensary or drugstore or even himself to patients.

Liaison with Public

Being a liaison between medical profession and people, a pharmacist should always keep himself abreast with the modern developments in pharmacy and other allied sciences by regularly reading books, journals, magazines and other periodicals, so that on the one hand, he may be in a position to advise the physician on pharmaceutical matters like those of colours, flavours, vehicles and newer forms of administration of medicines, on the other hand, he may be able to educate the people for maintaining healthy and sanitary conditions of living.

Thus a pharmacist can contribute his share in the nation-building activities of the country. A pharmacist should at all times endeavour to promote knowledge and contribute his quota in the advancement of learning.

A pharmacist should never disclose any information which he has acquired during his professional activities to any third party or person unless requires by law to do so. He should never betray the confidence which his patrons repose in him or which he has won by virtue of his eminent character and conduct.

Pharmacist in Relation to his Profession
Professional Vigilance

It is not only sufficient for a pharmacist to be law-abiding and to deter from doing things derogatory to society and his profession, but is also his duty to make others fulfil the provisions of the pharmaceutical and other laws and regulations. He should not be afraid of bringing or causing a miscreant to be brought to book, may be a member of his own profession. Whereas it is obligatory for a pharmacist to extend help and cooperation to a fellow member in his legitimate needs, scientific, technical or otherwise, he is to be, at the same time, vigilant to weed the undesirable out of the profession and thus help to maintain its fair name and traditions.

Law-abiding Citizens

A pharmacist engaged in profession has to be an enlightened citizen endowed with a fair knowledge of the land and he should strive to countenance and defend them. He should be particularly conversant with the enactments pertaining to food, drug, pharmacy, health, sanitation and the like and endeavour to abide by them in every phase of his life. A pharmacist is a unit whole and his life cannot be divided into compartments.

Relationship with Professional Organisations

In order to inculcate a corporate life in his own professional colleagues, a pharmacist should join and advance the cause of all such organisations, the aims and objects of which are conducive to scientific moral and cultural well-being of pharmacists and at the same time are in no way contrary to the code of pharmaceutical ethics.

Decorum and Propriety

A pharmacist should always refrain from doing all such acts and deeds which are not in consonance with the decorum and propriety of pharmaceutical profession or which are likely to bring discredit or upgrade to the profession or to himself.

Code of Pharmacy Ethics as Described in Pharmacy Practice Regulation

- Every person at the time of registration has to submit the signed declaration form (given at the end).
- The person who has registered is entitled to practice as 'Registered Pharmacist'; engage in the practice of profession of pharmacy; and recover the dues or fees as entitled.
- The name of the owner of the pharmacy business should be displayed at or near the main entrance. The name of the registered pharmacist along with registration number, qualification and photo need to be displayed adjacent to dispensing area. The registered pharmacist needs to comply with the dress code of wearing clean white over coat or apron with a badge displaying the name and registration number.
- The owner of the pharmacy business needs to appoint registered pharmacist. The appointment gets revoked automatically if the appointed person ceases to become registered pharmacist.
- The registered person should be an upright person instructed in the art of medicine. He/she should keep himself/herself pure in character, diligent in caring the sick, should be modest, sober,

patient, prompt in discharging duties without anxiety; conducting himself with propriety in his business and in all action of life. The registered pharmacist should uphold the dignity and honour of the profession.

- The registered pharmacist should not aid or abet or commit any act relating to advertisement, rebates and commission, secret remedies and human rights which may be construed as unethical.

Declaration

1. I solemnly pledge myself to consecrate my life to service of humanity.
2. Even under threat, I will not use my pharmacy knowledge contrary to the laws of Humanity.
3. I will maintain the utmost respect for human life from the time of conception.
4. I will not permit considerations of religion, nationality, race, party politics or social standing to intervene between my duty and my patient.
5. I will practice my profession with conscience and dignity.
6. The health of my patient will be my first consideration.
7. I will respect the secrets which are confined in me.
8. I will give to my teachers the respect and gratitude which is their due.
9. I will maintain by all means in my power, the honour and noble traditions of pharmacy profession.
10. I will treat my colleagues with all respect and dignity.
11. I shall abide by the code of ethics as laid down by the Pharmacy Council of India.

I certify that I have read and agree to abide by the declarations made above.

I make these promises solemnly, freely and upon my honour.

International Scenario

- The first code of ethics of American Pharmaceutical Association was published in 1852.
- The first code of ethics of Royal Pharmaceutical Society of United Kingdom was published in 1944.
- The International Pharmaceutical Federation (FIP) issued a code of ethics for pharmacy in 1997. Then it was revised in 2004. The General Principles of FIP's Guidelines (http://www.fip.org) accessed on 14 August 2011:

1. The Association of Pharmacists of the country should produce a code of ethics setting up their professional obligations and to take steps to ensure that the pharmacists comply with code of ethics.
2. The obligations of the pharmacists should include:
   - To act with fairness and equity in the allocation of any health resources made available to them.
   - To ensure that their priorities are the safety, well being and best interests of those to whom they provide professional services and that they act at all times with integrity in their dealings with them.
   - To collaborate with other health professionals to ensure that the best possible quality of healthcare is provided both to individuals and the community at large.
   - To respect the rights of individual patients to participate in decisions about their treatment with medicinal products and to encourage them to do so.
   - To recognise and respect the cultural differences, beliefs and values of patients, particularly as they may affect a patient's attitude to suggested treatment.
   - To respect and protect the confidentiality of information acquired in the course of providing professional services and ensure that information about an individual is not disclosed to others except with the informed consent of that individual or in specified exceptional circumstances.

- To act in accordance with professional standards and scientific principles.
- To act with honesty and integrity in their relationships with other health professionals, including pharmacist colleagues, and not engage in any behaviour or activity likely to bring the profession into disrepute or undermine public confidence in the profession.
- To ensure that they keep their knowledge and professional skills up-to-date through continuing professional development.
- To comply with legislation and accepted codes and standards of practice in the provision of all professional services and pharmaceutical products and ensure the integrity of the supply chain for medicines by purchasing only from reputable sources.
- To ensure that members of support staff to whom tasks are delegated have the competencies necessary for the efficient and effective undertaking of these tasks.
- To ensure that all information provided to patients, other members of the public and other health professionals is accurate and objective, and is given in a manner designed to ensure that it is understood.
- To treat all those who seek their services with courtesy and respect.
- To ensure the continuity of provision of professional services in the event of conflict with personal moral beliefs or closure of a pharmacy. In the event of labour disputes, to make every effort to ensure that people continue to have access to pharmaceutical services.

Pharmaceutical Marketing (Promotion)—Code of Practices

"Advertising is the art of convincing people to spend money they don't have for something they don't need."

— Will Rogers

After reading this chapter, you should be able to understand and appreciate:
- Pharmaceutical promotion methods
- Ethical and business conflicts in pharmaceutical promotion
- Regulations for pharmaceutical promotion in other countries

The medicines (a still broader term pharmaceuticals) play a crucial role in the attainment or maintenance of health. Hence it is vital that they are used rationally. As gatekeepers to the healthcare, the doctors and pharmacists need to ensure rational use of medicines through appropriate prescribing and dispensing respectively. Unfortunately there are growing concerns on industry's influence on prescribing and dispensing decisions through promotional tools. This influence can lead to less than optimum medication choice.

The terminology of pharmaceutical sales has changed over years: sales to marketing to promotion. Currently it is accepted as promotion. The pharmaceutical promotion has been defined as all informal and persuasive activities by the manufacturers, the effect of which is to induce the prescription, supply, purchase and/or use of medicinal drugs. The pharmaceutical promotion is the communication process that generates demand for medicines. Pharmaceuticals and medicines are equivalents and used interchangeably. Though the patients are the real customers they have no choice. It is either doctors or pharmacists decide their choice. In true sense,

the customers for medicines are either doctors who prescribe or pharmacists who sell. Nowadays, the general public are also targeted by the pharmaceutical promoters through direct to consumer advertising. Basically four types of techniques are used for pharmaceutical promotion: Personal Selling, Advertising, Sales Promotion and Publicity. In personal selling, the professional service representatives (PSR) or medical representatives (MR) visit the doctor for generation of prescriptions for their products. The PSR or MR visits the retailers (community pharmacies) too. Advertising is a paid non-personal presentation of idea, message, theme or details about products to consumers through media like Newspaper, TV, magazine, news bulletin, etc. The Direct to Consumer Advertising through electronic mass media is very powerful technique influencing the general public. However, the advertisements are regulated under Drugs and Magic Remedies (Objectionable Advertisement) Act. Promotion through advertisement seems to be cheaper but there is no assurance of generating sales. The sales promotion directly enhances sales through push or pull strategy.

Providing additional incentive or rebate to retailers, display contest for retailers, gift to physicians and retailers are a few examples of this technique. Publicity is again direct presentation of ideas, theme or message to consumers through media without expenses. The news in TV and newspaper, publication of articles in journals, organizing health camps are examples of this type of drug promotion. However, there are reports of paid news, ghost writing, etc. causing concern of these techniques.

The valuable and legitimate contribution to society by the pharmaceutical industries is well appreciated. But as business enterprises, their profits are heavily dependent on marketing. The greater the volume of medicines sold, the greater the return on investments. The promotion can lead to overprescribing as well as poor quality prescribing and medicine use which in turn lead to an increased risk of adverse effects and higher healthcare costs. Growing amount of money is being spent on drug promotion. In 2002, almost US dollar 21 billion was spent on promotion in the USA alone.

Essential Commodities (Control of Unethical Practices in Marketing of Drugs) Order 2017

This proposed regulation is likely to be notified soon. A few salient points:

- Prohibits companies from offering doctors cash, gift and paid vacations.
- Penalty for violation—at the lowest level is to suspend the marketing of drug.

The order is a welcome move: The earlier attempts by Medical Council of India to regulate the practice of doctors was found ineffective. The patients and their relatives pay from their own source. The order is likely to check the unethical practices of pharmaceutical companies by making mandatory disclosure of information on marketing expenditure.

Drug Promotion in other Countries

Although the Governments in other countries have legislated authority to control pharma-ceutical promotion, most have ceded nearly all day-to-day control over some or all aspects of pharmaceutical promotion to the voluntary national industry associations, called self-regulation.

In the United Kingdom, the Medicines Act has regulation of pharmaceutical promotion and Health Minister is responsible for enforcement. However, this responsibility is delegated to the Association of British Pharmaceutical Industry (ABPI). The justification for this delegation is the industries' expertise and willingness and the Department of Health's ability to save money and staff time. In one case reported in 2006 in The Guardian, ABPI ruled that the scale of the hospitality to doctors who might be influenced to prescribe Abbott Laboratories drugs breached its code of practice. It suspended the company from its board of management for six months. It was alleged that the company's drug representative had taken 27 doctors to the greyhound track in Manchester in January 2004 and 36 others in September. It was also complaint that two employees had taken a senior doctor to lap dancing club.

In the US, the government directly regulates pharmaceutical promotion. USFDA has separate division, Division of Drug Marketing, Advertising and Communication (DDMAC). Though it cannot insists on pre-approval of advertisements, the companies need to submit advertisements when they begin to campaign. If the advertisement violates the US Laws, DDMAC sends an "Untitled Letter" to the company asking it to stop running the advertisement immediately and explain why the advertisement was found to be illegal. For more serious offences, the "Warning Letter" to the company and "Dear Health Professionals" to all doctors are issued. These letters are posted on the FDA's website: http://www.fda.gov/cder/warn/warn2006.htm.

In US, there is Physicians Sunshine Act 2010 which is intended to increase transparency of financial relationships between healthcare providers and pharmaceutical manufacturers.

Two international regulatory standards exist: IFPMA (International Federation of Pharmaceutical Manufacturers' Association) Code of Pharmaceutical Marketing Practices (Latest Version 2007) and World Health Organization (WHO) Ethical Criteria for Medicinal Drug Promotion (1988). The WHO criteria do not have legal standing, but they are the guiding force for the National Governments developing legislations and as standard for voluntary code development. It covers the following aspects of drug promotion:

- Advertising to the physicians and other health professionals;
- Advertisements in all forms to the general public;
- Medical representatives;
- Free samples;
- Symposia and other scientific meetings;
- Post marketing scientific studies, surveillance and dissemination of information.
- Packaging and labelling;
- Information for patients: Package inserts, leaflets and booklets;
- Promotion of exported drugs.

There are reports of expensive gifts even distributing cheques and cash to doctors and their families. In order to reduce the unethical marketing practice of pharmaceutical companies, the Department of Pharmaceuticals (DoP) of Government of India released Uniform Code for Pharmaceutical Marketing Practices (UCPMP) on June 02, 2011. The code seeks to curb any kind of gifts to doctors, restricts hospitality and meetings, prescribes guidelines around promotional materials including drug samples and expects detailed implementation would be monitored through empowered committee at each association. Initially for the first six months, it is just a code of conduct and later planned to make it a law regulating the marketing practices.

The pharmaceutical associations are opposing several clauses of UCPMP urging the government to delete citing them as unreasonable and difficult to implement.

They have been pleading for deleting the clause on hospitality, sponsorship and meetings. The associations urge that it is difficult to keep tab on events other than medical which may be coinciding with company's scheduling of the meetings. The associations are also opposing two other clauses related to: Samples, and sponsoring or organizing entertainment, porting or leisure events.

There are reports that the pharmaceutical industries in India are currently spending 30–40% of the cost of the product for promoting their products. Now with successful implementation of the code, these promotional costs should come down resulting in reduction of drug prices. Most importantly we are hopeful that with the stoppage of incentives doctors will start prescribing affordable generics to the patients.

The Department of Pharmaceuticals proposes to introduce UCPMP under Essential Commodities Act to make it more deterrent. The voluntary code does not have provision to punish the violators. The many companies are reported to have not been adhering to the marketing code.

The details of the UCPMP are given below:

General Points

1. A medicinal product must not be promoted prior to receipt of the product authorization, authorizing its sale or supply.

2. The promotion of a medicinal product must be consistent with the terms of the product authorization.

3. Information about medicinal products must be up-to-date, verifiable and accurately reflect current knowledge or responsible opinion.

4. Information about medicinal products must be accurate, balanced, fair, objective, and must not mislead either directly or by implication.

5. Information must be capable of substantiation—substantiation that is requested must be provided without delay at the request of members of the medical and pharmacy professions including the

members of those professions employed in the pharmaceutical industry.

Claims and Comparisons

1. Claims for the usefulness of a medicinal product must be based on an up-to-date evaluation of all the evidence.
2. The word "safe" must not be used without qualification and it must not be stated categorically that a medicine has no side effects, toxic hazards or risk of addiction.
3. The word "new" must not be used to describe any medicinal product which has been generally available, or therapeutic indication which has been generally promoted in India for more than 12 months.
4. Comparisons of medicinal products must be factual, fair and capable of substantiation. In presenting a comparison, care must be taken to ensure that it does not mislead by distortion, by undue emphasis, omission or in any other way.
5. Brand names of products of other companies must not be used in comparison unless the prior consent of the companies concerned has been obtained.
6. Other companies, their products, services or promotions must not be disparaged either directly or by implication.
7. The clinical and/or scientific opinions of members of healthcare professionals must not be disparaged either directly or by implication.

Textual and Audio-Visual Promotional Material

1. All promotional material issued by a product authorisation holder or with his authority, must be consistent with the requirements of this Code.
2. Where the purpose of promotional material is to provide persons qualified to prescribe or supply with sufficient information upon which to reach a decision for prescribing or for use, then the following minimum information, must be given clearly and legibly and must be an integral part of the advertisement:

i. The relevant product authorisation number and the name and address of the holder of the authorisation or the business name and address of the part of the business responsible for placing the medicinal product on the market;
ii. The name of the product, and a list of the active ingredients, using the common name, placed immediately adjacent to the most prominent display of the name of the product;
iii. Recommended dosage, method of use and, where not obvious, method of administration;
iv. Adverse reactions, warnings and precautions for use and relevant contraindications of the product;
v. A statement that additional information is available on request;
vi. The date on which the above particulars were generated or last updated.

3. Promotional material such as mailings and journal advertisements must not be designed to disguise their real nature. Where a pharmaceutical company pays for or otherwise secures or arranges the publication of promotional material in journals, such promotional material must not resemble editorial matter.
4. All promotional materials appearing in journals, the publication of which is paid for or secured or arranged by a company and referring by brand name to any product of that company, must comply with Clause 3.3 of this Code as appropriate, irrespective of the editorial control of the material published.
5. Promotional material must conform, both in text and illustration, to canons of good taste and must be expressed so as to recognize the professional standing of the recipients and not be likely to cause offence.
6. The names or photographs of healthcare professionals must not be used in promotional material.
7. Promotional material must not imitate the devices, copy, slogans or general layout adopted by other companies in a way that is likely to mislead or confuse.

8. Where appropriate (for example, in technical and other informative material), the date of printing or the last review of promotional material must be stated.

9. Extremes of format, size or cost of promotional material must be avoided.

10. Postcards, other exposed mailings, envelopes or wrappers must not carry matter which might be regarded as advertising to the lay public or which could be considered unsuitable for public view.

11. Audio-visual material must be accompanied by all appropriate printed material so that all relevant requirements of the Code are complied with.

Medical Representatives

1. The term "medical representative" means sales representatives, including personnel retained by way of contract with third parties, and any other company representatives who call on healthcare professionals, pharmacies, hospitals or other healthcare facilities in connection with the promotion of medicinal products.

2. Medical representatives must at all times maintain a high standard of ethical conduct in the discharge of their duties. They must comply with all relevant requirements of the Code.

3. Medical representatives must not employ any inducement or subterfuge to gain an interview. They must not pay, under any guise, for access to a healthcare professional.

4. Companies are responsible for the activities of all their employees and must ensure that employees who are concerned in any way with the drafting or approval of promotional material (including employees of third parties contracted on behalf of the company) are fully conversant and compliant with the requirements of the Code.

5. Other third parties working for or on behalf of pharmaceutical companies, (including advertising companies executives, business consultants and market research companies), and those that do not act on behalf of companies (such as joint ventures and licensees) commissioned to engage in activities covered by the Code should also have a good working knowledge of the Code.

Samples

1. Not to supply free samples of medicinal products to any person who is not qualified to prescribe such product.

2. Where samples of products are distributed by a medical representative, the sample must be handed directly to a person qualified to prescribe such product or to a person authorised to receive the sample on their behalf.

3. The following conditions should be observed in the provision of samples to a person qualified to prescribe such product:
   i. Such samples are provided on an exceptional basis only (refer (ii) to (vii) below) and for the purpose of acquiring experience in dealing with such a product;
   ii. Such sample packs shall be limited to prescribed dosages for three patients;
   iii. Any supply of such samples must be in response to a signed and dated request from the recipient;
   iv. An adequate system of control and accountability must be maintained in respect of the supply of such samples;
   v. Each sample pack shall not be larger than the smallest pack presented in the market;
   vi. Each sample should be marked "free medical sample—not for sale" or bear another legend of analogous meaning;
   vii. Each sample should be accompanied by a copy of the most up-to-date version of the Product Characteristics relating to that product.

4. A person should not supply a sample of a medicinal product which is an antidepressant, hypnotic, sedative or tranquillizer.

5. The companies will maintain a detail record of free samples distributed to healthcare practitioners.

Gift

1. No gifts, pecuniary advantages or benefits in kind may be supplied, offered or promised to persons qualified to prescribe or supply by a pharmaceutical company.
2. Gifts for the personal benefit of healthcare professionals (such as tickets to entertainment events) also are not be offered or provided.

The GOI proposes to make rules restricting gifts and trips offered to doctors and pharmacists to 1,000 rupees ($15). While there are regulations in place in other countries, India is in the process of making the rules. At present only voluntary code exists. There are reports of unethical selling practices such as offering gifts ranging from electrical appliances to foreign junkets to encourage doctors and pharmacists to prescribe and stock certain medications.

Other features of the proposed regulations:

- Forbids marketing companies from making misleading claims around the curative abilities and efficacy of drugs.
- Restricts the number of trail samples (physician samples) offered to doctors.

Penalty for non-adherence to rules: Marketing ban on the company for more than a year depending on the degree of the violation, and the confiscation of "all packets of the highest selling brand of drugs". There is provision of payment of cash fine in lieu of marketing ban—500,000 rupees and 100,000,000 rupees depending on the severity.

- Companies are permitted to organize screening camps or awareness campaigns at public health centres, but it bars advertising by stealth and mandates that doctors involved in such events be paid commensurate to their average daily income.
- Implementing officer—there is provision of appointing 'Ethics Compliance Officer' with a rank of Joint Secretary.

[ET Health World, 2nd August 2017]

Hospitality, Sponsorship and Meetings

1. Companies may legitimately provide assistance that is directly related to the bonafide continuing education of the healthcare professionals and which genuinely facilitates attendance of the healthcare professional for the duration of the educational aspect of the event held in India. Such support and assistance must, however, always be such as to leave healthcare professionals' independence of judgement.
2. Where appropriate and depending on the time, location and length of the meeting, support to healthcare professionals may cover actual travel expenses, meals, refreshments, accommodation and registration fees. The events have to be organized in India only and all expenses mentioned above, must be incurred only for the events held in India.
3. Companies must not organise meetings to coincide with sporting, entertainment or other leisure events or activities. Venues that are renowned for their entertainment or leisure facilities or are extravagant must not be used.
4. Any hospitality offered to healthcare professionals must:
   i. Be reasonable in level and be likely to appear to independent third parties, to be reasonable;
   ii. Be secondary and strictly limited to the main purpose of the event at which it is offered;
   iii. Not exceed the level that recipients would normally be prepared to pay for themselves;
   iv. Not to be extended to spouses or other accompanying persons, unless they are healthcare professionals who qualify as participants in their own right. Travel expenses are not to be paid for spouses or other accompanying persons, unless they are healthcare professionals who qualify as participants in their own right;
   v. Not include sponsoring, securing, organising directly or indirectly any entertainment, sporting or leisure events.

5. Funding of healthcare professionals to compensate them for the time spent in attending the event is not permitted.

6. All promotional, scientific or professional meetings, congresses, conferences, symposia, and other similar events (including advisory board meetings, visits to research or manufacturing facilities, and planning, training or investigator meetings for clinical trials and non-interventional studies) (each, an "event") organized or sponsored by or on behalf of a company must be held at an appropriate venue in the country that is conducive to the main purpose of the event.

7. The companies must maintain a detail record of expenditure incurred on these events.

Mode of Operation

1. All the Indian Pharmaceutical Manufacturer associations will have UCMP uploaded on their website.

2. All the associations will upload the detail procedure (as stated in Para 10) of lodging complaints.

3. All the associations will have a detail of complaints received, i.e. the nature of complaint, the company against whom the complaint has been made, the action taken by the association including the present status in the complaint, uploaded on their website for three years. Whenever proceedings in a complaint are completed, a copy of proceedings and decisions will be sent by the concerned Association to the Department of Pharmaceuticals, on the following address:

Under Secretary(PI),

Room No-347, A-wing, Shastri Bhawan, New Delhi 110001

4. If a complaint received in a particular association is not concerned to its member, the receiving associations will input the details of the complaint but in the column of action taken, it will mention that the complaint has been transferred to such and such association as the respondent company is not its member.

Committee for Complaint Handling

1. There should be a complaint handling committee named "Committee for Pharma Marketing Practices "in all the associations.

2. The committee should have a panel of 5 member companies, represented by the Executive Head of the companies or a nominee from the Executive Head, but not below the rank of Director in the Board of Company.

3. Based on the complaint, specially, the company involved (either as complainant or as respondent), the Secretary General/Chairman/President (to be decided by the Executive Body of the Association) of the association will decide three members from the panel of 5 for handling the complaint.

4. There will be a review committee for which there will be a panel of seven member companies of the association and based on the company involved, Secretary General/Chairman/President of the Association will nominate five members for review committee including the three members of the complaint committee, who dealt with the complaint.

Procedure of Lodging a Complaint

1. All correspondences should be addressed to the "Committee for Code of Pharma Marketing", Secretary General/Chairman/President, "Name of Association".

2. All complaints about anyone activity should to the extent practicable be made at one time.

3. Complaints must be in writing and for each case THE COMPLAINANT should:
   i. Identify himself (whether a company or an individual) with a full mailing address (fax number, if possible, mobile, telephone nos.). When the complaint is from a pharmaceutical company, the complaint must be signed or authorized in writing by the company's managing director or chief executive or equivalent and must state those clauses of the Code which are alleged to have been breached.

ii. Identify the company which is alleged to be in breach of the Code, and the name of any company personnel, product or products which are specifically involved.

iii. Give the details of the activity which is alleged to be in breach of the Code.

iv. Give the date of the alleged breach of the Code which must have occurred during the last two months of the date of making the complaint.

v. Provide supporting evidence of the alleged breach(es).

4. A non-refundable charge of ₹ 1,000/-by any complainant. The associations will elaborate how this payment is to be made.

5. The name of the complainant has to be kept confidential by the association.

6. When it appears from media reports (other than letters to the editor of a publication) that a company may have breached the Code, the matter will be treated as a complaint. The author of the article, or the editor where no author is named, will be treated as the complainant not the person who has brought this report in the notice of the committee. If the editor or author declines involvement, this is stated in the case report

7. A published letter from which it appears that a company may have breached the Code will be dealt with as a complaint with the author being treated as the complainant.

8. Any complaint received by the Department of Pharmaceuticals will also be forwarded to the concerned Association for necessary action. In such cases, the concerned association will further take up the matter with the complainant directly.

Procedure of handling complaint

1. Once lodged a complaint, the complainant cannot withdraw it and it has to be dealt with by the committee.

2. The complaints will be received by the Secretary General/Chairman/President of the concerned associations.

3. The Secretary General/Chairman/President will mark the complaint to the seniormost (by designation) member of the panel as Chairman, also indicate the names of other two members of the committee.

4. The decision will be made by the majority.

5. When the committee receives information from which it appears that a company may have contravened the Code, the managing director or chief executive or equivalent of the company concerned will be requested to provide a complete response to the matters of complaint.

6. To assist companies in ensuring that a complete response is submitted, the committee may suggest relevant supporting material to be supplied. It is the responsibility of the respondent to ensure that a full response is submitted.

7. The company against which the complaint is made should provide supporting evidence if it thinks that the Code has not been breached.

8. Upon receipt of information from the committee, the respondent company has ten working days in which to submit its comments and supporting documents to the committee.

9. The committee should render a decision within 30 days of receipt of the complaint with supporting documentation and shall promptly notify the parties of its decision, and the reasons therefore, in writing and by registered mail.

10. Where the committee rules no breach of the Code because it considers the matter of complaint is not within the scope of the Code the complainant will be so advised in writing.

11. Where the committee rules that there is a breach of the Code, the complainant and the respondent company are so advised in writing and are given the reasons for the decision.

12. If a party to the complaint is dissatisfied with the decision of the Committee, it may request for review its decision. Any party requesting a review of a decision of

the Committee shall notify the Secretary General/Chairman/President of the Association.

13. If no request for a review of the Committee's decision is made within the period specified, the decision of the Committee shall be final and binding, and adherence to the decision shall be a condition of continued membership of the Association.

14. Once it is established that a breach of code has been made by a company, the committee can take one of the following decisions against the alleged company:

   i. To suspend or expel the company from the Association.

   ii. To reprimand the company and publish details of that reprimand.

   iii. To require the company to issue a corrective statement; details of the proposed content and mode and timing of dissemination of the corrective statement must be provided to the committee for approval and the same shall be put on the website of the Association.

   iv. To ask the company to take steps to recover items given in connection with the promotion of a medicine provided to health professionals and members of the public and the like; details of the action taken must be provided in writing to the Committee which will be uploaded on the website of the Association.

Review of Decisions of the Complaints

1. The complainant or the respondent company may go for review against a ruling of the committee.

2. Once asked for a review, the complainant/respondent cannot ask for the withdrawal.

3. A review by the complainant must be lodged within ten working days of notification of the ruling of the Committee.

4. Where the respondent company appeals, it must give notice of appeal within five working days of notification of the ruling

of the committee and must lodge the review within ten working days of notification of the ruling of the Committee.

5. If a complaint concerns a matter closely similar to one which has been the subject of a previous adjudication, it may be allowed to proceed at the discretion of the committee if new evidence is adduced by the complainant or if the passage of time or a change in circumstances raises doubts as to whether the same decision would be made in respect of the current complaint. If a complainant does not accept a decision of the committee, he may ask for the matter to be referred to the review committee and the decision of the review committee will be final.

6. If, in the view of the committee, a complaint does not show that there may have been a breach of the Code, the complainant shall be so advised. If the complainant does not accept that view, he may ask for review.

7. Where review is asked by the complainant, the respondent company has five working days to comment on the reasons given by the complainant for the review and these comments will be circulated to the members of the review committee. The complainant has five working days to comment on the respondent company's comments upon the reasons.

8. Where review is asked by the respondent company, the complainant has five working days to comment on the reasons given by the respondent company for the review and these comments will be circulated to the respondent company and the review committee. The respondent company has five working days to comment on the complainant comments upon the reasons.

9. If the promotional material or activity at issue is considered by the committee to be likely to prejudice public health and/or patient safety, and/or it represents a serious breach of the Code, the committee must decide whether, if there is subsequently review by the respondent company, the use of the promotional material or the activity would continue

during the period of review. If suspension of the promotional material or the activity during the period of review would be required, the company must be so notified when it is advised of the committee's ruling of a breach of the Code.

10. In case the respondent company accepts the breach of code, it has five working days to provide a written undertaking that the promotional activity or use of the material in question and any similar material (if not already discontinued or no longer in use) will cease forthwith and that all possible steps will be taken to avoid a similar breach of the Code in future. This undertaking must be signed by the managing director or chief executive or equivalent of the company or with his authority and must be accompanied by details of the actions taken by the company to implement the undertaking, including the date on which the promotional material was finally used or appeared and/or the last date on which the promotional activity took place.

OPPI Code of Pharmaceutical Marketing Practices (January 2007): The Organization of Pharmaceutical Producers of India (OPPI) is an organization of Pharmaceutical Manufacturers of India consisting of companies with international collaboration and large Indian companies. OPPI members adhere to the code of pharmaceutical marketing practices of International Federation of Pharmaceutical Manufacturers and Associations (IFPMA). The General Principles of OPPI Code are:

- Basis of Interaction: The interaction is intended to benefit patients and enhance practice of medicines.
- Independence of Healthcare Professionals: No financial benefit or benefit in kind may be provided or offered to a healthcare professional in exchange for prescribing, recommending, purchasing, supplying or administering products or for a commitment to continue to do so.

- Appropriate Use: Promotion should encourage the appropriate use of pharmaceutical products.
- Regulation: Relevant laws and regulations should be observed and adhered to.
- Transparency: Promotion should not be disguised.

The OPPI code does not cover the following activities:

- Promotion of prescription only pharmaceutical products directly to the general public.
- Promotion of self-medication products that are provided over the counter without prescription.
- Pricing or other trade terms for the supply of pharmaceutical products.
- The engagement of a healthcare professional to provide genuine consultancy or other genuine services to member company.
- The conduct of clinical trials (governed by GCP).
- The provision of non-promotional information by member companies.

Medical Council of India (MCI) Guidelines on Industry–Physician Relationship

The MCI is a quasi-judicial body and its code, though not law, is ethically binding on all practitioners of modern medicines in India. The guidelines issued by the MCI covers the relationship between the pharmaceutical industries and the medical profession; and clinical trials sponsored by the industry. It covers the issue of gifting and sponsorship. The MCI announced the list of punishments which are graded based on financial quantum of the gifts received. Those who have received more than one lakh rupees will be deregistered for more than a year. This is viewed as the first initiative in the whole world that the quantum of punishment has been specified.

In dealing with pharmaceutical and allied health sector industry, a medical practitioner shall follow and adhere to the stipulations given below (2009 Notification):

a. **Gifts:** Not to receive any gift from any pharmaceutical or allied healthcare industry and their sales people or representatives.

b. **Travel facilities:** Not to accept any travel facility inside the country or outside, including rail, air, ship, cruise tickets, paid vacations, etc. from any pharmaceutical or allied healthcare industry or their representatives for self and family members for vacation or for attending conference, seminars, workshops, CME programme, etc. as a delegate.

c. **Hospitality:** Not to accept individually any hospitality like hotel accommodation for self and family members under any pretext.

d. **Cash or monetary grants:** Not to receive any cash or monetary grants from any pharmaceutical and allied healthcare industry for individual purpose in individual capacity under any pretext. Funding for medical research, study, etc. can only be received through approved institutions by modalities laid down by law/rules/guidelines adopted by such approved institutions, in a transparent manner. It shall always be fully disclosed.

e. **Medical research:** A medical practitioner may carry out, participate in, work in research projects funded by pharmaceutical and allied healthcare industries. A medical practitioner is obliged to know that the fulfilment of the following items (i) to (vii) will be an imperative for undertaking any research assignment/project funded by industry—for being proper and ethical. Thus, in accepting such a position a medical practitioner shall:

   i. Ensure that the particular research proposal(s) has the due permission from the competent concerned authorities;

   ii. Ensure that such a research project(s) has the clearance of national/state/institutional ethics committee/bodies;

   iii. Ensure that it fulfils all the legal requirements prescribed for medical research;

   iv. Ensure that the source and amount of funding is publicly disclosed at the beginning itself;

   v. Ensure that proper care and facilities are provided to human volunteers, if they are necessary for the research projects;

   vi. Ensure that undue animal experimentations are not done and when these are necessary they are done in a scientific and humane way;

   vii. Ensure that while accepting such an assignment a medical practitioner shall have the freedom to publish the results of the research in the greater interest of the society by inserting such a clause in the MoU or any other document/agreement for any such assignment.

f. **Maintaining Professional Autonomy:** Always ensure that there shall never be any compromise either with his/her own professional autonomy and/or with the autonomy and freedom of the medical institution.

g. **Affiliation:** A medical practitioner may work for pharmaceutical and allied healthcare industries in advisory capacities, as consultants, as researchers, as treating doctors or in any other professional capacity. In doing so, a medical practitioner shall always:

   i. Ensure that his professional integrity and freedom are maintained;

   ii. Ensure that patients interest are not compromised in any way;

   iii. Ensure that such affiliation are within the law;

   iv. Ensure that such affiliations/employments are fully transparent and disclosed.

h. **Endorsement:** Not to endorse any drug or product of the industry publicly. Any study conducted on the efficacy or otherwise of such products shall be presented to and/or through appropriate scientific bodies or published in appropriate scientific journals in a proper way.

Code of Criminal Procedure

"Knowing is not enough, you must apply. Willing is not enough, you must do."

— *Goethe*

After reading this chapter, you should be able to understand and appreciate
- The power of Magistrate
- Procedure followed for searching a place:
  1. Entered by person to be arrested
  2. Suspected to contain stolen property, forged documents, etc.
  3. Closed premises

SOME RELEVANT POINTS

Power of Magistrate

1. The Court of a Chief Judicial Magistrate may pass any sentence authorized by law (except a sentence of death or imprisonment for life or imprisonment exceeding 7 years).
2. The Court of a First Class Magistrate may pass a sentence of imprisonment for a term not exceeding 3 years or of fine not exceeding 10 thousand rupees or both.
3. Second Class Magistrate may pass a sentence of imprisonment for a term not exceeding 1 year, or fine not exceeding 5 thousand rupees, or both.

Chief Metropolitan Magistrate and Chief Judicial Magistrate have equal powers. Similarly, Metropolitan Magistrate and Magistrate of the first class have equal powers.

Searching of Place Entered by Person to be Arrested

1. Person in charge of a place or residing, to which a person to be arrested has entered, must allow free ingress and offer reasonable facilities for a search to the officer acting under a warrant of arrest or police officer.
2. If required, the police officer may break upon outer or inner door to get an entry to such places. If the occupant of the apartment is a female (not the person to be arrested) and according to custom does not appear in public, the officer needs to allow the female to withdraw and then break open to enter.
3. Any police officer or other authorized person for making arrest may break upon the door or windows to liberate him, if detained.

Searching of places suspected to contain stolen property, forged documents (used for deposit, sale or production of objectionable articles):

The District Magistrate, Sub-divisional Magistrate, or Magistrate of the first class may authorize any police officer above the rank of a constable: to enter such place (if required with assistance), to search in a manner specified in warrant, to take possession of property, etc.; to convey such property before a Magistrate or guard the same on the spot till offender is taken before a Magistrate or dispose of it in some place of safety, and to take custody of the person suspected to be involved and carry before a Magistrate.

Searching of a Closed Place

In addition to the provision discussed under searching of a place, the authorized person need to call upon two or more independent and respectable inhabitants of the locality of the place to be searched who would be a witness. A necessary order in writing may be issued by the officer concerned. The person who refuses or neglects to attend and witness a search is deemed to have committed an offence.

The search should be made in the presence of three persons and the documents containing seized things need to be signed by the witness.

The occupant of the place or his authorized person should be permitted to enter the searching place and he is entitled the copy of the document prepared along with the witness signature.

17

The Tamil Nadu Shops and Establishments Act

"One of the greatest delusions in the world is the hope that the evils in the world are to be cured by Legislation."

— *Thomas Brackett Reed*

After reading this chapter, you should be able to understand and appreciate:
- Provisions of the Act protecting the interest of employees working in shops and commercial establishments
- Administrative procedure for implementing the Act
- Provision of Model Act

The Weekly Holidays Act 1942 had a very limited scope regulating the conditions of work of employees in shops, commercial undertakings, restaurants, etc. It was just restricted to providing holidays and did not have provisions regulating other matters affecting the employees such as hours of work, payment of wages, health and safety. There was a comprehensive need in Madras Province on these matters on the lines of similar enactments in force in other provinces. The bill was brought to bring all these matters under a regulation with a plan to implement in phases. In the first instances, it was proposed to cover the City of Madras and all Municipalities and extend the provisions to other parts of the Province. This led to the enactment of Madras Shops and Establishment Act 1947 and with the assent of Governor-General published in the Gazette on 10th February 1948. The Rules made in later called Madras Shops and Establishment Rules 1948. With change of name from Madras Province to Tamil Nadu, the Act and Rules were rephrased as Tamil Nadu Shops and Establishment Act and the Rules.

Every state has enacted such laws to protect the employees working in shops and commercial establishments. Here in this text, a model Act is discussed. In 2016, GOI proposed the model Shops and Establishment Act. The states may consider for enforcement either by adopting the Central Law or by amending the existing law of the state. The salient features of this model law is given in the Box. It is expected that the new model would bring about uniformity in the legislation ensuring uniform working conditions across the country and facilitate the ease of doing business and generate employment opportunities.

The Model Shops and Establishment (Regulation of Employment and Conditions of Services) Bill 2016

Salient Points
- It covers only establishments employing ten or more workers except manufacturing units;
- It provides opportunity for freedom to operate 365 days in a year and with flexibility of opening/closing time of establishment;

- It provides for women to be employed on night shifts with adequate security and facilities such as rest room, ladies toilet, adequate protection of their dignity and transportation;
- There would be no discrimination against women in the matter of recruitment, training, transfer or promotion;
- It provides for on-line one common registration through a simplified procedure;
- It provides for provision of clean and safe drinking water;
- It provides for opportunities to have common group facilities in lavatory, crèche, first aid and canteen, if not feasible by one establishment;
- It provides for five paid festival holidays in addition to National holidays; and
- The Act proposes exemption of highly skilled workers (workers in IT, bio-technology and R & D division).

The Labour and Employment Department of Government of Tamil Nadu is the administrative department for the Act and the Rules. The Commissioner of Labour of Chennai and Deputy Commissioners of Labour of other places are the authorities for implementation of the Act.

The objective of the Act is to regulate the conditions of work in shops, commercial establishments, restaurants, theatres, and other establishments. It extends to the whole state of Tamil Nadu. The salient points are described below:

Shops

Opening and Closing Hours of Shops: No shop is permitted to open on any day earlier than 6 am or closed on any day later than 10 pm.

Selling outside the shops prohibited after closing hour: No sale of goods after the closing hours is permitted. However, this does not apply to Newspapers.

Daily and Weekly Hours of Work in Shops: The working hours should not be more than 8 hours in any day and 48 hours in any week. However, the persons may be allowed to work in excess of the time limit described on payment of overtime wages but the total period of working hours should not exceed 10 hours in any day and 54 hours per week in aggregate. At a stretch a person is not allowed to work for more than 4 hours in any day unless given a rest of at least 1 hour. The periods of work for persons employed in shops should be arranged in such a way that the period would not exceed 12 hours inclusive of rest.

Dispensaries working during night are exempted from this provision provided the employed persons are paid the twice the wages as overtime for working more than 8 hours a day or more than 48 hours in any week. The persons employed in petrol bunks and storage depots for petrol and petroleum products are also exempted provided the spread over working hours should not exceed 16 hours in a day with an interval of not less than 30 minutes for meals. The night work should be given in turn and the overtime wages are the double the rate of ordinary wages.

Closing of Shops and Grant of Holidays: Every shop should remain entirely closed on one day of the week as decided by the shopkeeper and permanently exhibited in a conspicuous place in the shop. The day so decided should not be altered more often than once in three months. The wages of the holiday is not to be deducted. *The Chemists Shops holding valid drug license and dealing with drugs, surgical appliances, bandages or other medical requisites are exempted from this weekly holiday.*

Establishments Other than Shops

Opening and Closing Hours of Commercial Establishments: No commercial establishments situated in the state is permitted to open on any day earlier than 8 am or closed not later than 8 pm. For theatres and place of public amusement: Opening time is not earlier than 9 am and closing time not later than 1.30 am.

Daily and Weekly Hours of Work of Commercial Establishments: The working hours should not be more than 8 hours in any day and 48 hours in any week. However, the persons may be allowed to work in excess of the time limit described on payment of overtime wages but the total period of working hours should not exceed 10 hours in any day and 54 hours per week in aggregate. At a stretch a person is not allowed to work for more than 4 hours in any day unless given a rest of at least 1 hour. The periods of work for persons employed in shops should be arranged in such a way that the period would not exceed 12 hours inclusive of rest.

The persons employed in petrol bunks and storage depots for petrol and petroleum products are also exempted provided the spread over working hours should not exceed 16 hours in a day with an interval of not less than 30 minutes for meals. The night work should be given in turn and the overtime wages are the double the rate of ordinary wages. The persons employed in theatre should be given the aggregating rest period of 2 hours in a day with no interval of rest is less than 15 minutes at a time.

Employment of Children and Young Persons: The children are not allowed to work in any establishment. The young person's working hours are fixed at between 6 am and 7 pm. The young persons are not allowed to work for more than 7 hours in any day and 42 hours in a week. They are not allowed to work overtime.

Health and Safety

Cleanliness of the premises: The premises of establishments should be clean and free from effluvia arising from any drain or privy. All inside walls of the rooms and all ceiling of such rooms, all passages and staircases should be lime washed or color washed at intervals of not more than 12 months. All beams, rafters, doors, window frames and other woodwork with exception of the floor should be either lime washed or color washed at intervals of not more than 12 months. They should be painted or varnished at an interval of not more than 7 years.

The cleanliness provision of painting is not applicable to rooms used for storage of articles, walls or ceilings of rooms made of galvanized iron, flat tiles, asbestos sheets, glazed bricks, glass, slate, bamboo thatch, cement plaster or polished chunam and ceiling of rooms in which lowest part is at least 6 meters from the floor.

Rubbish, filth or debris should not be allowed to accumulate or to remain on any part of the establishment for more than 24 hours and should be appropriately disposed. All filth and other decomposing matter should be kept in covered receptacles.

All drains carrying waste or sewage should be constructed of masonry or other impermeable materials and should be regularly flushed at least twice daily and where possible, connected with some drainage line.

The establishments and the compound surrounding should be maintained in a strictly sanitary and clean condition. The floor should be swept or cleaned at least once daily and the ceilings should be dusted at least once a month.

The employer should enforce the proper use of latrines and urinals and prevent pollution of the surface of the ground in the vicinity by excreta or urine. They should make suitable arrangement for regular cleaning and conserving of urinals and latrines.

The drinking water distribution place should be kept clean and drained.

Ventilation of the premises: The rooms should have ventilation provision of ventilation opening in the proportion of 0.5 square meter for each worker employed and opening should be suitable to admit a continued supply for fresh air.

Lighting of the Premises: The premises should be sufficiently lighted during all working hours. If the inspector find the ventilation and lighting are not adequate, he may serve an order, in writing, specifying the measures should be adopted.

Precautions against Fire: The employer should adopt such precautions against danger by fire to the life of persons employed.

Appeal: The Commissioner of Labour is the Appellate Authority against the order of inspector.

Holidays with Wages

Holidays and Sick Leave: On completion of 12 months of continuous service, the employee is entitled to have 12 days holidays with wages in subsequent period of 12 months. These holidays with wages can be accumulated up to a maximum period of 24 days. If the employee leaves employment or he is discharged, before being allowed to avail the leaves, the employer has to pay the amount payable in respect of holidays.

During the first 12 months of the continuous service, the employee is entitled for two types of leaves with wages: Casual leave —12 days and sick leave—12 days. While the employee is discharged but is entitled to have leave, the employer has to pay the amount payable for the period of leave entitled.

Pay during Annual Holidays: The wages for the period of annual leave is to be paid at a rate equivalent to the daily average of his wages for the days on which he actually worked during preceding three months exclusive of overtime earnings.

Wages

The employer is responsible for the payment of wages and fixes the period of wages. He has to maintain a register in prescribed form. The wage period should not exceed one month. The wages are to be paid before the expiry of the fifth day after the last day of the wage period. The payment of wages is to be made on a working day.

When the employment is terminated, the wages should be paid before the expiry of the second working day from the day on which employment is terminated.

The wages should be paid in full without deduction. [However, the following deductions are permissible: Fines, deductions for absence, deductions for damage occur due to his negligence, deductions for house accommodation provided by employer, recovery of advance, income tax, subscription to the provident fund, contribution to the cooperative societies or insurance scheme, or any other savings scheme with written authorization].

Fines: The fine cannot be imposed without previous approval of state government or Authority. The Acts and Omissions for which fine can be imposed should be clearly exhibited. A list in English and Translation in a language of the majority of the employees should be displayed at or near entrance of the establishment. The fines cannot be imposed on person not completed his fifteenth year. The employee should be given opportunity of show cause against the fine before imposing a fine on him. Every fine is deemed to have imposed on the day of act or omission. The fine is to be recovered within 60 days of date of imposition. After 60 days, it cannot be recovered.

Notice of Dismissal: The employment cannot be terminated if the person is in employment continuously for a period of minimum of six months except for a reasonable cause and without giving at least one month's notice or wages in lieu of. This notice is not necessary where the services of such persons are dispensed with on charge of misconduct supported by satisfactory evidence recorded at an enquiry held for the purpose.

The person so terminated has the option to appeal to the Authority within 30 days of the receipt of termination order. The Deputy Commissioner of the Labour is the Appellate Authority. While hearing the appeal, the Deputy Commissioner of Labour should record briefly the evidence produced before him and pass order accordingly.

Appointment, Powers and Duties of Inspectors

The state government appoints inspectors who are empowered to enter into any premises at all reasonable times with assistants to examine the premise, prescribed registers, records as necessary. Person with direct or indirect interest in any establishment cannot be appointed as inspector. The inspector ensures the proper maintenance of the records, registers, compliance of the intervals for rests, holidays and limits of hours of work, proper payment of overtime works, non-employment of children.

The employer is required to maintain a register of employment in the prescribed form. He has to provide the service book to the employees.

The authentic extract from the records of any school, village munsif, panchayat or municipality serve as record of age. In the absence of these abstracts, at least a certificate from the Registered Medical Practitioner giving the age in prescribed form is acceptable for deciding the age of the employee.

The name of board of the establishment is to be written in Tamil. Wherever other languages are to be used, the version of English should be the second followed by other languages. The Tamil version should be written predominantly in the board by providing more space than for other languages.

Every inspector is deemed to be a public servant.

Penalties for Offences: The employer, who contravenes the provision with respect to opening and closing hours, working hours and holidays, employment of children and young persons, health and safety, is punishable with fine extending up to ₹ 25 for the first offence. In the second and subsequent offence, the fine is extendable up to ₹ 250. Offence relating to selling of goods at outside the shop after the closing hours invites a penalty of ₹ 10 for the first offence. This extends to ₹ 100 in the second and subsequent cases.

Persons willfully obstructs the inspector or other persons assisting the inspector from discharging the functions or duties are punishable with fine extending up to ₹ 250.

Appendices

Terms in regulations are legally binding and therefore have restricted meaning. The meanings are expressed in simplified form for easy understanding.

Drugs and Cosmetics Act

Term	Meaning
Adulterated drug	a. If it consists, in whole or in part, of any filthy, putrid or decomposed substance; or b. If it has been prepared, packed or stored under insanitary conditions, whereby it may have been contaminated with filth or whereby it may have been rendered injurious to health; or c. If its container is composed in whole or in part, of any poisonous or deleterious substance which may render the contents injurious to health; or d. If it bears or contains, for purposes of colouring only, a colour other than one which is prescribed; or e. If it contains any harmful or toxic substance which may render it injurious to health; or f. If any substance has been mixed therewith so as to reduce its quality or strength.
Ayurvedic, Siddha or Unani drugs	All medicines intended for internal or external use for or in the diagnosis, or treatment, mitigation or prevention of disease or disorder in human beings or animals, and manufactured exclusively in accordance with the formulae described in, the authoritative books of [Ayurvedic, Siddha and Unani Tibb systems of medicine].
Cosmetic	Any article intended to be rubbed, poured, sprinkled or sprayed on, or introduced into, or otherwise applied to, the human body or any part thereof for cleansing, beautifying, promoting attractiveness, or altering the appearance, and includes any article intended for use as a component of cosmetic.
Drugs	1. All medicines for internal or external use of human beings or animals and all substances intended to be used for/or in the diagnosis, treatment, mitigation or prevention of any disease or disorder in human beings or animals, including preparations applied on human body for the purpose of repelling insects like mosquitoes. 2. Substances (other than food) intended to affect the structure or any function of the human body or intended to be used for the destruction of [vermin] or insects which cause disease in human beings or animals, as may be specified from time to time by the central government. 3. All substances intended for use as components of a drug including empty gelatin capsules. 4. Devices intended for internal or external use in the diagnosis, treatment, mitigation or prevention of disease or disorder in human beings or animals, as may be specified from time to time by the central government.

(Contd...)

243

(Contd...)

Term	Meaning
Medical device	*In vitro* diagnostics and surgical dressings, surgical bandages, surgical staples, surgical sutures, blood and blood components collection bags; mechanical contraceptives (condoms, intrauterine devices, tubal rings), disinfectants and insecticides.
Medical Device Officer	Drugs Inspector designated as Medical Device Officer.
Medical Device Testing Officer	Government Analyst designated as Medical Device Testing Officer
Manufacture	Any process or part of a process for making, altering, ornamenting, finishing, packing, labelling, breaking up or otherwise treating or adopting any drug [or cosmetic] with a view to its sale or distribution but does not include the compounding or dispensing of any drug, or the packing of any drug or cosmetic, in the ordinary course of retail business.
Misbranded cosmetic	a. If it contains a colour which is not prescribed; or b. If it is not labelled in a prescribed manner; or c. If the label or container or anything accompanying the cosmetic bears any statement which is false or misleading in any particular.
Misbranded drug	a. If it is so coloured, coated, powdered or polished that damage is concealed or if it is made to appear of better or greater therapeutic value than it really is; or b. If it is not labelled in the prescribed manner; or c. If its label or container or anything accompanying the drug bears any statement, design or device which makes any false claim for the drug or which is false or misleading.
National Accreditation Body	National Accreditation Board for Certification Bodies under Quality Council of India, Ministry of Commerce and Industry
Notified Body	The empowered organization to carry out auditing of manufacturing sites of Class A and Class B medical devices to verify the conformity with Quality Management System and other applicable standards.
Spurious cosmetic	a. If it is imported under the name which belongs to another cosmetic; or b. If it is an imitation of, or is a substitute for, another cosmetic or resembles another cosmetic in a manner likely to deceive or bears upon it or upon its label or container the name of another cosmetic, unless it is plainly or conspicuously marked so as to reveal its true character and its lack of identity with such other cosmetic; or c. If the label or the container bears the name of an individual or company purporting to be the manufacturer of the cosmetic, which individual or company is fictitious or does not exist; or d. If it purports to be the product of a manufacturer of whom it is not truly a product.
Spurious drug	a. If it is imported under a name which belongs to another drug; or b. If it is an imitation of, or a substitute for, another drug or resembles another drug in a manner likely to deceive or bears upon it or upon its label or container the name of another drug unless it is plainly and conspicuously marked so as to reveal its true character and its lack of identity with such other drug; or c. If the label or the container bears the name of an individual or company purporting to be the manufacturer of the drug, which individual or company is fictitious or does not exist; or

(Contd...)

(Contd...)

Term	Meaning
	d. If it has been substituted wholly or in part by another drug or substance; or
	e If it purports to be the product of a manufacturer of whom it is not truly a product.
Patent or proprietary medicines (ASU)	All formulations containing only such ingredients mentioned in the formulae described in the authoritative books of Ayurveda, Siddha or Unani Tibb systems of medicine (but does not include a medicine which is administered by parenteral route and also a formulation included in the authoritative books).
Patent or proprietary medicine (other than ASU)	A drug which is a remedy or prescription presented in a form ready for internal or external administration of human beings or animals and which is not included in the edition of the Indian Pharmacopoeia for the time being or any other Pharmacopoeia authorised in this behalf by the central government after consultation with the Drugs Technical Advisory Board.
Central License Approving Authority	Drugs Controller General, India
Homeopathic medicine	Any drug which is recorded in Homeopathic provings or therapeutic efficacy of which has been established through long clinical experience as recorded in authoritative Homeopathic literature of India and abroad and which is prepared according to the techniques of Homeopathic pharmacy and covers combination of ingredients of such Homeopathic medicines but does not include a medicine which is administered by parenteral route.
Registered Homeopathic medical practitioner	A person who is registered in the Central Register or State Register of Homeopathy.
Registered medical practitioner	A person: 1. Holding a qualification granted, specified or notified under Section 3 of the Indian Medical Degrees Act, 1916, or specified in the schedules to the Indian Medical Council Act, 1956; or 2. Registered or eligible for registration in a medical register of a State meant for the registration of persons practising the modern scientific system of medicine excluding the Homeopathic system of medicine; or 3. Registered in a medical register, other than a register for the registration of Homeopathic practitioner, of a State, and is declared by a general or special order made by the state government; or 4. Registered or eligible for registration in the register of dentists for a State under the Dentists Act, 1948; or 5. Who is engaged in the practice of veterinary medicine and who possesses qualifications approved by the state government.
Repacking	The process of breaking up any drug from a bulk container into small packages and the labelling of each such package with a view to its sale and distribution, but does not include the compounding or dispensing or the packing of any drug in the ordinary course of retail business.
Loan License	A license issued to an applicant who does not have his own arrangements for manufacturing but who intends to avail himself of the manufacturing facilities owned by a licensee.

Pharmacy Act

Term	Meaning
Central Council	Pharmacy Council of India
Central Register	Register of pharmacists maintained by the Pharmacy Council of India
Executive Committee	Executive committee of central council or state council
Medical Practitioner	A person • Holding a qualification granted by the authority Under Indian Medical Degrees Act, 1916 or specified in the schedules to Indian Medical Council Act 1956; • Registered or eligible for registration in a medical register of a state (Modern system of medicines); • Registered or eligible for registration in the register of dentists for a state; who is engaged in the practice of veterinary medicine and who possess qualification approved by the state government.
Registered pharmacist	A person whose name is for the time being entered in the register of the state in which he is for the time being residing or carrying on his profession or business of pharmacy.
State Council	State Council of Pharmacy or Joint State Council of Pharmacy.

Narcotic Drugs and Psychotropic Substances Act

Term	Meaning
Addict	Person addicted to any narcotic drug or psychotropic substance.
Board	Central Board of Excise and Customs
Cannabis	• Charas: Separated resin, in whatever form, whether crude or purified; from the cannabis plant. It includes concentrated preparation and resin known as hashish oil or liquid hashish; • Ganja: The flowering or fruiting tops of cannabis plant (excluding the seeds and leaves when not accompanied by the tops); and • Any mixture, with or without any natural material, of any of the above forms of cannabis or drink prepared therefrom.
Coca derivative	• Crude cocaine—any extract of coca leaf which can be used directly or indirectly for the manufacture of cocaine; • Ecgonine and all the derivatives of ecgonine from which it can be recovered • Cocaine-methyl ester of benzoyl-ecgonine and its salts; and • All preparations containing more than 0.1 percent of cocaine.
Coca leaf	• The leaf of the coca plant except a leaf from which all ecgonine, cocaine any other ecgonine alkaloids have been removed; • Any mixture with or without any natural material; but does not include any preparation containing not more than 0.1 percent of cocaine.
Coca plant	Plant of any species of the genus Erythroxylon.
Essential Narcotic Drugs	Methyl morphine, Ethyl morphine and their salts (including Donine) (Except the preparations containing not more than 100 mg per dosage unit); Fentinyl and its preparations; Dihydrocodeinone, its salts and preparations; 4:4–diphenyl-6-dimethylamino–heptanone-3, its salts and preparations; Morphine, its salts and preparations containing more than 2% morphine; and dihydroxy codeinone, its salts and preparations.
Manufacture	• All processes other than production by which such drugs or substances may be obtained;

(Contd...)

(Contd...)

Term	Meaning
	• Refining of such drugs or substances; • Transformation of such drugs or substances; and • Making of preparation (other than in pharmacy or prescription) with or containing such drugs or substances.
Manufactured drugs	• All coca derivatives, medicinal cannabis, opium derivatives and poppy straw concentrate; • Any other narcotic or preparation which the central government declares.
Medicinal cannabis	Medicinal hemp (any extract or tincture of cannabis).
Narcotic drug	Coca leaf, cannabis, opium, poppy straw and includes all manufactured drugs.
Opium	• The coagulated juice of opium poppy; • Any mixture, with or without any natural material, of the coagulated juice of the opium poppy (does not include preparation containing not more than 0.2 percent of morphine)
Opium derivative	• Medicinal opium—opium which has undergone the processes necessary to make it for medicinal use as per Indian Pharmacopoeia or any other recognized pharmacopoeia in the form of powder, granules or mixed with neutral materials; • Prepared opium—any product of opium designed to transform into an extract suitable for smoking and dross or other residue remaining after opium is smoked; • Phenanthrene alkaloids—morphine, codeine, thebaine and their salts; • Diacetylmorphine—diamorphine or heroin and its salts; and • All preparations containing more than 0.2 percent of morphine or containing any diacetylmorphine.
Opium poppy	• The plant of the species *Papaver somniferum* L.; and • The plant of any other species of *Papaver* from which opium or any phenanthrene alkaloid can be extracted and which the central government notifies.
Poppy straw	All parts (except the seeds) of the opium poppy after harvesting in the original form or cut, crushed or powdered and whether or not juice has been extracted.
Poppy straw concentrate	Any material arising when poppy straw has entered into a process for the concentration of its alkaloids.
Production	Separation of opium, poppy straw, coca leaves or cannabis from the plants from which they are obtained.
Psychotropic substance	Any substance, natural or synthetic, or any other material or any salt or preparation of such substance or material included in the list of psychotropic substances specified in the schedule.

Patent Act

Term	Meaning
Product patent	It refers the final product and it precludes others from manufacturing the product.
Process patent	It covers only the method by which one makes the product. The process patent does not preclude others from entering the market with the same product as long as the individual or company is able to devise an alternate means of manufacture.
Controller	Controller General of Patents, Designs and Trademarks
Invention	A new product or process involving an inventive step and capable of industrial application
Inventive step	A feature of an invention that involves technical advance as compared to the existing knowledge or having economic significance or both and that makes the invention not obvious to a person skilled in the art.
New invention	Any invention or technology which has not been anticipated by publication in any document or used in the country or elsewhere in the world before the date of filing of patent application with complete specification, i.e. the subject matter has not fallen in public domain or that it does not form part of the state-of-the-art.

Drug Price Control Order

Term	Meaning
Active Pharmaceutical ingredient/bulk drug	Pharmaceutical, chemical, biological or plant product including its salts, esters, isomers, analogues and derivatives which is used as such or as an ingredient in any formulation
Brand	Name, term, design, symbol, trademark or any other feature that identifies one seller's drug as distinct from those of other sellers
Ceiling price	Price fixed by the government
Formulation	Medicine processed out of/or containing one or more drugs with or without use of any pharmaceutical aids, for internal or external use for/or in the diagnosis, treatment, mitigation or prevention of disease
Manufacturer	Person who manufactures, imports and markets drugs for distribution or sale in the country
Market share	Ratio of domestic sales value (on the basis of moving annual turnover) of a brand or a generic version of a medicine and the sum of total domestic sales value of the all brands and generic versions of that medicine sold in the domestic market having same strength and dosage form
Maximum retail price	Ceiling price or the retail price plus local taxes and duties as applicable, at which the drug shall be sold to the ultimate consumer and where such price is mentioned on the pack
Moving annual turnover	Cumulative sales value for twelve months in domestic market, where the sales value of that month is added and the corresponding sales of the same month in the previous year are subtracted
National List of Essential Medicines	NLEM as revised and updated
New drug	Formulation launched by an existing manufacturer of a drug of specified dosages and strengths as listed in the NLEM by combining the drug with another drug either listed or not listed in the NLEM or a formulation launched by changing the strength or dosages or both of the same drug of specified dosages and strengths as listed in the NLEM
Non-scheduled formulation	Formulation, the dosage and strengths of which are not specified in the First Schedule
Price to retailer	Price of a drug at which it is sold to a retailer which includes duties and does not include local taxes
Scheduled formulation	Formulations included in the first schedule
Wholesale price index	Annual wholesale price index of all commodities as announced by the Department of Industrial Policy and Promotion, Government of India, from time to time.

Drugs and Magic Remedies (Objectionable Advertisement) Act

Term	Meaning
Advertisement	Any notice, circular, label, wrapper, or other document, and any announcement made orally or by any means of producing or transmitting light, sound or smoke.
Drug	I. A medicine for internal or external use of human beings or animals;
	II. Any substance intended to be used for or in the diagnosis, cure, mitigation, treatment or prevention of disease in human beings or animals;

(Contd...)

(Contd…)

Term	Meaning
	III. Any article other than food, intended to affect or influence in anyway the structure or any organic function of the body of human beings or animals;
	IV. Any article intended for use as component of any medicine, substance or article as described above.
Magic remedy	A talisman, mantra, kavacha, and any other charm of any kind which is alleged to possess miraculous powers for or in the diagnosis, cure, mitigation, treatment or prevention of any disease in human beings or animals or affecting or influencing in anyway the structure or any organic function of the body of human beings or animals
Registered medical practitioner	A person who holds a qualification granted by an authority under Indian Medical Degree Act 1916 or specified in the schedules of Indian Medical Councils Act 1956 or who is entitled to be registered as registered medical practitioner under any law being in force in the state.
Taking part in the publication of any advertisement	The printing of advertisement, publication of advertisement outside the territories to which the act extends or at the instance of a person residing within the said territories.

The Medicinal and Toilet Preparations (Excise Duty) Act

Term	Meaning
Alcohol	Ethyl alcohol of any strength and purity
Bonded manufactory	The premises or any part of the premises approved and licensed for the manufacture and storage of medicinal and toilet preparations containing alcohol, opium, Indian hemp and other narcotic drugs or narcotics on which duty has not been paid.
Coca derivative	i. Crude cocaine, that is, an extract of coca leaf which can be used directly or indirectly, for the manufacture of cocaine,
	ii. Ecgonine, that is, laevo-ecgonine having the chemical formula, $C_9H_{15}NO_3H_2O$, and all the derivatives of laevo-ecgonine from which it can be recovered, and
	iii. Cocaine, that is, methyl-benzoyl-laevo-ecgonine having the chemical formula, $C_1H_2NO_4$ and its salts;
Coca-leaf	i. The leaf and young twigs of any coca plant, that is, of the Erythoxylo coca (Lamk.) and the Erythroxylon novo-granatense (Hiern.) and their varieties, and of any other species of this genus which the central government may, by notification in the official gazette, declare to be coca plants for the purposes of this Act, and
	ii. Any mixture thereof, with or without neutral materials.
Denatured spirit or denoted alcohol	Alcohol of any strength which has been rendered unfit for human consumption by the addition of substances approved by the central government or by the state government with the approval of the central government.
Derivative of opium	i. Medicinal opium, that is, opium which has undergone the processes necessary to adopt it for medicinal use
	ii. Prepared opium, that is, any product of opium obtained by any series of operations designed to transform opium into an extract suitable for smoking and the dross or other residue remaining after opium is smoked
	iii. Morphine (the principal alkaloid of opium having the chemical formula $C_{17}H_{19}NO_8$ and its salts, and its derivatives)
Indian hemp	i. The leaves, small stalks and flowering or fruiting tops of the Indian hemp plant (*Cannabis sativa* L). including all forms known as bhang, sidhi or ganja;

(Contd…)

(Contd...)

Term	Meaning
	ii. Charas (the resin obtained from the Indian hemp plant, which has not been submitted to any manipulation other than those necessary for packing and transport; iii Any mixture, with or without neutral materials, of any of the above forms of Indian hemp or any drink prepared therefrom
Medicinal preparations	All drugs which are a remedy or "prescription" prepared for internal or external use of human beings or animals and all substances intended to be used for or in the treatment, mitigation or prevention of disease in human beings or animals.
Narcotic drugs	Substance which is coca leaf, or coca derivative or opium or derivative of opium, or Indian hemp and shall include any other substance, capable of causing or producing in human beings dependence, tolerance and withdrawal syndromes and which the central government may declare to be a narcotic drug.
Non-bonded manufactory	The premise or any part of the premises approved and licensed for the manufacture and storage of medicinal and toilet preparations containing alcohol, opium, Indian hemp and other narcotic drugs or narcotics on which duty has been paid.
Opium	1. The capsules of the poppy (*Papaver somniferum* L), whether in their original form or cut, crushed or powdered and whether or not juice has been extracted therefrom 2. The spontaneously coagulated juice of such capsules which has not been submitted to any manipulations other than those necessary for packing and transport; and 3. Any mixture, with or without neutral materials of any of the above forms of opium.
Prove	To test the strength of alcohol by hydrometer or other suitable instrument
Quarter	A period of three months beginning with 1st January, 1st April, 1st July, or 1st October
Rectified spirit	Plain un-denatured alcohol of a strength not less than 50.00 over proof and includes absolute alcohol
Restricted preparation	Every medicinal preparation specified in the schedule and includes every preparation declared by the central government as restricted preparation
Spirit store	That portion of the bonded or non-bonded manufactory which is set apart for the storage of alcohol, opium, Indian hemp and other narcotic drugs or narcotic purchased free of duty or at prescribed rates of duty
Toilet preparation	Any preparation which is intended for use in the toilet of the human body or in perfuming apparel of any description, or any substances intended to cleanse, improve or alter the complexion, skin, hair or teeth, and includes deodorants and perfumes.
Unrestricted preparation	Any medicinal preparation containing alcohol but other than a restricted preparation or a spurious preparation

Medical Termination of Pregnancy Act

Term	Meaning
Admission register	Register maintained for recording the details of women undergoing MTP
Guardian	A person having the care of the person of a minor or a lunatic
Hospital	Hospital established or maintained by central government or government of union territory
Mentally ill person	Person who is in need of treatment by reason of any mental disorder other than mental retardation
Minor	A person who has not attained majority under the provisions of the Indian Majority Act, 1875 [not attained 18 years of age]
Registered medical practitioner	A medical practitioner who possesses any recognized medical qualification under Indian Medical Council Act, whose name has been entered in a State Medical Register and who has required experience or training in gynaecology and obstetrics

Prevention of Cruelty to Animals Act

Term	Meaning
Animal	Any living creature other than a human being.
Animal welfare organisation	Welfare organizations for animals registered under Societies Registration Act and recognised by Animal Welfare Board of India.
Experiment	Any programme or project involving use of animal(s) for the acquisition of knowledge of a biological, physiological, ethological, physical or chemical nature. This includes the use of animal(s) in the production of reagents and products such as antigens and antibodies, routine diagnosis testing activity and establishment of transgenic shocks, for the purpose of saving or prolonging life or alleviating suffering, or significant gains in the wellbeing for the people of the country or for combating any disease of human beings, animals or plants.
Local authority	A municipal committee, State Animal Welfare Board, District Board.
Society	Society for Prevention of Cruelty to Animals.

Clinical Establishment Act

Term	Meaning
Clinical Establishment	Hospital, maternity home, nursing home, dispensary, clinic, sanatorium, or any other institution that offers services, facilities requiring diagnosis, treatment or care for illness, injury, deformity, abnormality or pregnancy in any recognized system of medicine. It also includes laboratory and diagnostic centre or any other place where pathological, bacteriological, genetic, radiological, chemical, biological investigations or other services with aid of laboratory or other medical equipment are carried out.
National Council	20-member body under ex-officio chairman DGHS, MOHFW, Government of India
State Council	A multi-member body in the state with Health Secretary as Chairman
District Registration Authority	A multi member authority at district level responsible for registration.

Right to Information Act

Term	Meaning
Competent authority	1. Speaker in the case of the House of the People or the Legislative Assembly of a state or a union territory having such Assembly and the Chairman in the case of the Council of States or Legislative Council of a State; 2. Chief Justice of India in the case of the Supreme Court 3. Chief Justice of the High Court in the case of a High Court 4. President or the Governor, 5. Other Authorities Appointed by the Government.
Information	Any material in any form, including records, documents, memos, e-mails, opinions, advices, press releases, circulars, orders, logbooks, contracts, reports, papers, samples, models, data material held in any electronic form and information relating to any private body which can be accessed by a public authority under any other law for the time being in force.
Record	• Any document, manuscript and file; • Any microfilm, microfiche and facsimile copy of a document;

(Contd...)

(Contd...)

Term	Meaning
	• Any reproduction of image or images embodied in such microfilm (whether enlarged or not); and • Any other material produced by a computer or any other device.
Right to information	The right to information accessible under this Act which is held by or under the control of any public authority and includes the right to: • Inspection of work, documents, records; • Taking notes, extracts or certified copies of documents or records; • Taking certified samples of material; • Obtaining information in the form of diskettes, floppies, tapes, video cassettes or in any other electronic mode or through printouts where such information is stored in a computer or in any other device.

Code of Marketing Practice for Indian Pharmaceutical Industry

Term	Meaning
Medical representative	Sales representatives, including personnel retained by way of contract with third parties, and any other company representatives who call on healthcare professionals, pharmacies, hospitals or other healthcare facilities in connection with the promotion of medicinal products.

Tamil Nadu Shops and Establishment Act

Term	Meaning
Children	Persons not completed 14 years.
Establishment	Shop, commercial establishment, restaurant, eating house, residential hotel, theatre, place of public amusement or entertainment.
Commercial establishment	Establishment which is not a shop but carries business of advertising, commission, forwarding or commercial agency, clerical department of a factory or industrial undertaking, insurance company, joint stock company, bank, broker's office, Chambers of Commerce, Trade Unions registered under Trade Union Act, The Employers' Federation of Southern India, Southern India Millowners' Association, United Planters' Association of Southern India, Lodging Houses.
Day	24 hours beginning at midnight. [When the work extends beyond midnight, the day means the period of 24 hours beginning from the time when employment commences.]
Shop	Premise where any trade or business is carried out or where services are rendered to customers. [Offices, store rooms, godowns, warehouses excluding restaurants, eating house or commercial establishments]
Wages	Remuneration (in terms of money) for employment or work done and includes bonus. [it does not include house accommodation, supply of light, water, medical attendance, contribution to pension or provident fund, travel allowance and gratuity payable on retirement].
Week	A period of 7 days beginning at midnight on Saturday.
Young person	A person who is not child but not completed 17 years.

B. SCHEDULE H OF DRUGS AND COSMETICS RULES

The Schedule contains 536 drugs as of 16th March 2006. These drugs are required to be sold on the prescription of Registered Medical Practitioner only. As the law is not implemented strictly, these drugs are sold even without prescription. The unrestricted sale of antibiotics is one of the major reasons of irrational use and that leads to development of antibiotic resistance. In order to restrict the sale and use of high-ended antibiotics, the government has notified a new Schedule H1. The H1 schedule contains the 3rd and 4th Generation antibiotics, anti-TB drugs and some habit forming drugs.

The Rules relating to Schedule H and Schedule H1 are given here.

Labeling requirements: These instructions are in addition to the general labeling requirements for medicinal products.

- If the product contains a substance specified in Schedule H, it should be labeled with the symbol Rx and conspicuously displayed on the left top corner of the label. The label should have the following words:
  - *Schedule H Drug—Warning*: To be sold by retail on the prescription of Registered Medical Practitioner only.
- If the product contains a substance specified in Schedule H and also comes under the purview of Narcotic Drugs and Psychotropic Substances Act, it should be labeled with the symbol NRx in Red and conspicuously displayed on the left top corner of the label. The label should have the following words:
  - *Schedule H Drug—Warning*: To be sold by retail on the prescription of Registered Medical Practitioner only.
- If the product contains a drug substance specified in Schedule H1, it should be labeled with the symbol Rx in Red and conspicuously displayed on the left top corner of the label. The label should have the following words in a Box with Red Border:

Schedule H1 Drug—Warning

- It is dangerous to take this preparation except in accordance with the medical advice.
- Not to be sold by retail without the prescription of a Registered Medical Practitioner.

Dispensing and Supply

- The supply of drugs specified in Schedule H, Schedule H1, or Schedule X to the Registered Medical Practitioner, Hospital, Dispensary and Nursing Home should be made against the signed order in writing which needs to be preserved by the licensee for a period of 2 years.
- The supply of drugs specified in Schedule H1 should be recorded in a separate register at the time of supply giving the name and address of the prescriber, the name of the patient, name of the drug and the quantity supplied. Such records are required to be maintained for three years and are open for inspection.
- *Condition of Dispensing*: The person dispensing a prescription containing Schedule H, Schedule H1, and Schedule X has to comply with the following requirements in addition to other requirements:
  - The prescription MUST not be dispensed more than once, unless stated by the prescriber;
  - At the time of dispensing, 'The name and address of the seller, and date of dispensing' should be noted on the prescription above the signature of prescriber.
- Brand substitution is not permissible.
- The advertisement cannot be made except with previous sanction of central government.

C. SCHEDULE M OF DRUGS AND COSMETICS RULES

Good Manufacturing Practices and Requirements of Premises, Plant and Equipment for Pharmaceutical Products

Quality of medicinal products (also called medicines, or pharmaceuticals) is always a public concern. Though quality of medicines is difficult to define, it is often synonymous with conformity to specifications regarding identity, strength, purity and other characteristics as specified by recognized government or authorities. Testing of quality of medicines at the end of manufacturing, known as quality control operation, has been in practice for long time. Quality control of representative samples of finished products cannot guarantee or assure the quality of products. Often the quality control testing is destructive. It cannot test all the samples manufactured. The quality needs to be built into the product.

To ensure high standard for medicinal products' quality, the first GMP regulations were promulgated in 1963 in USA. They are revised in 1978 and have been updated regularly. The World Health Organization (WHO) too developed GMP as a part of its obligation "to develop, establish and promote international standards with respect to food, biological, pharmaceutical and similar products". The first WHO GMP was developed during 1967–69 and revised in 1975. They are subsequently revised periodically. In India, GMP, were given statutory status much later in 1988 and were incorporated as schedule M under Drugs and Cosmetics rules 1945. This was later again revised in 2001 but implemented only in 2005 after stiff resistance from many small-scale manufacturers.

USA, Japan, Germany, France and UK have highly developed detailed GMP regulations. There are other GMP guidelines too: GMP of the Association of South East Asian Nations. GMP aims primarily at diminishing the risks inherent in pharmaceutical production, such as cross-contamination (in particular of unexpected contaminants) and mix-ups (confusion). GMPs for manufactured products cover all areas of manufacturing, including premises, equipment, materials, cleaning, personnel, and documentation and many other matters related to production and quality control.

The Schedule M specifies the Good Manufacturing Practices and requirements of premises, plant and equipment for pharmaceutical products. It comes with a note in the beginning: Each licensee shall evolve appropriate methodology, systems, and procedures which shall be documented and maintained from inspection and reference; and the manufacturing premises shall be used exclusively for production of drugs and no other manufacturing activity shall be undertaken.

Schedule M-I specifies the GMP and Requirements of Premises, Plant and Equipment for Homeopathic Medicines.

Schedule M-II specifies the Requirements of Factory Premises for Manufacture of Cosmetics.

Schedule M-III specifies the Requirements of Quality Management System for notified Medical Devices and *in vitro* diagnostics. Now there is separate rule for Medical Devices.

The Schedule M has the Following Parts

Part–1: Good Manufacturing Practices for Premises and Materials;

Part–1A: Specific Requirements for Manufacture of Sterile Products, Parenteral Preparations and Sterile Ophthalmic Preparations;

Part–1B: Specific Requirements for Manufacture of Oral Solid Dosage Forms (Tablets and Capsules);

Part–1C: Specific requirements for Manufacture of Oral Liquids (Syrups, Elixirs, Emulsions, and Suspensions);

Part–1D: Specific requirements for Manufacture of Topical Products, External Preparations (Creams, Lotions, Ointments, Pastes, Emulsions, Solutions, Dusting Powders and Identical products);

Part–1E: Specific requirements for Manufacture of Metered Dose Inhalers;

Part–1F: Specific requirements of premises, plant and materials for Manufacture of Active Pharmaceutical Ingredient;

Part–II: Requirements of Plant and Equipments.

This part of the text just describes the salient points of Part–1 of Schedule M. The readers may refer the original schedule to know more about other aspects.

1. **General Requirements:**
    1.1: *Location and Surrounding*: The factory should be located in such environment that the risk of contamination from open sewage, drain, public lavatory or any factory producing disagreeable or obnoxious odour, fumes, dust, smoke, chemical or biological emissions.

    1.2: *Building and premises*: The building should be designed, constructed, adapted and maintained to meet the manufacturing operation under hygienic condition. The guidelines for premises for manufacturing, processing, warehousing, packaging, labelling and testing are specified. It should conform to the regulations laid down in Factories Act.

    1.3: *Water system*: The validated water treatment system is a necessity. Prepared purified water is to be used for all operations except washing and cleaning.

    1.4: *Disposal of waste*: The disposal of waste of the factory should be in consistence with the requirements of State Environmental Pollution Control Board and Biomedical Waste (Management and Handling) Rules.

2. **Warehousing Area:** The warehouse is to be designed and adapted to ensure good storage conditions for all types of materials like starting and packaging materials, intermediates, bulk and finished products, products in quarantine.

3. **Production Area:** The unidirectional flow of materials in production area is recommended. Separate dedicated and self-contained facilities should be made available for pharmaceutical products like penicillin, sex hormones and cytotoxic agents. This would avoid cross-contamination.

4. **Ancillary Area:** Rest and refreshment rooms, toilets, etc. must not have direct link to manufacturing and storage area.

5. **Quality Control Area:** The area of quality control must be independent of production area and there should be separate area for each type of analysis: Physicochemical, biological, microbiological and radio-isotopes.

6. **Personnel:** The personnel involved in manufacture, quality assurance, quality control must be in adequate number and suitably qualified. These operations should be conducted under supervision of Competent Technical Staff. The employed persons need to be trained appropriate to their duties and responsibilities.

7. **Health, Clothing and Sanitation:** The personnel need to be protected from ill effects of handling chemicals. They may be tested for penicillin sensitivity. Those handling sex hormones, cytotoxic substance should be periodically examined for adverse effects. Adequate hygiene must be required to be maintained. Smoking, eating, drinking, etc. are not permitted in production areas.

8. **Manufacturing Operations and Control:** All operations including weighing, measuring should be carried out under the direct supervision of approved technical staff. Adequate precautions need to be taken to prevent mix up and cross-contamination. Proper records and Standard Operating Procedure should be maintained.

   Products not prepared under aseptic condition are required to be free from pathogens like *Salmonella, E. coli.*

9. **Sanitation in the Manufacturing Premise:** The premises must be kept cleaned and maintained to make it free from accumulated waste, dust, debris. Routine sanitation should be carried out.

10. **Raw Materials:** The raw materials inventory should be properly maintained with adequate labeling as under test, approved, and rejected. All raw materials should be purchased from approved sources under valid vouchers.

    The quarantined materials must be checked by quality control staff before moving them further in production line.

11. **Equipment:** The equipments must be of appropriate size and type for carrying out the desired operation. The equipments need to be designed in such a way to minimize risk of errors and permit effective cleaning and maintenance.

12. **Documentation and Records:** Appropriate documentation needs to be maintained to define the specifications for all materials, method of manufacture and control, to ensure that the personnel concerned with manufacture to know the information necessary to decide whether or not to release a batch of drug for sale. The documents should be designed, prepared, reviewed, and controlled to make them in compliance with regulation.

    They should be approved, signed with date by the approved and authorized staff. Records and Sops are to be maintained for at least one year after the expiry date of the finished product.

13. **Labels and other Printed Materials:** The labels should be printed in bright colours and should be legible. They are essential for identification. Different coded labels should be used to indicate the status of product: Under Test, Approved, Passed or Rejected.

14. **Quality Assurance:** The system of quality assurance should ensure that the pharmaceutical products are designed and developed in a way that takes account of GMP, GLP and GCP.

15. **Self-inspection and Quality Audit:** A self-inspection team with quality audit procedure in place may help for assessment of all or part of a system with a specific purpose of improving it. They would also be able to assess the compliance with GMP.

16. **Quality Control System:** Quality Control System manned by the qualified and experienced staff should be in place to ensure that the necessary and relevant tests are actually carried out and that the materials are not released for use, sale or supply unless their quality is judged to be satisfactory, SOPs should be available for sampling, inspecting and testing of raw materials, intermediate bulk, finished product and packaging materials.

17. **Specifications:** Raw materials and packaging materials, product containers, in-process and bulk products, finished product, should have appropriate specification and in compliance with regulatory requirements.

18. **Master Formula Records:** The master formula records of all manufacturing procedures for each product and batch size should be prepared and endorsed by the competent technical staff (Head of Production and Quality Control).

19. **Packing Records:** Packaging instructions for each product, pack size, and type should be available.

20. **Batch Packaging Records:** A batch packaging record should be kept for each batch or part of batch processed.

21. **Batch Processing Record:** Batch processing record for each product is to be maintained. The method of preparation of such records included in the master formula shall be designed to avoid transcription error.

22. **SOPs and Records: There should be SOP for each activity or operation:** Receipt of materials, sampling, batch manufacturing, testing, records of analysis, reference samples, etc.

23. **Reference Samples:** Each lot of every active ingredient, in a quantity sufficient to carry out all the tests except sterility and pyrogen/bacterial endotoxin, should be retained for a period of 3 months after the date of expiry of the last batch produced from that active ingredient.

    Samples of finished products should also be retained in the same or simulated container in which the drug is marketed.

24. **Reprocessing and Recoveries:** Where reprocessing is necessary, written procedures should be established and approved by the quality assurance department who specifies the conditions and limitations of repeating chemical reactions. Reprocessing should be validated.

25. **Distribution Records:** Records of distribution should be maintained in a manner which would facilitate prompt and complete recall of the batch.

26. **Validation and Process Validation:** Validation should be conducted as per pre-defined protocols for processing, testing and cleaning. The validation reports giving results and conclusions should be prepared and maintained.

27. **Product Recalls:** There should be SOP for effective recall of distributed products: Recall from stockists, wholesaler, suppliers, in a shortest time period.

28. **Complaints and Adverse Reactions:** All complaints concerning product quality are to be carefully reviewed and recorded according to written procedure. Each complaint should be investigated/evaluated and records of investigation and remedial action taken to be recorded.

    Reports of serious adverse drug reactions with comments, from the use of the drug, are to be submitted to the Licensing Authority.

29. **Site Master File:** There should be development of document in the form of 'Site Master File' containing specific and factual GMP about the production and/or control of pharmaceutical manufacturing preparations carried out at the licensed premise. It should contain the description under the following headings:
    - General information,
    - Personnel,
    - Premise,
    - Equipment,
    - Sanitation,
    - Documentation,
    - Production,
    - Quality control,
    - Loan license manufacture and licensee,
    - Distribution, complaints and product recall,
    - Self inspection, and
    - Export of drugs.

Based on scientific and technological development, the GMP guidelines need revision. Worldwide concept of quality is changing. The quality domain has now widened from purity to impurity profile. To sum up, GMP is necessary even if there is a well-equipped quality control laboratory. The even extensive testing cannot detect all possible defects. Without GMP it is impossible to be sure that every unit of medicine is of same equality as the units tested in the laboratory. Often GMP certification is accepted as pre-qualification criteria for procuring medicines in public sector health facilities.

D. SCHEDULE Y OF DRUGS AND COSMETICS RULES

The clinical trial including Bioavailability and Bioequivalency in India is regulated under Drugs and Cosmetics Act 1940 and the Rules 1945. The principal rule that governs the clinical trial and bioequivalency is Schedule Y. The Schedule Y was first introduced in 1988 and subsequently amended. The Schedule was revised in 2005 synchronizing India's requirements with that of Global Ethical and Good Clinical Practices. This has been further revised in 2013 incorporating the provision for compensation in case of injury or harm, mandatory registration of ethics committee and required informed consent format.

There are 12 Appendices to this Schedule

Appendix–I: Data to be submitted along with the application to conduct clinical trials/ import/manufacture of new drugs for marketing in the country;

Appendix–IA: Data required to be submitted by an applicant for grant of permission to import and/or manufacture a new drug already approved in the country;

Appendix–II: Structure, Contents and Format for Clinical Study Reports;

Appendix–III: Animal Toxicology (Non-Clinical Studies);

Appendix–IV: Animal Pharmacology;

Appendix–V: Informed Consent;

Appendix–VI: Fixed Dose Combinations;

Appendix–VII: Undertaking by the Investigator;

Appendix–VIII: Ethics Committee including their Registration;

Appendix–IX: Stability Testing of New Drugs,

Appendix–X: Contents of the Proposed Protocol for conducting Clinical Trials;

Appendix–XI: Data Elements for Reporting Serious Adverse Events Occurring in a Clinical Trial; and

Appendix–XII: Compensation in case of Injury or Death during Clinical Trial.

APPENDIX–I

The data should be submitted under the following headings

1. Introduction;
2. Chemical and Pharmaceutical Information: Information on active ingredients, Drug Information; Physico-Chemical Data; Analytical Data; Complete Monograph; Validation; Stability Studies; and Data on Formulation.
3. Animal Pharmacology;
4. Animal Toxicology;

5. Human or Clinical Pharmacology (Phase I Study);
6. Therapeutic Exploratory Trials (Phase–II);
7. Therapeutic Confirmatory Trials (Phase–III);
8. Special Studies: Bioavailability and Bioequivalence; Geriatrics, Paediatrics, Pregnant or Nursing Women;
9. Regulatory Status in Other Countries: Marketed/Approved/Approved as Investigational New Drug, Withdrawn etc;
10. Prescribing Information: Full prescribing Information including draft Labels; and
11. Samples and Testing Protocol(s).

APPENDIX–IA

The data should be submitted under the following headings

1. Introduction;
2. *Chemical and Pharmaceutical Information*: Chemical Name and Code Number; Dosage Form and its Composition;
3. *Marketing Information*: Proposed Package Inserts/Promotional Literature and Draft label;
4. *Special Studies Conducted with Approval of Licencing authority*: Bioavailability and Bioequivalency; Comparative Dissolution Studies, Sub-Acute Animal Toxicities for Intravenous Infusions and Injectables.

APPENDIX–II

The data should be submitted under the following headings

1. Title Page;
2. Study Synopsis;
3. Statement of Compliance with Guidelines for Clinical Trials on Pharmaceutical Products— GCP Compliance;
4. List of Abbreviations and Definitions;
5. Table of Contents;
6. Ethics Committee;
7. Study Team;
8. Introduction
9. Study Objective;
10. Investigational Plan;
11. Trial Subjects;
12. Efficacy Evaluation;
13. Safety Evaluation;
14. Discussion and Overall Conclusions;
15. List of References; and
16. Appendices giving protocol and amendments, specimen case record form, protocol deviations, publications from the trial, etc.

APPENDIX–III

It describes the animal toxicity requirements for clinical trials and marketing. It gives the detail guidelines to be followed for pre-clinical testing adopting the Good Laboratory Practice.

APPENDIX–IV

It gives the detail guidelines to be followed in generating various pharmacological data in animals to support use of therapeutics in humans. The adoption of Good Laboratory Practices is mandatory.

APPENDIX–V

It gives the guideline for developing informed consent form. It also gives a format.

APPENDIX–VI

It divides the Fixed Dose Combinations into different categories and the requirement of safety and efficacy data required.

APPENDIX–VII

It describes what should be the 'Contents of the Undertaking by the Investigator'.

APPENDIX–VIII

Composition of ethics committee

- Minimum seven members; Chairman from outside the institute.
- Other members from medical, scientific, non-medical and non-scientific fields including lay public;
- Members should be well versed with Good Clinical Practices;
- Quorum should have at least five members with the following representation: Basic Medical Scientist, Clinician, Legal Expert, Social Scientist and Lay Person from the Community.

The Ethics Committee is required to be registered with CDSCO. The appendix provides 'Format for According Approval to Clinical Trial Protocol by the Ethics Committee'.

APPENDIX–IX

It provides at what condition and how long stability studies (Both Long Term and Accelerated) are to be conducted for new drugs. The long term study has different temperature conditions and duration should be for 12 months. For accelerated condition, the duration of the study is for 6 months.

APPENDIX–X

The protocol of the proposed study should contain

1. Title page;
2. Table of contents;
   a. Background and Introduction: Pre-Clinical and Clinical Experience;
   b. Study Rationale;
   c. Study Objectives;

d. Study Design;

e. Study Population;

f. Subject Eligibility—Inclusion and Exclusion Criteria;

g. Study Assessments;

h. Study Conduct;

i. Study Treatment;

j. Adverse Events;

k. Ethical Considerations;

l. Study Monitoring and Supervision;

m. Investigational Product Management;

n. Data Analysis;

o. Undertaking by the Investigator and

p. Appendices.

APPENDIX–XI

The serious adverse events reporting form should have the following elements

1. Patient Details;

2. Suspected Drug(s);

3. Other Treatment(s);

4. Details of Suspected Adverse Drug Reaction(s);

5. Outcome;

6. Details about the Investigator.

APPENDIX–XII

It provides the provision for payment of compensation in case of injury or death occurred during clinical trial. The financial compensation for clinical trial related injury or death could be in the form of: Payment for medical management; financial compensation to nominee; and financial compensation to the parents if the child is injured *in utero* due to parent's participation.

The Sponsor or Permission Holder for the Clinical Trial is responsible for payment of compensation.

Currently the following amounts of compensation is notified by the government: Minimum Rs 2 Lakh and maximum Rs 73.60 Lakh.

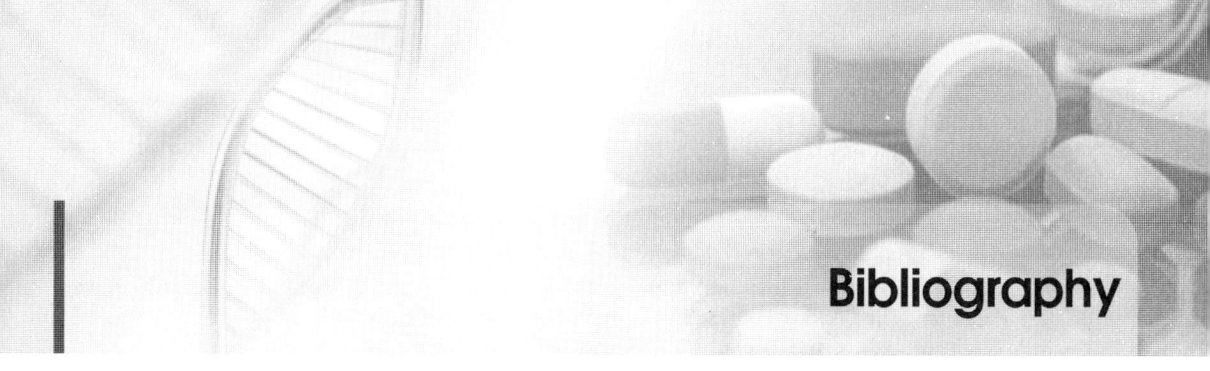

Bibliography

1. A Career in Pharmacy, IPA–PCI Booklet, November 2009.

2. A Lay Person's Guide to Medicines, LOCOST, Vadodara, 2006.

3. Akram Ahmad, Isha Patel, S. Parimalakrishnan, Guru Prasad Mohanta and Anantha Naik Nagappa, *Advertisement on Medicines /Treatment in Newspapers Violating Indian laws*, International journal of Current Pharmaceutical Review and Research, 6(1), 49–58, 2015.

4. Annual Report, 2008–2009, Department of Pharmaceuticals, Government of India, 2009.

5. Anurag Bhargav and S Srnivisan, Price Regulation of Essential Medicines, The Hindu, 17.10.2006.

6. Brooke Ronald Johnson Jr *et al*, A global database of abortion laws, policies, health standards and guidelines, Bulletin of World Health Organization, 2017; 95, 542–544.

7. Code of Pharmaceutical Marketing Practices, Organization of Pharmaceutical Producers of India, 2007.

8. Draft Pharmaceutical Policy 2017, Department of Pharmaceuticals, Government of India, 2017.

9. Drug Price Control Order, 1995, Government of India.

10. Drug Price Control Order, 2013, Department of Pharmaceuticals, Government of India.

11. Drugs and Cosmetics Act 1940 and the Rules 1945, Government of India, 2010.

12. G P Mohanta, Impact of New Patent Regime in Medicine Scenario, The Pharma Review, August 2006.

13. G P Mohanta, Laws and Regulations, The New Indian Express Supplement-Health, 22nd November 2005.

14. G P Mohanta, P K Manna, and R Manavalan, Impact of New Patent Regime in Public Health, Express Pharma Pulse, 28th April, 2005.

15. G P Mohanta, P K Manna, and R Manavalan, Product Patent Regime: A Threat or Boon, Express Pharma Pulse, 16th June 2005.

16. G P Mohanta, P K Manna, and R Manavalan, Some Policy Proposals (Pharmaceutical Policy 2006), Express Pharma, 16 March, 2006.

17. G P Mohanta, P K Manna, R Manavalan, *Medicine Pricing: Need for effective mechanism, Pharma Pulse, 13 May 2004.*

18. G P Mohanta, P K Manna, S Parimalakrishnan, and R Manavalan, Drug Legislation in India—a Closer Look, International Pharmacy Journal 18(1), 29–31, August 2004.

19. Guru Prasad Mohanta, Irrational and Counterfeit Medicines, Rational Drug Bulletin, 18(1), Jan–Mar, 2009.

20. Guru Prasad Mohanta, Textbook on Clinical Research: A Guide for Aspiring Professional and Professionals, Second Edition, PharmaMed Press, 2017.

21. Harkishan Singh, History of Drugs and Pharmacy Statues in Views and Reviews, Association of Pharmaceutical Teachers of India, 2009.

22. Indian Pharma Sector Dissected, Choice, June 6, 2017,

23. Joel Lexchin, Deception by Design—Pharmaceutical Promotion in Third World, Consumer International, 1995.

24. Kriti Dwivedi, Medical Termination of Pregnancy Act, 1971: An Overview; accessed at http://www.legalservicesindia.com/articles/pregact.htm on 8 May 2008.

25. Medical Termination of Pregnancy Act (MTP): www.equityasia.net/others/mtp.pdf, accessed on 8.5.2008.

26. Medicinal and Toilet Preparations (Excise Duties) Act 1955 and the Rules.

27. Medicines Regulation: Regulatory System in India, WHO Drug information, 31(3), 2017.

28. Molly Charles, Dave Bewley-Taylor and Amanda Neidpath, Drug Policy in India: Compounding Harm? Briefing Paper ten, The Beckley Foundation Drug Policy Programme, October 2005.

29. Narcotic Drugs and Psychotropic Substances Act 1985.

30. P K Dutta, Drug Control–Desk Reference, Second Edition, Eastern Law House, 1997.

31. Pharmaceutical Policy 2002, Department of Pharmaceuticals, Government of India.

32. Pharmacy Act 1948.

33. Pharmacy Practice Regulation 2015.

34. Praful Bidwai, One Step forward, Many Steps Back: Dismemberment of India's National Drug Policy, in Development Dialogue, Dag HammarskjÖld Foundation, 1995.

35. Report of Drug Price Control Review Committee, Department of Chemicals and Petrochemicals, Government of India, 1999.

36. Report of the Working Group on Drugs and Pharmaceuticals for the Eleventh Five Year Plan (2007–2012), Planning Commission of India, 1st December 2006.

37. Right to Information Act 2005, Government of India.

38. S C Basak, Changes in India's Patent Regime and Access to Medicines, Pharmabiz.com, July 17, 2005.

39. S Sakthivel, Access to Essential Drugs and Medicines, Financing and Delivery of Health Care Services in India, 2005.

40. S. Srinivas, T. Srikrishna, Anant Phadke, Drug Price Control order 2013—As Good as a Leaky Bucket, Economic and Political weekly, XLVIII, No. 26 & 27, June29, 2013.

41. Shanti Mendis *et al*, The availability and affordability of selected essential medicines for chronic diseases in six low and middle income countries, Bulletin of World Health Organization, 2007, 85(4).

42. Tamil Nadu Shops and Establishment Act 1947.

43. The Clinical Establishments (Registration and Regulation) Act 2010 and the Rules 2012.

44. The Drugs and Magic Remedies (Objectionable Advertisement) Act 1954.

45. The Patent Act 1970 and the Rules.

46. The Prevention of Cruelty to Animals Act 1960

47. The Report of the Committee on Drugs and Pharmaceutical Industry (Hathi Committee Report), Ministry of Petroleum and Chemicals, Government of India, April 1975.

48. The Third Round Up of Developments in Pharmaceutical Sector: Department of Pharmaceuticals, Government of India, July 2009.

49. The World Medicine Situation, WHO, 2004.

50. Times of India, Delhi Edition, 15.11.2007.

51. The Clinical Establishments (Registration and Regulation) Act 2010 and the Rules 2012.

52. Uniform Code for Pharmaceutical Marketing Practices (UCPMP), 2011 Department of Pharmaceuticals, Government of India.

53. WHO/HAI' s Understanding and Responding to Pharmaceutical Promotion—a Practical Guide, First Edition, 2011.

54. www.drugscontrol.org

55. www.pharmabiz.com

56. www://Drug-Rehabs.org accessed on 30.4.2008.

57. Zafrullah Chowdhury, The Politics of Essential Drugs, ZED Books, 1995.

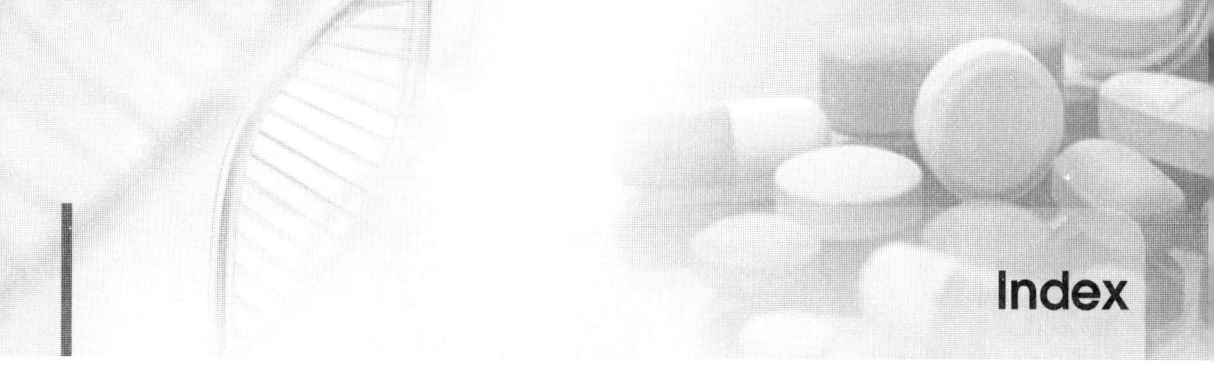

Index